Distance Learning and Online Education in Social Work

This edited collection focuses on the early development, gradual evolution, and present status of distance learning and online education in the social work profession. Relevant for social work students and educators in baccalaureate, masters and doctoral programs, this book is an authoritative statement authored by widely recognized educators on the cutting edge of technological innovation.

In addressing the future of web-based social work education, the collection demonstrates the power of distance learning and online technology. The chapters cover a comprehensive range of topics, including organizational and administrative aspects, teaching and practice, recent research and the challenge of creating intimacy and interaction. The volume provides a valuable set of insights into how distance learning and online education are transforming how social work is increasingly being taught today, and will surely be offered in the future.

This book was originally published in the *Journal of Teaching in Social Work*.

THE EDITORS

Paul A. Kurzman, Ph.D., ACSW holds a dual appointment as a Professor of Social Work at the Silberman School of Hunter College, USA, and as a Professor of Social Welfare at the Graduate School and University Center of The City University of New York, USA, where he teaches policy and practice in the MSW and PhD Programs and Chairs the World of Work Field of Practice Specialization. He also is the Editor-in-Chief of the *Journal of Teaching in Social Work* and a member of the Editorial Board of the *Journal of Workplace Behavioral Health.* Dr. Kurzman served for a record 26 years on the New York State Social Work Licensing Board, chaired the Board of the first *Register of Clinical Social Workers*, was elected the President of the Faculty of Hunter College, and appointed the Acting Dean of the School of Social Work. Professor Kurzman has held major leadership positions in the National Association of Social Workers, locally and nationally, including as President of the New York City Chapter, from which he recently received their Lifetime Achievement Award. He is an author or editor of eight prior books, including *Union Contributions to Labor Welfare Policy and Practice* (with R.P. Maiden), *Work and the Workplace: A Resource for Innovative Policy and Practice* (with S. Akabas), *Labor and Industrial Settings: Sites for Social Work Practice* (with S. Akabas & N. Kolben), *Psychosocial and Policy Issues in the World of Work*, *Work, Workers and Work Organizations: A View from Social Work* (with S. Akabas), *Harry Hopkins and the New Deal*, *Work and Well-Being: The Occupational Social Work Advantage* (with S. Akabas), and *The Mississippi Experience: Strategies for Welfare Rights Action.* Dr. Kurzman holds an MSW from Columbia University and a PhD from New York University. He can be reached at pkurzman@hunter.cuny.edu.

R. Paul Maiden, Ph.D., LCSW is a Professor and the Executive Vice-Dean of Academic and Student Affairs at the University of Southern California School of Social Work, USA, the largest graduate school of social work in the United States, with 3,200 MSW students at five academic centers. He spearheaded creation of the school's military social work program, launched the San Diego Academic Center, expanded the school's global immersion offerings, and led the development of its Virtual Academic Center, the first and only web-based MSW program serving a national and international student population. Dr. Maiden is also the Editor-in-Chief of the *Journal of Workplace Behavioral Health*, and has published extensively in the areas of employee assistance, substance abuse, work site domestic violence, managed behavioral health care, trauma management, and the evaluation of work-based human services. He has extensive international experience and has been the recipient of Senior Fulbright Scholar awards to Russia and South Africa. Dr. Maiden is an editor of nine prior books, including *The Older Worker and the Changing Labor Market: New Challenges for the Workplace* (with J. Gonyea), *EAPs in Higher Education* (with S. Phillips), *Union Contributions to Labor Welfare Policy and Practice* (with P. Kurzman), *Workplace Disaster Preparedness and Disaster Management* (with R. Paul & C. Thompson), *The Integration of Employee Assistance, Work/Life and Wellness* (with M. Attridge & P. Herlihy), *Global Perspectives on Occupational Social Work*, *Employee Assistance Services in the New South Africa*, *Accreditation of Employee Assistance Programs*, and *Total Quality Management in EAPs*. Dr. Maiden holds an MSW from the University of Tennessee, USA, and a PhD from the University of Maryland, USA. He can be reached at rmaiden@usc.edu.

Distance Learning and Online Education in Social Work

Edited by
Paul A. Kurzman and R. Paul Maiden

Routledge
Taylor & Francis Group
LONDON AND NEW YORK

First published 2014
by Routledge
2 Park Square, Milton Park, Abingdon, Oxon, OX14 4RN, UK

and by Routledge
711 Third Avenue, New York, NY 10017, USA

Routledge is an imprint of the Taylor & Francis Group, an informa business

British Library Cataloguing in Publication Data
A catalogue record for this book is available from the British Library

ISBN13: 978-1-138-01959-1

Typeset in Garamond
by Taylor & Francis Books

Publisher's Note
The publisher accepts responsibility for any inconsistencies that may have arisen during the conversion of this book from journal articles to book chapters, namely the possible inclusion of journal terminology.

Contents

Citation Information

The chapters in this book were originally published in the *Journal of Teaching in Social Work*, volume 33, issue 4-5 (November 2013). When citing this material, please use the original page numbering for each article, as follows:

Introduction
Introduction: The Evolution of Distance Learning and Online Education
Paul A. Kurzman
Journal of Teaching in Social Work, volume 33, issue 4-5 (November 2013)
pp. 331-338

Chapter 1
Launching the Virtual Academic Center: Issues and Challenges in Innovation
Marilyn Flynn, R. Paul Maiden, Wendy Smith, June Wiley, and Gary Wood
Journal of Teaching in Social Work, volume 33, issue 4-5 (November 2013)
pp. 339-356

Chapter 2
Cost Analysis of a Distance Education MSW Program
Rebecca L. Stotzer, Keith Fujikawa, Jill Sur, and Pam Arnsberger
Journal of Teaching in Social Work, volume 33, issue 4-5 (November 2013)
pp. 357-368

Chapter 3
Distance and Online Social Work Education: Novel Ethical Challenges
Frederic G. Reamer
Journal of Teaching in Social Work, volume 33, issue 4-5 (November 2013)
pp. 369-384

Chapter 5
Distance Guest Speakers in Online Synchronous Classrooms: Practical and Legal Considerations
Melanie Sage
Journal of Teaching in Social Work, volume 33, issue 4-5 (November 2013)
pp. 385-392

Chapter 6
Current Challenges in Social Work Distance Education: Responses from the Elluminati
William Pelech, Dan Wulff, Ellen Perrault, Jessica Ayala, Myra Baynton, Margaret Williams, Rachael Crowder, and Janki Shankar
Journal of Teaching in Social Work, volume 33, issue 4-5 (November 2013) pp. 393-407

Chapter 7
Teaching MSW Social Work Practice in a Blended Online Learning Environment
Shelley Levin, Doni Whitsett, and Gary Wood
Journal of Teaching in Social Work, volume 33, issue 4-5 (November 2013) pp. 408-420

Chapter 8
Teaching Direct Practice Skills Using Web-Based Simulations: Home Visiting in the Virtual World
Amy Blank Wilson, Suzanne Brown, Zoe Breen Wood, and Kathleen J. Farkas
Journal of Teaching in Social Work, volume 33, issue 4-5 (November 2013) pp. 421-437

Chapter 9
Establishing a Community of Inquiry through Hybrid Courses in Clinical Social Work Education
Maria Ferrera, Noam Ostrander, and Sonya Crabtree-Nelson
Journal of Teaching in Social Work, volume 33, issue 4-5 (November 2013) pp. 438-448

Chapter 10
Utilizing Video Conferencing to Introduce an International Perspective to Foundation Practice
Mary Ann Forgey, Hilda Loughran, and Johna Hansen
Journal of Teaching in Social Work, volume 33, issue 4-5 (November 2013) pp. 449-466

Chapter 11
A Comparison of Student Knowledge and Attitude toward Research: Are Main Campus Students Different from Those in a Hybrid Environment?
Rachel L. Buchanan and Deborah A. Mathews
Journal of Teaching in Social Work, volume 33, issue 4-5 (November 2013) pp. 467-480

Chapter 12
A National Research Survey of Technology Use in the BSW Teaching and Learning Process
Brittany Buquoi, Carli McClure, Joseph W. Kotrlik, Krisanna Machtmes, and J. C. Bunch
Journal of Teaching in Social Work, volume 33, issue 4-5 (November 2013) pp. 481-495

Chapter 13
Research on Webbed Connectivity in a Web-Based Learning Environment: Online Social Work Education
Dorinda Noble and Amy Catherine Russell
Journal of Teaching in Social Work, volume 33, issue 4-5 (November 2013)
pp. 496-513

Chapter 14
A Process Evaluation of an Online BSW Program: Getting the Student Perspective
Carolyn McAllister
Journal of Teaching in Social Work, volume 33, issue 4-5 (November 2013)
pp. 514-530

Chapter 15
Being an Elbow: A Phenomenological Autoethnography of Faculty-Student Collaboration for Accommodations
Regina T. P. Aguirre and Chad Duncan
Journal of Teaching in Social Work, volume 33, issue 4-5 (November 2013)
pp. 531-551

Chapter 16
Introducing Case Management to Students in a Virtual World: An Exploratory Study
Joanne Levine and Ruifang Hope Adams
Journal of Teaching in Social Work, volume 33, issue 4-5 (November 2013)
pp. 552-565

Chapter 17
Meeting Professional Competencies through Specialized Distance Education: The McMaster University Addiction Studies Program
Rick Csiernik and Christie McGaghran
Journal of Teaching in Social Work, volume 33, issue 4-5 (November 2013)
pp. 566-577

Chapter 18
Increasing MSW Students' Information Competencies through Online Tutorials, Application Exercises, and Course Assignments
John A. Kayser, Jennifer Bowers, Lin Jiang, and Marian Bussey
Journal of Teaching in Social Work, volume 33, issue 4-5 (November 2013)
pp. 578-593

Chapter 19
The Pathway Program: How a Collaborative, Distributed Learning Program Showed Us the Future of Social Work Education
Teresa Morris, Christine Mathias, Ronnie Swartz, Celeste A. Jones, and Meka Klungtvet-Morano
Journal of Teaching in Social Work, volume 33, issue 4-5 (November 2013)
pp. 594-606

Chapter 20
Conclusion: Toward the Future
R. Paul Maiden
Journal of Teaching in Social Work, volume 33, issue 4-5 (November 2013)
pp. 607-610

Please direct any queries you may have about the citations to
clsuk.permissions@cengage.com

Notes on Contributors

Ruifang Hope Adams, Ed.D. is an Assistant Professor of Information Technology in the MBA School for Graduate Studies of Empire State College of the State University of New York and can be reached at hope.adams@esc.edu.

Regina T. P. Aguirre, Ph.D., LMSW-AP is an Associate Professor at the School of Social Work of the University of Texas at Arlington and can be reached at rtpaguirre@uta.edu.

Pamela Arnsberger, Ph.D., LCSW is a Professor at the Myron B. Thompson School of Social Work of the University of Hawaii at Manoa and can be reached at arnsburg@hawaii.edu.

Jessica Ayala, Ph.D., RSW is a Senior Instructor and Director of Field Education at the Faculty of Social Work of the University of Calgary in Canada and can be reached at jayala@ucalgary.ca.

Myra Baynton, Ph.D, RSW, AASW is an Instructor, Practicum Coordinator and Faculty Liaison for the MSW Distance Program at the University of Calgary in Canada and can be reached at mbaynton@ucalgary.ca.

Jennifer Bowers, MA is an Associate Professor and Social Sciences Librarian at the University of Denver and can be reached at Jennifer.bowers@du.edu.

Suzanne Brown, Ph.D., LICSW is an Assistant Professor at the School of Social Work of Wayne State University and can be reached at Suzanne.brown@wayne.edu.

Rachel L. Buchanan, Ph.D. is an Assistant Professor and Online Program Director in the Department of Social Work at Salisbury University and can be reached at rlbuchanan@salisbury.edu.

J. C. Bunch, Ph.D. is an Assistant Professor of Agricultural Education in the School of Human Resource Education and Workforce Development at Louisiana State University and can be reached at jcbunch@lsu.edu.

Brittany Buquoi, Ph.D., LICSW is Director of Pscyhological Health at the Minnesota Army National Guard and can be reached at brittany.o.buquoi.ctr@mail.mil.

Marian Bussey, Ph.D., LCSW is an Associate Professor and Director of Assessment and Program Evaluation at the Graduate School of Social Work of the University of Denver and can be reached at marian.bussey@du.edu.

Sonya Crabtree-Nelson, Ph.D., LCSW is an Assistant Professor of Social Work at DePaul University in Chicago and can be reached at scrabtr3@depaul.edu.

Rachael Crowder, Ph.D., RSW is an Assistant Professor at the Faculty of Social Work of the University of Calgary in Canada and can be reached at rcrowder@ucalgary.ca.

Rick Csiernik, Ph.D., RSW is a Professor of Social Work at King's University College of the University of Western Ontario in Canada and can be reached at rcsiernik@uwo.ca.

Chad Duncan, MSW was a Graduate Student at the School of Social Work of the University of Texas at Arlington and can be reached at chad.duncan@mavs.uta.edu.

Kathleen J. Farkas, Ph.D., LISW, ACSW is Associate Professor and Chair of the Direct Practice Concentration at the Mandel School of Applied Social Sciences of Case Western Reserve University and can be reached at kathleen.farkas@case.edu.

Maria J. Ferrera, Ph.D., LCSW is an Assistant Professor of Social Work at DePaul University in Chicago and can be reached at mferrera@depaul.edu.

Marilyn L. Flynn, Ph.D. is Professor and Dean of the School of Social Work at the University of Southern California and can be reached at mflynn@usc.edu.

Mary Ann Forgey, Ph.D., LCSW is Associate Professor and Chair of the Online MSW Faculty Committee at the Fordham University Graduate School of Social Service and can be reached at forgey@fordham.edu.

Keith Y. Fujikawa, M.Ed. is an Administrative Officer at the Myron B. Thompson School of Social Work of the University of Hawaii at Manoa and can be reached at kfujikaw@hawaii.edu.

Johna Hansen, LCSW is a Doctoral Student at the Fordham University Graduate School of Social Service and can be reached at johansen@fordham.edu.

Lin Jiang, MS.Sc. is a Graduate Teaching Assistant and Doctoral Student at the University of Denver and can be reached at lin.jiang@du.edu.

Celeste A. Jones, Ph.D., ACSW, BCD is a Professor at the School of Social Work of California State University – Chico and President of the Board of the California Social Work Education Center and can be reached at cajones@csuchico.edu.

John A. Kayser, Ph.D., LCSW is a Professor at the Graduate School of Social Work at the University of Denver and can be reached at john.kayser@du.edu.

Meka Klungtvet-Morano, MSW is a Lecturer and Title IV-E Project Coordinator at the School of Social Work of the California State University – Chico and can be reached at mklungtvet-morano@csuchico.edu.

Joseph W. Kotrlik, Ph.D. is Atherton Alumni Professor Emeritus of Human Research Education and Workforce Development at the College of Human Sciences and Education of Louisiana State University and can be reached at kotrlik@lsu.edu.

Shelley Levin, Ph.D., LCSW is a Clinical Associate Professor at the School of Social Work of the University of Southern California and can be reached at slevin@usc.edu.

Joanne Levine, MPH, DSW, LCSW is an Associate Professor and Area Coordinator for Human Services at the Center for Distance Learning of Empire State College, State University of New York and can be reached at joanne.levine@esc.edu.

Hilda Longhran, Ph.D., CQSW, SWRB is a Senior Lecturer and Director of Social Work at University College Dublin in Ireland and can be reached at hilda.longhran@ucd.ie.

Krisanna Machtmes, Ph.D. is an Associate Professor of Educational Studies at the Patton College of Education of Ohio University and can be reached at machtmes@ohio.edu.

Deborah A. Mathews, Ph.D., LCSW, DCSW is Professor and Chair of the Department of Social Work at Salisbury University and can be reached at damathews@salisbury.edu.

Christine Mathias, MSW is Director of the Title IV-E Stipend Program at the California Social Work Education Center of the University of California at Berkeley School of Social Welfare and can be reached at cmathias@berkeley.edu.

Carolyn Anne McAllister, Ph.D. is an Assistant Professor, BASW Program Director and Distance Education Consultant at the School of Social Work of California State University – San Bernadino and can be reached at cmcallis@csusb.edu.

Carli McClure, MS is a Doctoral Student at Louisiana State University and Executive Account Manager for Trans Coastal Marketing in Baton Rouge and can be reached at cmcclure@tigers.lsu.edu.

Christie McGaghran, MA is a Program Manager of the Addiction Studies Program at the Centre for Continuing Education of McMaster University in Canada and can be reached at mcgagh@mcmaster.ca.

Teresa Morris, Ph.D. is a Professor Emerita at the School of Social Work of California State University – San Bernadino and currently Coordinator of the University's Pathway Distance Education Program and can be reached at tmorris@csusb.edu.

Dorinda N. Noble, Ph.D., LCSW is Professor and Director of the School of Social Work at Texas State University and can be reached at dn12@txstate.edu.

Norm Ostrander, Ph.D., LCSW is an Associate Professor and Director of the MSW Program in the Department of Social Work of DePaul University and can be reached at rostran1@depaul.edu.

William Pelech, Ph.D., RSW is an Associate Professor and Academic Associate Dean at the Faculty of Social Work of the University of Calgary in Canada and can be reached at pelech@ucalgary.ca.

Ellen Perrault, Ph.D., RSW is an Instructor and the e-Learning Director at the Faculty of Social Work of the University of Calgary in Canada and can be reached at Perrault@ucalgary.ca.

Frederic G. Reamer, Ph.D. is a Professor at the School of Social Work of Rhode Island College and can be reached at freamer@ric.edu.

Amy C. Russell, Ph.D., LMSW is an Assistant Professor and Director of the Richter Research Institute at the School of Social Work of Texas State University and can be reached at ar41@txstate.edu.

Melanie Sage, Ph.D., LICSW is an Assistant Professor and BSSW Program Director in the Department of Social Work of the University of North Dakota and can be reached at Melanie.sage@und.edu.

Janki Shankar, Ph.D, RSW is an Associate Professor at the Faculty of Social Work of the University of Calgary in Canada and can be reached at jshankar@ucalgary.edu.

Wendy B. Smith, Ph.D., LCSW, BCD is a Clinical Associate Professor and Associate Dean for Faculty Development at the School of Social Work of the University of Southern California and can be reached at wsmith@usc.edu.

Rebecca L. Stotzer, Ph.D. is an Associate Professor and Director of Distance Education at the Myron B. Thompson School of Social Work of the University of Hawaii at Manoa and can be reached at rstotzer@hawaii.edu.

Jill E. K. Sur, MSW is Program Coordinator of the MSW Distance Education Program at the Myron B. Thompson School of Social Work of the University of Hawaii at Manoa and can be reached at sur@hawaii.edu.

Ronnie Swartz, Ph.D., LCSW is Professor and Chair of the Department of Social Work and Co-Director of the Altruistic Personality and Prosocial Behavior Institute at Humboldt State University and can be reached at Swartz@humboldt.edu.

Doni P. Whitsett, Ph.D., LCSW, BCD is a Clinical Professor of Social Work and Associate Director of Faculty Development at the University of Southern California School of Social Work and can be reached at whitsett@usc.edu.

June L. Wiley, Ph.D. is a Clinical Associate Professor and Director of the Virtual Academic Center at the School of Social Work of the University of Southern California and can be reached at jwiley@usc.edu.

Margaret Williams, Ph.D., RSW is an Associate Professor and Director of Undergraduate Student Affairs at the University of Calgary in Canada and can be reached at Williamm@ucalgary.ca.

Amy Blank Wilson, Ph.D., LSW is an Assistant Professor and Chair of the Mental Health Specialization at the Mandel School of Applied Social Sciences of Case Western Reserve University and can be reached at amy.b.wilson@case.edu.

Gary J. Wood, Ph.D., LCSW is the Senior Vice President of Curriculum and Academic Relations at 2U, Inc. and can be reached at gwood@2U.com.

Zoe Breen Wood, Ph.D., LSW is an Assistant Professor of Social Work and Director of Educational Outcomes Assessment at the Mandel School of Applied Social Sciences of Case Western Reserve University and can be reached at zbw@case.edu.

Dan Wulff, Ph.D., RSW is an Associate Professor at the Faculty of Social Work of the University of Calgary in Canada and can be reached at dwulff@ucalgary.edu.

Acknowledgements

When we issued a Call for Papers for a book on *Distance Learning and Online Education in Social Work* we had not imagined the response it would receive. While we knew this to be a cutting-edge issue, which prompted our interest in taking the initiative, the sheer number of excellent manuscripts we received, for the journal special issue and hence the book, certainly did surprise us! Our belief that the time had come for a new and authoritative text on the subject had been validated, and we hope the peer-reviewed selection of these 20 superb chapters confirms that conviction to the reader. Representing the ideas of 57 contributing authors, the chapters herein present new information, novel experimentation, fresh conceptualization, and creative templates for what surely represents the thrust of professional social work education for the future.

As editors, we are very grateful for the can-do spirit and steady support of Jessica O. MacDonald, Associate Editor for Social Work and Public Health, Kimberley Smith, Associate Book Editor, Hazel Sharkey, Production Editor at Taylor & Francis Books, and Elizabeth T. Kerr, Production Editor at Routledge and the Taylor and Francis Group. Their patience and flexibility made a difference. And it is clear that this book would not have been possible without the quiet, steady and focused support of Ruth Flaherty, the Assistant Editor of the *Journal of Teaching in Social Work*, who carried out so many of the tasks of assignment and production with an always skillful and steady hand.

And to the contributors, whose insights and innovations are so articulately expressed here, we give thanks and tribute for their remarkable creativity and their insightful innovations. In this book, each of them individually, and all of them collectively, have made an indelible professional contribution to the future of social work education.

Paul A. Kurzman

R. Paul Maiden

January, 2014.

INTRODUCTION

The Evolution of Distance Learning and Online Education

PAUL A. KURZMAN
Silberman School of Social Work, Hunter College, CUNY, New York, New York, USA

THE ELECTRONIC REVOLUTION

Over the past 30 years, a revolution has taken place, but no troops took to the battlefield, and no shots were fired. This revolution has been electronic and has had a profound impact on citizens of all nations in ways that often were unexpected. The arena of higher education has not been exempt, and most of us would consider this reality to essentially be good news. It is now possible to offer college and university education to more people, at a greater convenience, and often at a lower cost. The advent of distance learning and online education has been heralded by most of us as a creator of new opportunities, especially in the area of higher and continuing education; and opportunity in a democracy is the coin of the realm.

Massive open online courses, frequently called MOOCs, have been created and have emerged as a way to deliver college instruction to anyone with access to a computer with an Internet connection. During fall semester 2011, about 6.7 million (or 32%) of students who were enrolled in higher education in the United States took at least one course online, while in fall 2002, only 1.6 million (10%) did so (Allen & Seaman, 2013). In spring 2013, a professor of classical Greek literature at Harvard University offered his popular course titled "Concepts of the Hero in Classical Greek Civilization" in a MOOC format, and the enrollment exceeded 31,000 (Heller, 2013).

MOOCs first landed in the spotlight in 2011 when a Stanford University professor offered a free artificial-intelligence course that attracted 160,000 students from 192 nations. In a *New York Times* series, aptly titled "Virtual U.,"

Tamar Lewin (2012) notes the rapidity of the expansion of MOOC courses and that currently millions of students are enrolled in such courses, offered by prestigious public and private universities, as well as by an emerging cohort of for-profit providers. Many of the elite private universities have joined forces with the three leading external providers—Udacity, EdX and Coursera—to pioneer as partners in joint ventures. EdX evolved featuring joint collaborations with Harvard and MIT, Coursera as a partnership with Stanford, Brown, and Princeton, and Udacity in league with Georgia Tech. As an example, Udacity is planning to launch an entirely MOOC-based online master's degree program in computer science (Lewin, 2013), and Coursera has experienced explosive growth, having already enrolled more than 2 million students. Founded by two Stanford computer science professors, Coursera now is offering online courses in the professional school of engineering at Columbia University and on systems biology at the Mount Sinai School of Medicine, further demonstrating the utility of distance learning for graduate profession education.

In addition, many of the largest accredited universities, all operating as for-profits, are principally (or entirely) offering their courses online via distance education. These universities include American Intercontinental, Strayer, National, Western International, and the University of Phoenix (Cronin & Bachorz, 2006). While their names may be less familiar and their reputations less renowned than many of the Ivy League partners named above, their collective impact in the realm of higher education should not be underestimated.

Lawrence Grossman, the vice-chair of Digital Promise, notes that in this digital age it would be shortsighted "to ignore the great potential that digital technologies have to improve, extend and transform teaching, learning and skills training" at all levels of education (Grossman, 2012, p. 2). In recognition of this reality, the U.S. Congress recently established and appropriated modest start-up funds for a nonprofit and independent national research center. What the National Science Foundation did for science and the National Institutes of Health did for health care, the new National Center for Research in Advanced Information and Digital Technologies is anticipated to do for teaching and education "in order to provide Americans with the knowledge and skills needed to compete in the global economy" (p. 2).

The Social Work Response

In the current issue of the *Encyclopedia of Social Work*, Ouellette and Westhuis (2008, p. 118) presciently observe that "The integration of technology for teaching the social work curriculum has the potential to make social work education, and ultimately direct practice, more effective, more widespread, and less expensive." With the advent of broadband availability, more powerful processors, secure interactive video transmission, simulcast broadcasting with ITV, versatile web conferencing software, high-end graphics, avatar assisted animation, and sophisticated web-based platforms, the options for online education (and therefore distance learning) today are extensive. Even field work education, sometimes considered to be the pedagogical exception to the rule, can be secured using a 3D virtual world where clients and students interact with one another visually via digitally generated avatars (Reamer, 2013).

Recent reviews of social work education tend to support the early embrace of technology in the delivery of baccalaureate and graduate education. A survey conducted by the Council on Social Work Education (CSWE) Commission on Accreditation in 2005 found that 41% of the respondents from BSW programs and 52% from MSW programs were delivering courses using some form of technology (Vernon, 2006). Further, a polling of 501 accredited BSW and MSW programs in 2008 discovered that 61% of BSW and 83% of MSW programs were willing to consider offering a degree by means of online courses (Vernon, Vakalahi, Pierce, Pittman-Munke & Adkins, 2009). Vernon and colleagues (p. 269) also found that "More than one-third of BSW programs and one-quarter of MSW programs did not require a face-to-face experience as an integral component of course work. Instead, these programs offered courses that were entirely online, without direct human contact."

According to the Commission on Accreditation of CSWE, there are distance education offerings by accredited programs at 22 master's and 5 baccalaureate level programs in the U.S. today (CSWE, 2013). Along with the two key national sister organizations, the National Association of Social Workers (NASW) and the Association of Social Work Boards (ASWB), the CSWE generally has been supportive of efforts (by the programs it accredits) to move toward increasing online and distance education options. For example, in 2007, the CSWE hosted a Distance Education Summit; has published many articles on the topic in its quarterly *Journal of Social Work Education*; offers many presentations on the topic at its Annual Program Meeting; and has made provisions for this educational innovation in its current *Educational Policy and Accreditation Standards* (EPAS) document. Moreover, the new 2008 EPAS focus on "core competencies" is very supportive, since online education is less interested in how students acquire a competency (i.e., the process) than in offering evidence that the competency was mastered. The NASW has provided support for this new pedagogy as well through an extensive focus on technology, distance learning, and online education in the most recent edition of its frequently cited *Encyclopedia of Social Work* publication; coverage in its widely read journal, *Social Work;* and through co-development (with the ASWB) of *Standards for Technology and Social Work Practice* (2005), an authoritative guidepost for professional education and practice.

Books and journals also have emerged on the subject during the past decade. In 2005, Professor Paul Abels at California State University-Long Beach published *Distance Education in Social Work* (Abels, 2005), and Professors Richard Beaulaurier (Florida International University) and Martha Haffey (Hunter College) assembled the text titled *Technology in Social Work Education* (Beaulaurier & Haffey, 2005). Over the course of the decade, new peer-reviewed social work journals appeared, such as the *Electronic Journal of Social Work*, and *Technology in Social Work Education and Curriculum*, as well as the *Journal of Technology in the Human Services, American Journal of Distance Education, Journal of Computers in the Human Services, Quarterly Review of Distance Education* and many more. In addition, the ASWB and the NASW were approving continuing education units required for licensure renewal and credential endorsement that were being offered entirely online by distance education firms such as CEUNITS.com and NetCE.com. Moreover, display advertisements, from CSWE-accredited programs, recently have begun to appear regularly in *NASW News* and in *Social Work Today*, promoting their online distance learning educational options. By 2013, it was clear that widespread recognition of this alternative pedagogical opportunity had been achieved.

Some of the social work program choices were being put forward early on by relatively new and proprietary institutions, such as Walden University, whose entirely online MSW program (in July 2013) was merely in pre-candidacy status with the CSWE; however, others, such as Brescia University in Kentucky, were offering a CSWE-accredited BSW degree entirely online. Nevertheless, wider recognition in the profession of the distance education option did not come until major, nationally ranked university programs, such as the University of Southern California and Rutgers University, announced their programs. Since both of these schools of social work are ranked among the "top 12" (of more than 200) accredited MSW programs in the country, everyone in the field of social work education began to take note. As mentioned, now 22 graduate schools (and five baccalaureate programs) provide a distance education option, although currently only a relatively small number offer a fully online degree choice in the manner pioneered by USC and Rutgers. Under present regulatory provisions, which were designed for courses taught in traditional brick-and-mortar classrooms, generally social work schools must initially register their accredited degree programs in every state where they are offered, which of course is a time consuming and expensive proposition.

The Pros and Cons

It is difficult to compare classroom-based social work education with that delivered largely (or entirely) online via the medium of distance education. To some extent, it is an "apples and oranges" comparison, since both modalities meet a need, and both lead to the award of an accredited professional degree and full eligibility for state licensure and professional employment. The latter simply offers an alternative route, and alternatives generally are honored and valued. One faculty member, with MSW and DSW degrees, stated her opinion quite clearly. She opined, "Well-designed online courses taught by professors at local universities can cultivate autonomous learning strategies and create opportunities for student-to-student engagement as well as student-to-professor engagement". She concluded, "This can provide the student who is juggling school, work and family responsibilities the means to complete college" (Rose, 2013, A-27). Providing that online faculty agree to eschew the "sage on the stage" orientation to teaching and are comfortable with a more modern "guide on the side" approach, many would argue that distance learning is an entirely viable framework for professional education. (Indeed, the Concord Law School in California offers a JD degree fully online that satisfies the legal education requirements for the California Bar Exam.) As the Pulitzer Prize–winning columnist and author Thomas L. Friedman (2013, p. A-18) observes, "There is one big thing happening that leaves me incredibly hopeful about the future, and that is the budding revolution in global online higher education." Indeed, there is a quintessentially democratic spirit embedded in the proposition that a potential student's remote location, limited transportation options, family commitments, or work obligations will not be a barrier to the pursuit of higher education and to the opportunities it almost always provides. In fact, these are social work values, articulated in our professional code of ethics. Unless research can uncover a statistically significant difference in student satisfaction, licensing exam pass rates, or post-graduation career achievement, we have no basis to assert that one way of pursuing the BSW or MSW degree is definitely better than another. Little summative research has been conducted to date, although a small but well-designed study of 183 MSW graduates of the University of Tennessee's distance education and traditional degree pathways found no significant difference in final attainment in the 10 EPAS core competency area ratings or in GPA (Cummings & Chaffin, 2012).

Nonetheless, the critics are many and vocal. Some argue that the movement toward online education has primarily been motivated by profit making and led by proprietary educational corporations such as Coursera and Udacity, along with for-profit universities like Phoenix, Walden, and American Intercontinental. While there is no question that several proprietary firms and institutions of higher education have taken the lead, it also presently is true that prestigious public and nonprofit colleges and universities have mounted the leading master's and baccalaureate online options. They include such nationally regarded schools of social work as Fordham, Case Western Reserve, USC, Rutgers, and the universities of Indiana, Alabama, and Tennessee. Although some firms in the emerging industry may primarily be focused on profit, and sometimes accused of fraud, currently such does not seem to be the experience with online and distance education for the social work profession. The quandaries and conundrums for us may be of a difference order.

Seventy-five years ago, the noted educator John Dewey (1938) stated that learning is based on discovery guided by mentoring, rather than on the transmission of information. Therefore, he argued that students need engagement with their teachers to feel comfortable, confident, and successful. As the provost of a prominent university quite recently put it, "No PowerPoint presentation or elegant online lecture can make up for the surprise, the frisson, the spontaneous give-and-take of a spirited, open-ended dialogue with another person" (Brooks, 2013, p. A-27). A faculty member and prolific author adds his own concern about the relative "sterility" of the distance learning medium. "A real course," he suggests, "creates intellectual joy, at least in some. I don't think an Internet course ever will. Internet learning promises to make intellectual life more sterile and abstract than it already is—and also, for teachers and students alike, far more lonely" (Edmundson, 2012, p. 11).

The Future

Certainly it is clear that distance learning and online education for the social work profession are here to stay. They are not temporary, passing, or ephemeral phenomena that will dissipate and decline within the decade. From a Parsonian structural-functional perspective, they perform a function and, therefore, structures will continue to be put in place to ensure their survival. Indeed, we would expect that these educational modalities will expand in the future and become far more common in the preparation for professional practice than they are today. We have begun to discuss and witness their evolution in this paper, and the reader will see a great deal of further evidence in the superb papers that follow. As one social work authority in this arena has commented, "There is no doubt that new developments in technology will continue at a rapid pace that will make teaching with technology even more effective and widespread." She therefore wisely adds that there is a pressing need "to develop a coherent body of knowledge to support the delivery of teaching in technology-enhanced learning environments for future social work education" (Coe Regan, 2008, p. 218).

We must recognize the medium has limitations, including a higher general rate of attrition and the frequently unstated expectation of a very well-organized, disciplined, and motivated student. Field practicum, sometimes referred to as the signature pedagogy of the profession, often may be more difficult to execute well at a distance. Yet the online revolution offers intriguing opportunities for broadening and extending access to social work education. Whenever possible, perhaps use of a hybrid format, with online education complemented and supplemented by faculty mentoring and personal contact, would lead toward an optimal protocol. But as the noted political sage Douglas Schoen (2010, p. 198) reminds us:

> Our society and all of its institutions are in continuous processes of transformation. We cannot expect new stable states that will endure for our own lifetimes . . . . We [reflective practitioners] must learn to understand, guide, influence and manage these transformations.

It is our hope that the chapters that follow will help us to begin this journey of understanding together.

REFERENCES

Abels, P. (Ed.). (2005). *Distance education in social work.* New York, NY: Springer.

Allen, I. E., & Seaman, J. (2013). *Changing course: Ten years of tracking online education in the U.S.* Newburyport, MA: The Sloan Consortium.

Beaulaurier, R. & Haffey, M. (Eds.). (2005). *Technology in social work education.* Binghamton, NY: Haworth

Brooks, A.C. (2013). My valuable, cheap college degree. *The New York Times*, February 1, p. A–27.

Coe Regan, J. A. (2008). Technology in social work education. In T. Mizrahi & L. Davis (Eds.), *Encyclopedia of social work* (20th ed., vol. 4, pp. 217–218). Washington, DC: NASW Press.

Cronin, J. M., & Bachorz, P. M. (2006). The rising phoenix and what it means for higher education. *Journal of Education, 186*(1), 11–21.

Council on Social Work Education. (2013). Distance education. Retrieved at www.cswe.org/accreditation/information/DistanceEducation.aspx

Cummings, S. M., & Chaffin, K. (2012). Comparison of outcomes of a distance education and a traditional MSW program. Paper presented at the 58th Annual Program Meeting of the Council on Social Work Education, November 11, 2012, Washington, DC.

Dewey, J. (1938). *Logic: The theory of inquiry.* New York, NY: Henry Holt.

Edmundson, M. (2012). The trouble with online education. *The International Herald Tribune*, January 18, p. 11.

Friedman, T. L. (2013). Revolution hits the universities. *The New York Times*, January 27, p. A–18.

Grossman, L. K. (2012). Reading, 'riting, 'rithmetic, and R & D. Letter to the editor. *The Nation*, February 6, p. 2.

Heller, N. (2013). LaptopU: Has the future of college moved online? *The New Yorker*, May 20, pp. 80–91.

Lewin, T. (2012). College of future could be "come one, come all." *The New York Times*, November 20, pp. A-1 & A-16.

Lewin, T. (2013). Master's degree is new frontier of study online. *The New York Times.* August 18, pp. A-1 & A-18.

National Association of Social Workers & Association of Social Work Boards. (2005). Standards for Technology and Social Work Practice. Retrieved at www.aswb.org/Technology SWPractice.pdf

Ouellette, P.M. & Westhuis, D. (2008). Social work education: Electronic technologies. In T. Mizrahi & L. Davis (Eds.), *Encyclopedia of social work* (20th ed., vol. 4, pp. 118–120). Washington, DC: NASW Press.

Reamer, F.G. (2013). Social work in a digital age: Ethical and risk management challenges. *Social Work, 58*(2), 163–172.

Rose, L. H. (2013). Letter to the editor. *The New York Times*, April 29, p. A–27.

Schoen, D. E. (2010). *The Political Fix*. New York, NY: Time Books.

Vernon, R. (2006). CSWE commission on accreditation distance education survey. Unpublished manuscript. Alexandria, VA: CSWE.

Vernon, R., Vakalahi, H., Pierce, D., Pittman-Munke, P., & Adkins, L. F. (2009). Distance education in social work: Current and emerging trends. *Journal of Social Work Education, 45*(2), 263–276.

Part 1: Organizational and Administrative Perspectives

Launching the Virtual Academic Center: Issues and Challenges in Innovation

MARILYN FLYNN, R. PAUL MAIDEN, WENDY SMITH, and JUNE WILEY
School of Social Work, University of Southern California, Los Angeles, California, USA

GARY WOOD
Social Work Curriculum and Faculty Relations, 2U, Inc., Los Angeles, California, USA

In October 2010, the University of Southern California School of Social Work entered the online education environment with the launch of the first national web-based MSW program. After an initial enrollment of 80 students, in just 3 years this state-of-the-art MSW, offered in a technology-advanced synchronous and asynchronous format, has generated an enrollment of 2,000 students residing in 38 states. The development and rapid growth of the Virtual Academic Center has not been without significant challenges, the most substantial of which has been the creation of a national field education program. This paper describes the MSW courses taught in the online environment, and pedagogical hurdles faced in order to maintain the educational quality that is the hallmark of the School's campus-based MSW program.

CHALLENGES FACING SOCIAL WORK EDUCATION

The business model for schools of social work is not a pleasant one to contemplate. Almost all programs are tuition-driven, with modest to nonexistent endowments and relatively little revenue from research. While the traditional sciences and medical schools have clinical practices, patents, consultancies, and donors with relatively deep pockets, social work has carried out little experimentation with new methods of revenue development. In the long run, this reality threatens the future of professional education on university campuses, especially at major research institutions, because we generally are not seen as central to the university's mission.

The profession to some extent has also resisted the incursion of online education—a major mechanism for potential program expansion. Concerns about quality of students, fidelity of content, and socialization to the profession seem to be deep-rooted. There has been a sense that online education is, for social work, inherently substandard and useful only in extremis as a secondary mechanism when all traditional means are not feasible. And even where online programs have been introduced, they usually have ironically been limited to state boundaries or have chosen to exclude students who live near campus. They are generally small. At the same time, larger university systems and some of the nation's most exclusive institutions are flooding the educational world with new opportunities for learning and teaching in virtual environments. Leadership is coming from many intellectual domains.

Finally, all involved in higher education are confronting a future decline in the number of students of college-going age, due to reduced childbearing and the demographic shifts this has produced. While the ramifications have not fully spun out nor have they fully touched graduate education yet, the drop is impending. The problem of maintaining demand, recruiting new students from untapped sources, along with the influence of social work programs themselves on campus are all impending, fundamentally serious issues.

It was within this context that the School of Social Work at the University of Southern California decided to take an unprecedented leap in developing a virtual academic center (VAC). Our decision was unique in several respects. First, we elected to form a 10-year, exclusive, binding agreement with an East Coast firm that would link our program in a unique way with the for-profit sector. The firm, 2U, agreed to recruit students, market our program, build a customized platform, help to convert our curriculum, assist with monitoring and evaluation, support for initial outreach for identification of field placements, and partner with us in the provision of scholarships. They also pledged not to work with any other school of social work.

Second, we took a step that is familiar in the business world but almost unprecedented in academia: to move to scale in an unprecedented period of 24 months. This decision was based on a fundamental change in the business model for the school, designed to build financial resilience and support expansion of research activity in the face of declining federal resources. We monitored retention rates, academic performance, and other variables closely as we grew, and we revised administrative structures as we learned.

Graduate students in our online program reside in more than 40 states (also U.S. Territories and abroad). We became the first social work program fully available locally throughout the United States and Canada. This scope of outreach brought with it expected and unanticipated consequences for course content, interactions among students, and a true reexamination of what is meant by diversity in the classroom. While medicine and many other professions have long been inherently national in internship training and practice, social work has remained preeminently local in character. This shift has for us been transformative.

Implications for the School's concept of faculty membership were profound. We introduced new approaches to recruiting and screening faculty, new communications technology to allow our "virtual" faculty to participate in faculty meetings and school events, and new faculty support roles at the associate dean level. We adopted new rules for faculty governance that permitted "virtual" faculty to be elected to certain committees and established webinars to promote the School's culture. These and other measures reflected a choice not to marginalize our virtual faculty but to integrate them to the fullest extent possible.

One of the most important actions in moving toward this unprecedented change in our School's academic profile was insistence on full and formal faculty approval. While some programs in social work and sister disciplines have side-stepped this process, we did not. Leadership from the most prestigious senior faculty was needed if the VAC were to reflect the best aspects of our teaching. We anticipated that many of our tenure line faculty would teach in the online environment and bring the best aspects of that experience back to our traditional classes. In the long run, we imagined a fluid and ever-extending connection among various settings for immersive learning, with the online program representing only one of many forms of engagement for students and faculty. After deep and concerned examination of issues, the faculty voted to endorse start-up of the VAC, has continued to monitor it closely through the elected Curriculum Council, and has gravitated toward use of the platform in research collaborations as well as in instruction.

The School understood from the onset that field internships would require creative thinking and new forms of outreach. Field faculty were hesitant, concerned that traditional methods of cultivating agency relationships would no longer be possible. At the same time, almost everyone has recognized that older patterns of field placement—especially the one-to-one apprenticeship model—are breaking down due to economic forces, competition from other disciplines, overwhelming client demand in some sectors, and similar factors. Independent of other reasons for moving toward the VAC, the School was poised to re-imagine its methods and structures for field education. The online program offered an impetus that the School used to test a variety of innovations. This included use of simulated clients for students awaiting placement, "teaching institution" agreements with large service providers, providing external field instructors for clinical supervision in non-traditional settings, and most recently, online field experience to prepare students for agency roles. Planning for the VAC thus allowed the School to address one of the profession's most vexing issues.

In sum, introduction of an online program at the University of Southern California was not simply an offset to our basic campus program but a revolution in our business model, field education program, faculty governance system, and classroom environment—both virtual and on campus and with our student body. It was intended to generate new revenues for research expansion and has in fact transformed the nature of the School's research infrastructure support, adding six new post-doctoral positions and a host of new interdisciplinary research clusters. In launching the VAC, the School attempted to address some of the intractable difficulties that educational institutions are facing in the twenty-first century. This aspiration led us to implement a program conceptualization that was sweeping, exceptional, and replete with unknowns. It also has led us to discovery, invention, and transformation, which are, we believe, the basic elements of creativity and success.

Launching the Virtual Academic Center

In October 2010, the School of Social Work launched its innovative web-based MSW program with an initial first cohort of 80 students. The VAC is now welcoming its fifteenth cohort, with 2,000 students enrolled. Students at first came mainly from California, with a significant enrollment growth in other states when the School was approved by the respective state departments of higher education to offer the USC MSW degree to residents of those states. The geographic composition of the VAC now is approximately 30% from California, with the remaining from other states and the U.S. Territories, Canada, and Western Europe—primarily Germany due to the concentration of military installations: Landstuhl, Ramstein, Baumholder.

The VAC also was subject to a full accreditation review by the Western Association of Schools and Colleges (WASC) which also serves as the accrediting body for the University of Southern California. WASC accreditation was necessary as the MSW is offered in its entirety through the VAC and therefore constituted a new program offering. The School now is approved to offer the degree through the VAC in 49 states (New Hampshire has not approved any online programs to date). There are currently student enrollments from 40+ states, including Alaska and Hawaii. The School also accepts applicants from U.S. Territories with the caveat that a viable field placement must be secured prior to starting the program. The VAC has four admission cycles and enrollment targets per academic year, which include both regular and advanced standing admissions (for highly qualified applicants with a BSW). The admission cycles and enrollment projections are August (260 regular and 24 additional advanced standing admits); September (340 MSW), January (300 regular and 30 advanced standing); and, May (280 regular and 12 advanced standing). (It is important to note that the School of Social Work introduced the advanced standing option less than 2 years ago.) The admission requirements are stringent, requiring an overall undergraduate GPA of

3.2 and a BSW course GPA of 3.5. All students applying for admission to advanced standing must take a six–unit "bridge" program prior to admission to the MSW program, achieving a GPA of 3.0 or better. Those unable to do so are admitted to the regular 2-year MSW program. The advanced standing program is nearing the end of a 2-year pilot phase. Once reviewed by the School's Curriculum Council, it is anticipated that USC will open the enrollment and admit all qualified applicants. The advanced standing program was introduced simultaneously in the School's four other campus based programs (University Park, USC's main campus; Skirball Academic Center in West Los Angeles; Orange County Academic Center; and, the San Diego Academic Center). However, the admission of advanced standing students into the VAC outstrips the four campus-based centers by approximately a four-to-one ratio.

Foundation, Concentration, and Elective Offerings in the VAC

Planning, development, and implementation of the VAC were carried out with the intent that courses offered in the School's campus-based academic centers eventually would all be offered in the VAC. The 60 courses in the School's MSW program include foundation, concentration, and elective course offerings. Course conversions for web-based instruction started with the MSW foundation courses followed by the concentration and elective course offerings. The School offers five concentrations in the advanced year: Community Organization, Planning and Administration (COPA); Families and Children; Health; Mental Health and Social Work and Business in a Global Society. There are also four sub-concentrations: Aging Studies; Military Social Work and Veteran Services; Public Child Welfare; and, School Social Work. A decision was made in the early stages of VAC development to launch the most high-demand concentrations first. These are Families and Children, Mental Health, and Military Social Work. The next major wave of course conversions focused in the Health and COPA concentrations (and related electives) followed by Social Work and Business, School Social Work, Aging Studies, and Public Child Welfare. There are some 50 course offerings in the VAC with another 6 in the conversion queue.

MSW curriculum offerings also include a number of highly specialized or unique classes that do not always attract viable enrollment to justify offering them on a regular basis. However, they are courses important to the faculty who developed them and are well received by the students who take them. They include Spirituality and Social Work, Human Sexuality in Social Work Practice, Social Work Practice with African American Families, Social Work Practice with Latino Populations, and two LGBT courses. These special offerings are going to be added to the VAC, thereby more than doubling the potential student draw.

The School recently realigned its "ground and cloud" semester terms to enable campus-based students to take VAC courses. This change also enables VAC students residing in close proximity to one of the School's campuses to take traditional campus-based courses. It is noteworthy that the School has experienced a substantial increase in enrollment of campus-admitted students in VAC courses in the summer. This enables such students to participate in the School's summer global immersion offerings and also permits many non-residential students to return to their home states for the summer months.

Profiling the Virtual Student

Prior to the development of the VAC, the School always had a predominantly full-time student population with an 80:20 full-time to part-time ratio. The median age across the four campus-based academic centers is approximately 28.

The initial VAC enrollment target for full-time students was set at 75%, but the highest achieved in the first few cohorts was 70%. However, the full-time to part-time ratio has declined dramatically over the course of 15 cohorts. Seventy percent of the current student enrollment consists of part-time students who are completing the degree over a 3- to 4-year span. Their median age is 33 years. This variation between the campus-based centers and the VAC is substantial and presents a challenge in terms of acculturating VAC students to the university, the school, and the "Trojan Family." USC is a culture-rich environment for students, faculty, and alumni. However, it has been challenging to inculcate part-time students into the USC culture, which is made more difficult with students who reside in the virtual campus. In retrospect, the full-time to part-time enrollment ratios capsized for a number of reasons. The students in the VAC are older and have more other obligations such as employment and families; these necessitate a part-time pursuit of the degree. Cost of the program is also another deterrent to attending full-time and part-time working students tend to accrue less tuition-related debt. (The tuition in the VAC is the same rate as for the campus-based programs.) Finally, in the last year or so, we have experienced a dramatic rise in the number of admitted students who are ineligible for the federal Direct Grad Plus loan program due to a poor credit rating or late repayment of consumer debt. This fact has forced many students to drop from full- to part-time status since they cannot secure adequate financial assistance to cover the cost of tuition.

INTEGRATION AND CONVERSION OF ON-GROUND CURRICULUM

From its inception, the MSW degree earned through the VAC and the curriculum that comprises its course of study were intended to be identical to those offered at the School's campus-based academic centers. Of particular concern in the development of the VAC was the optimization of students' engagement and interaction with curriculum content, instructors, and one another—known in the literature, respectively, as *cognitive presence, teaching presence*, and *social presence* (Swan, 2003). The VAC can be described broadly as consisting of four essential components, intended to closely parallel the experiences of campus-based students, each of which contributes to building cognitive, teaching, and social presence. Students access these components through the VAC's learning management system (LMS), which was developed and is now maintained and enhanced by the School's partner company 2U. Inc. Each of the four components—asynchronous content, live synchronous classes, social networking, and field practicum—is described below.

Asynchronous Content Development

Asynchronous, or pre-produced, curriculum is content that faculty developed as learning experiences for students to engage in independently. Asynchronous content may consist of written text, media-rich video slide presentations, video presentations or interviews of faculty or guest experts, self-check quizzes, forums (threaded online discussions, often called discussion boards), and commercially available third-party videos, such as might be shown in campus classrooms. Specific asynchronous content is developed for each course; students are expected to have completed each week's content prior to meeting in the live synchronous class session. Students in all sections of the same course study the same asynchronous content. As in campus-based classes, reading assignments are considered homework, to be done *in addition to* pursuit of the asynchronous and synchronous content. Asynchronous content promotes a high degree of cognitive presence due to engagement with course content, contributing little to social or teaching presence. The asynchronous format is completed independently by students, without interaction with others, with the exception of forum posts that offer discussion of issues with colleagues, albeit not in real time.

Live Synchronous Class Sessions

In addition to pursuing asynchronous content, students attend weekly live class sessions for each of their classes. The live class is a real-time audio/video session in which an instructor and a maximum of 12 students log onto a web-based classroom where they can hear and see one another as they participate in discussion and other activities. As they do on campus, students register for classes by specific day of the week and time, adjusting for time zones. For each weekly unit of each class, equally the live session comprises 50% and the asynchronous content 50%. Students are expected to attend class each week, with the expectation as noted that they already will have completed that week's asynchronous content.

The live classroom provides the instructor with a wide variety of instructional tools, including the ability to use PowerPoint presentations and white boards, display documents, conduct discussions, divide students into smaller breakout rooms for role play, poll the class, and allow students to make individual or group presentations. During live synchronous class time, students and instructor explore, deepen, and apply the week's asynchronous content, maximizing teaching and social presence through interaction between instructor and peers. Taken together, the integrated asynchronous and synchronous components provide a *blended online learning* model. Office hours with instructors also take place in the same online classroom setting, individually or in small groups, determined by need.

Social Networking

Built into the LMS is a series of social networking devices, including communication walls, personal profiles, and student-initiated social groups. Any student or faculty member can start a new social group, and there are currently 510 active social groups with 2,448 total members. This online community is intended to parallel the outside-of-classroom experience that students generally have on campus, adding to the felt social presence.

Field Practicum

Developing the field education program has been one of the most challenging aspects of the VAC, particularly when the program expanded beyond Southern California. Community, agency, and collegial relationships across the United States in urban, metropolitan, and rural areas have and continue to be cultivated. Thousands of agency field visits have been conducted both on-site and virtually, memoranda of understanding (MOUs) negotiated and signed, field learning contracts developed and students placed in foundation and concentration year placement in close proximity to where they reside. The School now has in excess of 3,700 field education partnerships across the country. In many instances, viable agency placements were located but the setting did not employ an MSW. To respond to this gap, the School instituted an external field instructor model to ensure weekly supervision of all students while in placement. Regular supervision typically is conducted virtually on the LMS. However one of 15 full-time VAC regional field faculty, residing in four multi-state regions, conducts in-person, on-site field agency visits as needed.

Students' practicum experiences follow the traditional on campus model of providing placements concurrently during each semester. Students attend placement as they do at the campus-based academic centers, working in agencies and receiving supervision from a field instructor. For VAC students, the agencies, of course, are in their own communities, which often are not in greater Southern California.

After realizing the potential of creating high-quality standardized asynchronous training material (that also could be used on campus), some initial field training on evidence-based practice was developed. Currently, all students on campus and in the VAC receive asynchronous and live training in motivational interviewing *before* arriving at their first field placement. This practicum modality is continuously being refined and expanded to include new technology on virtual client engagement and the development of avatars that can simulate a range of client presenting problems. This format enables students to practice their interview and assessment skills prior to live client engagement.

While building a national model of field education has been a significant logistical challenge in the VAC, the actual foundation and concentration year field experience closely parallels field education at the school's other four campus based academic centers. (USC students placed in hundreds of agencies across the country also frequently encounter MSW field students from other universities in the local area.) For the most part, the agencies are quite receptive to hosting USC students along with MSW students from area schools of social work, and recent graduation statistics indicate that 27% of the graduates have been hired in the agency where they completed their field placement.

VAC COURSE CONVERSION TIMELINE

The initial identification of courses to be converted to become web-based was straightforward since the first year of the MSW degree is a fixed curricular structure with no elective choices. It was essential, therefore, that all these foundation level courses be converted. Foundation courses in Human Behavior in the Social Environment, Policy, Practice, Research and Field (11 courses in all) constituted the core of the first two waves of courses to be developed, first semester and then second semester, respectively. Additional support offerings also were constructed: an initial student orientation and a new faculty orientation.

The third and fourth waves of course conversions involved two of the program's five concentrations—Mental Health and Families and Children—as well as the courses in the military sub-concentration. The advanced concentration year of study consists of three core concentration-specific courses, three electives, a leadership course taken by all students, and field practicum. Mental Health and Families and Children concentrations were converted first because they represented the two most popular concentrations at the academic centers. COPA, Health, and Social Work and Business in a Global Society were developed in the following years, eventually leading to the availability of all five of the School concentrations in the VAC. Elective offerings were selected for conversion based on the demand, with an eye toward selecting courses with cross-concentration appeal. With the conversion of foundation, all five concentrations, and the electives, over 50 courses were constructed on the platform within a 3.5-year period.

Faculty Course Conversion Process

The course conversion process for faculty involved taking existing courses that were taught on the ground and preparing them for use in a virtual environment. Rather than alter or redevelop course content, conversion focused on ensuring that the online version of the course adhered as closely as possible to the version currently taught. Each course was assigned a lead faculty member who was responsible for converting the course and teaching it the first semester.

The first step for faculty was to rethink their courses in terms of which content and learning activities could be carried out asynchronously and which would require a synchronous environment. Activities that expected students to interact with one another (or the instructor) were slated for live synchronous sessions. Learning activities, such as group discussion, role plays, or making group presentations, had to be conducted in synchronous time. Watching a video or faculty slide presentation could be completed by students independently and thus were primed for asynchronous development. Re-conceptualizing courses into two different yet interlocking segments initially was a challenge for instructors—especially for those faculty members who converted courses first, when there were no existing models or examples. Naturally, faculty members who converted later courses, after having taught in the VAC, had the advantage of experiencing how asynchronous and synchronous segments work together.

Together with design and production consultants at 2U, the School's partner firm, faculty planned each of the 15 weeks of the semester for their courses, determining asynchronous and synchronous content. Asynchronous content then was developed. Faculty presentations were filmed to be made into synchronous slide presentations; existing paper-based case studies were scripted and brought to life with professional video enactments; a narrative was completed for written text screens; forum question prompts were planned for student discussion; and self-check quiz questions were written. Production of the asynchronous content was arduous and time consuming for faculty, requiring 3 months or longer of focused effort.

Faculty also had to develop a means to share synchronous learning activities with colleagues who would be teaching other sections of the course. Faculty accomplished this in a variety of ways, including developing written guides and meeting with assigned faculty on a regular basis.

Recruitment and Hiring VAC Teaching Faculty

Durrington, Berryhill, and Swafford (2006) assert that the demand for distance education has become nearly a universal expectation among students, resulting in an increased need for faculty who can teach in a web-based environment. While social work's history in higher education dates back to 1898 at Columbia University, the establishment of online social work programs is a relatively new phenomenon for the profession (http://www.nasw.org). This innovative approach to teaching has thereby created a challenge for higher education institutions who need to recruit individuals who are willing to teach in an online environment and who are enthusiastic about how technology can be used to further advance student learning.

Now with the proposal to launch the VAC vetted by social work faculty and approved by senior administration of the University, the need to staff the VAC became the next task to be achieved. Schnitzer and Crosby (2003) indicate that the process of recruiting and preparing adjuncts for teaching in a distance learning program "is a sequential strategy consisting of recruitment, screening, hiring, training, course preparation, support and mentoring, and evaluation." Consistent with Schnitzer and Crosby's premise, it was recognized early in the establishment of the VAC that having a gifted cadre of faculty to teach in the program was critical. To achieve the goal of having VAC instructors prepared to teach, employment advertisements were placed in higher education and professional journal print publications and on an electronic employment website. Applicants were required to submit their CV's on the university's human resources website. A secondary concern arose regarding how to interview candidates whose education and experience matched the hiring criteria but who were located a great distance from the campus. While telephone interviews could have been conducted, the use of technology was determined to be a better alternative, consistent with the overall approach of a virtual program. A computer-based electronic interview format was selected, which enabled the VAC administrators to create the interview questions for prospective candidates that they could respond to via their computers in their locale. The features of the technology also would permit on-ground faculty, along with administrators, to view the candidates' responses and to share their comments about the interviewee with other faculty engaged in the process. Because these electronic interviews can be done from the candidates' homes or offices, they reduce the time and costs associated with bringing the applicants to the campus. Additionally, using the format of the electronic interview creates the opportunity for faculty and administrators to assess the individual's presence on camera, which is useful in determining how the candidate might handle the live synchronous component of the virtual classroom.

Training and Evaluating the New VAC Faculty

With the hiring process completed and the new instructor placed on the class schedule, getting the faculty trained on the software prior to the class start was the next element to be accomplished. Because a majority of the new instructors were unfamiliar with the specific technology and living in different time zones across the country, one-to-one training was deemed most feasible. To ensure that the training would be easily recalled, it was determined that scheduling the training close to the cohort start date would be most beneficial. The training included teaching the basics of the LMS and its more advanced features such as creating small groups for class discussion. While an individual with little experience with technology might be fearful of learning how to use the technology, the one-to-one sessions assisted the instructor in practicing the features of the platform with our technology support personnel, minimizing their anxiety. A by-product of the training was the opportunity for rapport building with the technology personnel who would be available for assistance throughout the semester.

Following the need to have faculty trained to use the software, it was recognized that similarly to the on-ground program, curricular oversight and mentoring of new VAC instructors by lead faculty would also need to occur. In the VAC, as on-ground, the lead faculty facilitated regularly scheduled virtual meetings to share content-specific teaching resources, provide suggestions, and update instructors about curricular matters. These meetings also helped to create a sense of community between the VAC and on-ground faculty. In addition, VAC faculty participated in the monthly School of Social Work all-faculty meetings through the use of video streaming.

In conjunction with the one-to-one training on the platform and the mentoring provided to VAC faculty, instructors also were given copies of the syllabus, the textbooks, and access to the course prior to its start. The syllabus and textbooks were mailed directly to their residence, and electronic access to the course was provided several weeks in advance, thus creating another opportunity for faculty to be acquainted and comfortable with the materials and the setting that would be part of the weekly synchronous session. To further acquaint faculty with other strategies for success, opportunities to "compare notes" with other faculty have been created via a virtual faculty lounge designated specifically for VAC faculty.

The importance of the flawless functioning of the technology and its proficient use by the instructor were essential. This optimal combination was realized by the work of the technology support staff, which trained faculty to use the software and were available to troubleshoot problems for both instructors and students. As mentioned previously, faculty in the VAC was trained well in advance of their class start. Having the additional support that a technology team can provide during "live" class sessions was vital for the success of the classes and ultimately, the program. The technology support staff were also responsible for any technical revisions that needed to be made to the asynchronous course material, and supported faculty during the first 3 weeks.

Schnitzer and Crosby (2003) state that evaluation must be an element of the "sequential strategy" in a distance learning program. As a mechanism of quality control, an evaluation process was established for the VAC. During the 15-week semester, two evaluations occur—one just prior to the mid-point of the semester and one at the end of the course, the final evaluation. The mid-point evaluation permitted students to assess the instructors' performance at a point where corrective measures could be taken by them, if necessary, to refine aspects of their teaching to enhance the students' learning. Completed on the VAC platform, these evaluations were sent directly to the instructor so that the individual could access the feedback quickly, reviewing the comments from their computer; they were also encouraged to discuss the feedback with their students in order to reinforce the value of the feedback. The mid-semester evaluations also were reviewed by the School's senior administrators, and guidance was provided when scores and comments were below the acceptable range of performance. Unlike the mid-semester evaluations, the final evaluations were tabulated by a research firm contracted by the School to provide a statistical analysis of the overall performance of the instructor, and respond to related questions of pedagogy. Upon receiving the tabulated responses, the associate dean of faculty development scheduled meetings with the instructors whose scores were marginal. These meetings entailed a discussion of the report, strategies for improvement, or whether the instructor's performance indicated that virtual teaching may not be compatible with the instructor's skill set. The instructor could be assigned an additional class in the upcoming semester, based on the feedback provided to the VAC director by the executive vice dean and associate dean for faculty development.

The innovative VAC and associated technology advancements constitute a monumental shift in social work pedagogy. It encompasses innovation, vision, and magnitude. To educate students in this new format necessitates having faculty who can envision how learning can successfully occur in a virtual environment as well as the skill and enthusiasm to work in such a nontraditional venue. To ensure that occurs, the process identified above regarding faculty recruitment, hiring, training, and evaluation continue to be essential to the success of the program.

Faculty Development

The role of the online instructor is not limited to instruction but also influences the extent and nature of connectedness and community that students should feel in a web-based learning environment. Indeed, as Gibson & Blackwell (2005) put it, "The online instructor is the single most important person in making the student's experience a positive or negative one . . ." (p. 2). As they teach their classes, instructors embody and communicate the culture of the host institution as well as the values and knowledge base of their discipline. As we moved into the world of virtual education and our numbers of students and faculty rose,[1] we pondered the best way to help our instructors meet the demands of their multi-dimensional role.

Faculty training, support, and development are widely recognized as essential to ensuring instructional quality and retention of both students and faculty in online programs (Puzziferro-Schnitzer, 2005; De Gagne & McGill, 2010; Lackey, 2011; Orr, Williams, & Pennington, 2009; Rovai & Jordan, 2004; Tipple, 2010). Types of faculty support include orientation, mentoring, online discussion forums and, more recently, communities of practice (Brooks, 2010; Gibson & Blackwell, 2005; Puzziferro-Schnitzer, 2005; Lackey, 2011; Peters & Boylston, 2006); however, studies of effectiveness of any of these approaches is sparse. Faculty support and development are offered in many campus-based programs, but far-flung online faculty arguably has an even greater need for institutional assistance in attaining a sense of community and connection, with peers, administrators, and the institution itself. The more isolated nature of online education means that instructors, like their students, might benefit from live-time interaction with and social presence of faculty colleagues and institutional representatives.

Faculty in the VAC needs practical assistance and social connectedness. When it is not possible to encounter one another in the hall, attend committee and faculty meetings in the same physical space, or stop by a colleague's office, virtual spaces can provide the venues for community building. The sense of community is relationally maintained and activated through continuous virtual interactions. Our awareness of the centrality of face-to-face (or sometimes, voice-to-voice) experience in community building strongly influenced our faculty development initiatives.

Our approach to supporting faculty in the VAC centers was on three interrelated dimensions: the individual faculty member (his or her knowledge and expertise, teaching experience and style, professional/academic goals); the instructional, pedagogical, and curricular aims and needs of the School; and the community and culture of the VAC as an element of the School and the University. Our multi-pronged faculty development program includes orientation for new faculty, individual face-to-face (and telephonic) instructional support, mentoring of lead instructors for multi-sectioned courses, observation of live synchronous class sessions and feedback, oversight of instructional quality via mid-semester and final student evaluations, instruction-related synchronous webinars, and instruction-related asynchronous modules. Consultation is provided to VAC administration, lead faculty, and individual instructors regarding student-instructor issues or

---

[1] Since opening in the fall of 2010, the number of faculty members teaching in the Virtual Academic Center has more than doubled, from a total of 95 full- and part-time to the current 217. The greatest increase has been among adjunct faculty: 74 in the first year, 151 in the second year, 182 in the third year. (Full-time faculty, the majority of whom are clinical teaching and field faculty, who numbered 21 in the first year, are now at 27.)

conflicts. Mentoring and support for scholarly activities and academic career planning is also provided.

Orientation for New Faculty

On-ground orientation is offered to new faculty each semester. All new VAC faculty are brought to campus for this event as well as to meet their foundation and concentration colleagues. Those hired as full-time clinical faculty, whether local or living at a distance, are required to attend, and adjuncts living in the Southern California area often do as well. All new VAC faculty receive training and orientation to the virtual platform and view an online faculty orientation, with modules introducing them to the University and the School and to School instructional practices and policies. The material duplicates and augments the on-ground orientation and is available at the faculty member's convenience. As of fall 2013, new VAC faculty also participate in a live-time online face-to-face welcome and orientation with members of the School administration.

Instructional Mentoring and Support

Those who teach in the VAC encounter the same challenges as instructors on the ground: mastering the material, creating engaging lesson plans that help students to achieve learning outcomes, classroom management, grading, and so on. In addition, they may be new to online teaching or to our blended model of online teaching that includes asynchronous and synchronous dimensions and to the integration of these into a meaningful and effective learning experience. Instructors often find that the journey to realizing their potential as teachers is not a smooth or linear one. Sometimes they are aware of their difficulties and seek consultation, either with their lead instructor or with the associate dean of faculty development; often problems come to notice by means of low ratings, descriptive comments on student evaluations, or student complaints. Systematic review of the course evaluations is used to identify instructors who might benefit from instructional mentoring or consultation. The associate dean offers to meet with these instructors to provide consultation or classroom observation (via recordings) and feedback. A survey of instructors at varying ranks and levels of experience during the past 2 years, both on-ground and online, indicates that 69% found the consultation very helpful, and 31% found it somewhat helpful. The opportunity to discuss their classroom experiences, difficulties, and strategies in detail was cited as the most useful aspect of the consultation.

Webinars and Modules

Faculty needs for information, practical help, and community in part are addressed through our program of webinars and pre-recorded modules, which are continuing to evolve. Current modules provide orientation to the VAC, information on student support services, library resources, and working with students with disabilities. Instruction-related webinars include "Increasing Instructor Effectiveness in a Web-based Learning Environment," "Student Learning in a Web-based Environment," and "instruction clinics" in which faculty bring questions and concerns for consultation with peers and the associate dean. Additional webinars and pre-recorded sessions are under development for the coming academic year.

The literature suggests that there has been little improvement over the last 10 years in increasing the instructional and technical training needed by faculty to teach online successfully (Lackey, 2011). Therefore, we seek to create faculty support structures that not only answer these needs but contribute to a sense of belonging to a learning and teaching community. Our students look to their professors (and ultimately, to their classmates) as embodiments of the School and the professional communities and culture; our instructors reflect the knowledge and experience they bring but also the pedagogical values and community feeling that we build together as a profession.

FUTURE DEVELOPMENTS IN THE VAC

The VAC has been operational for 3 years and has achieved a steady enrollment of 1,800 to 2,000 students. The School is now exploring other areas of expansion and development. There are three new initiatives currently in development that likely will be launched over the next 2 years.

One of these is the "agency-embedded" cohort model. The School has begun developing agreements with large multi-purpose family service, mental health, and substance abuse agencies to enroll cohorts of 20 ± agency employees in the VAC. This "grow your own MSW workforce" provides a mechanism for agencies to partner with USC to enroll qualified full-time employees in an eight-semester VAC part-time program. Agency employees will be enrolled in VAC courses along with other MSW students across the country. Both the School and the agency will provide partial tuition subsidies that will limit the amount of federal financial aid needed to complete the degree. Further, given the size, multiple locations, and range of agency services, employees (via a work study model) will be able to complete both foundation- and concentration-year field placements at their place of employment, with two substantially different field learning experiences. The agency thereby can cultivate a more highly qualified work force without employees needing a leave of absence to pursue a professional degree.

A second area of growth for the VAC will be global enrollment. This objective is being driven primarily by the School's highly successful and sought after Military and Veterans Services specialization. From its inception, the VAC has been marketed for its "portability." VAC courses can be taken anywhere in the world. The only restriction is time zone. Active duty, National Guard, and Reserve personnel (and their dependents) presently constitute a substantial number of students enrolled in the VAC. The campus-based centers (San Diego in particular) also enroll many active duty and military veterans. Some of the School's active-duty students are subject to assignments of 2 to 3 years at U.S. military installations in Europe and Asia. Others are subject to temporary duty assignments (TDY) overseas of 6 months or more. The VAC enables students enrolled in one of the School's campus-based academic centers to request a temporary transfer to the VAC to meet TDY obligations or long-term reassignments to military installations throughout the United States and abroad. The only restriction for transfers to the VAC and relocation overseas is that a viable field placement must be secured and a field agency MOU in place before such a program transfer request is approved. The School has now dedicated resources for international field placement development to accommodate this growing demand and also is experiencing growing interest among foreign students for pursuit of an MSW through the VAC. A small number have been admitted and currently are matriculating through the program. However, similar to the School's military students stationed abroad, the cadre of foreign students, while granted admission, are not allowed to start the program until a viable field placement has been secured and appropriate MSW supervision has been arranged.

Finally, in fall 2015, the School will launch a professional doctoral degree in its VAC. The DSW will have two distinct tracks, one in management and leadership and a second in advanced evidenced-based clinical practice. The DSW degree offering will differ from the MSW program in that each track in the DSW program will be delivered via a hybrid model that will involve a series of campus based summer institutes and pre-conference seminars prior to major national conferences, such as the Network for Social Work Managers, Society for Clinical Social Work, and Council on Social Work Education.

CONCLUSIONS

The challenges of launching a VAC have been substantial. The naysayers of online education, those stating "you cannot teach social work practice in an online environment," are not in the distant past, but USC and other schools of social work have demonstrated that one can indeed teach practice skills online and it can be done effectively, because technological advances have increased rapidly in the past few years. From a social work education perspective, one of the most important of these has been the development of the synchronous, live interactive technology that has bridged the divide among social work educators and MSW students who are engaged together in online education. However, quality development must be the absolute focus of attention in creating and teaching courses in the virtual environment. Developing asynchronous instruction only or relying solely on blackboard is an inferior and insufficient approach to online social work course development. The investment is substantial, but harnessing the best in what technology has to offer is essential to social work skill development, the continued advancement of social work pedagogy, and the production of well-educated and highly qualified professional social work practitioners.

REFERENCES

Brooks, C. (2010). Toward 'hybridized faculty development for the twenty-first century: Blending online communities of practice and face-to-face meetings in instructional and professional support programs. *Innovations in Education and Teaching International*, *47*(3), 261–270.

De Gagne, J., & McGill, B. (2010). Faculty development in online education. *Journal of Online Higher Education*, *1*(7), 1–13.

Durrington, V. A., Berryhill, A. & Swafford, J. (2006). Strategies for enhancing student interactivity in an online environment. *College Teaching*, *54*(1), 190–193. Retrieved from http://www.redorbit.com/news/technology/433631/strategies_for_enhancing_student_interactivity_in_an_online_environment

Gibson, J., & Blackwell, C. (2005). Education without boundaries: Faculty training and support. *Journal of College Teaching and Learning*, *2*(1), 1–6.

Lackey, K. (2011). Faculty development: An analysis of current and effective training strategies for preparing faculty to teach online. *Online Journal of Distance Learning Administration, 14*(4). Retrieved from http://www.westga.edu/distance/ojdla/wnter144/lackey144.html

Orr, R., Williams, M., & Pennington, K. (2009). Institutional efforts to support faculty in online teaching. *Innovative Higher Education*, *34*, 257–268.

Peters, M., & Boylston, M. (2006). Mentoring adjunct faculty: Innovative solutions. *Nurse Educator*, *31*(2), 61–64.

Puzziferro-Schnitzer, M. (2005). Supporting online adjunct faculty: A virtual mentoring program. *Journal of Asynchronous Learning Networks*, *9*(2), 39–43.

Rovai, A., & Jordan, H. (2004). Blended learning and sense of community: A comparative analysis with traditional and fully online graduate courses. *International Review of Research in Open and Distance Learning*, *5*(2). Retrieved from http://www.irrodl.org/index.php/irrodl/article/viewArticle/192/274

Schnitzer, M., & Crosby, L. S. (2003). Recruitment and development of online adjunct instructors. *Online Journal of Distance Learning Administration*, *VI*(II). Retrieved from http://www.westga.edu/~distance/ojdla/summer62/crosby_schnitzer62.html

Swan, K. (2003). Learning effectiveness: What the research tells us. In J. Bourne & J. C. Moore (Eds.), *Elements of Quality Online Education, Practice and Direction* (pp. 13–45). Needham, MA: Sloan Center for Online Education.

Tipple, R. (2010). Effective leadership of online adjunct faculty. *Online Journal of Distance Learning Administration*, *13*(1). Retrieved from http://www.westga.edu/distance/ojdla/wnter144/lackey144.html

Cost Analysis of a Distance Education MSW Program

REBECCA L. STOTZER, KEITH FUJIKAWA, JILL SUR, and PAM ARNSBERGER

Myron B. Thompson School of Social Work, University of Hawai'i at Mānoa, Honolulu, Hawai'i, USA

The use of technology to facilitate education and the provision of an entire higher education degree has exploded in the last two decades. Social work educators have been a part of that trend and have started to utilize distance education (DE) technologies. There is a growing literature regarding the efficacy of DE instruction in social work, and scholars are actively developing best practices. However, there is little research in general to support the cost of DE, no cost studies in social work, and none comparing costs of DE delivery to costs associated with a face-to-face program. This study hopes to fill this gap by providing an analysis of the direct costs of an MSW DE program in comparison to similar costs of a face-to-face program.

The use of technology to facilitate education has exploded in the last two decades (U.S. Department of Education, National Center for Education Statistics, 2008). Social work education has also been a part of that trend and has started to utilize distance education technologies for course delivery (Vernon, Vakalahi, Pierce, Pittman-Munke, & Adkins, 2009). Research on educational efficacy for distance education (DE) students compared to students receiving face-to-face instruction have indicated that DE courses are not necessarily better *or* worse than face-to-face courses, just different (e.g., Mason, Helton, & Dziegielewski, 2010; Coe Regan & Youn, 2008; Bernard et al., 2004; Csiernik, Furze, Dromgole, & Rishchynski, 2006; York, 2008).

However, even without evidence ensuring educational quality, many schools of social work started making the move toward DE. For some, this initiative was about educational opportunity and equity for students located in remote or rural locations (Wilson, 1999), while others have argued that costs were a significant factor in the decision-making process (McCormack, 1996). Yet, there is little research to support the cost-effectiveness of distance education (Bray, Harris, & Major, 2007), no cost studies in social work, and none comparing costs of DE delivery to costs associated with a face-to-face program. This paper fills this gap by providing a case study of the direct costs of an MSW DE program in comparison to similar costs of a traditional face-to-face program.

DISTANCE EDUCATION COSTS

Inglis, Ling, and Joosten (2002) argued that DE costs are recoverable at different rates depending on the nature of the DE program and its offerings. The authors divide DE courses into two main categories: (1) classroom-based learning and (2) resource-based learning. Classroom-based learning most closely mimics traditional forms of education, with constant interaction between the teacher and students as well as students interacting with other students, and learning is based in large part on that interaction. In contrast, resource-based learning focuses on a student's interactions with self-paced instructional materials. The United States has generally adopted the "remote classroom" model utilizing a variety of interactive technologies such as interactive television, online classrooms, or asynchronous class management systems through bulletin boards and chat discussions (Inglis, 2007). Given that the costs of moving toward technology are best recovered by economies of scale (having large numbers of students accessing the same technology to distribute the cost), Inglis argues that DE is unlikely to recover costs effectively in a classroom-based learning style of distance education delivery (Inglis, 2003; Ingliss et al., 2002). Turoff (1996) has argued that it is possible to have an entire "virtual university" at costs relative to traditional programs but warns against increasing class sizes, decreasing instructor pay, or other compromises to quality in order to more effectively recover costs.

Social work education is less likely to adopt the more cost-effective strategy of the resource-based learning model due to the importance of interaction and the development of interpersonal and practice skills in the curriculum. This focus on the classroom-based learning style will decrease the probability that DE social work programs will be profitable. In addition, the Council on Social Work Education requires low teacher-to-student ratios for accreditation, which impacts DE cost containment (Kreuger & Stretch, 2000). Forster and Washington (2000) argue that adopting DE in social work may not in fact reduce costs; adoption just shifts money to technology costs. Van Dusen (2000, pg. v., Introd.) has argued that "distance education is unlikely to affect institutional cost savings over the short or middle term," and Potashnik (1998) notes that the cost of conducting DE classes goes down as the number of students rises; however, the cost of services for students will also rise, balancing out the overall costs of distance education.

In fact, rather than being a source of additional revenue, some studies have found that DE programs run at a loss (Bledsoe, 2008; Taylor, Parker, & Tebeaux, 2001). Increased expenses have led to administrative pressures to add more students to DE classes, thereby reducing personnel overhead by increasing classroom size. In contrast, current DE best practice suggests that lower student-to-teacher ratios are necessary to maintain quality (Forster & Washington, 2000). Also, similar to campus-based public programs, course fees generally do not cover the costs of DE, even when DE students pay additional fees (Taylor et al., 2001). Losses may also be related to over-expansion and DE adoption for the sake of the technology itself or for an unproven perception of market-based profit motive (Krueger & Stretch, 2000; Wilson, 1999). Some scholars have argued that costs will decline over time after the initial investment in upgrades and program/course startups (Office of Institutional Research, Northern Virginia Community College, 2002). Other scholars have argued that the costs will never come down to a reasonable level because of the need to maintain low teacher-to-student ratios for accreditation and the need to constantly upgrade and update technology and due to persistent technology maintenance costs (Krueger & Stretch, 2000).

These arguments back and forth in the literature about the cost-effectiveness of DE highlight the need for more cost studies of DE (Rumble, 2001a), particularly for social work, given its historic reliance on a more expensive interactive style of DE delivery. This study attempts to address this issue by examining the direct costs associated with a DE MSW delivered throughout the State of Hawai'i when compared to its equivalent campus-based program. The goal of this research was to uncover the relative direct costs of these two delivery modalities.

The University of Hawai'i Model

As noted above, the delivery method, technology, and number of students in the DE program all have an impact on cost. This analysis will provide an examination of the *direct* cost of DE for a rural DE program when compared to a traditional face-to-face model. Direct costs are those that are immediately attributable to the program (e.g., travel to the island of Kaua'i for a practicum site visit). Direct costs attributable to each program do not include those costs that are shared (e.g., salaries for the dean, the fiscal officer), costs that are separate from educational programs (e.g., research, grants, special short-term projects), or costs that are financed by the University and not billed to individual schools/departments (e.g., electricity, rent). Thus, this analysis will not be able to provide an *absolute* cost of the comparative MSW programs but will offer the first attempt to quantify these differences in direct expenditures in order to help administrators better calculate the fiscal implications of engaging in a DE program.

Given that expenditures are directly related to administrative decisions about program design and to better understand the comparison of costs, it is critical to first understand the model of DE being used.

The Myron B. Thompson School of Social Work (SSW) is located in a top-tier research university and is the only school in the Pacific that offers BSW, MSW, and doctor of philosophy in social welfare (PhD) degrees. However, only the MSW is offered via DE, and only students located on "neighbor islands" (those outside of the island of O'ahu) currently are eligible to enroll. The campus-based MSW program serves O'ahu-based students, admitting roughly 190 students a year. All students must successfully complete a total of 57 credits to graduate with an MSW (30 credits if admitted as advanced standing). Each year, the SSW serves a total of roughly 160 MSW students in the campus-based program. Only 30 DE students are admitted in each admission year, with two cohorts running concurrently. DE students must follow either the 3-year plan or the advanced standing plan (1–2 years, depending on year of admission). Unlike other schools that have chosen to increase their DE class sizes, the UHSSW has chosen to limit DE class size to ensure high-quality instruction for the program.

The current DE option is a technology-based program, utilizing course management software, interactive television, and online synchronous classrooms. This current technology-enhanced version of the DE MSW option accepted its first cohort of students in 2007. The two cohorts ran simultaneously, and at the time of this study, two cohorts had graduated. Unlike the findings in prior research that indicated high dropout rates in DE programs (Haga & Heikamp, 2000), Cohorts 1 and 2 combined had a drop-out rate of only 7.4%.

School of social work personnel

At the main campus, there are three committed tenure-track faculty, one tenure-track DE director, one faculty project coordinator, one administrative assistant, one part-time practicum coordinator, and part-time support from the central UH campus-based SSW student services office committed to DE. In addition, one site coordinator is located at each neighbor island site (five sites total) to provide commitment and coordination in delivering the program. All of these positions were added to the existing faculty and staff to run the DE program. In contrast, the campus-based Manoa program has approximately 20 faculty, one dean, and five staff. Staff and faculty travel to see DE students is highly encouraged, and mandatory site visits to each practicum site are conducted by practicum personnel or faculty each semester. Thus, students have frequent face-to-face contact with faculty and staff that are primarily located on O'ahu.

Distance education administrative infrastructure—Outreach College

DE courses are administered through UH Outreach College. This college is an entity that originally focused on community extension programs and has grown to include some academic programs that are off-campus. Tuition paid by students into Outreach College is treated separately from other tuition funds and goes directly to the schools/departments that generated the tuition. However, because Outreach College is providing a high level of administrative infrastructure—processing tuition payments, financial aid, billing and payments from Outreach Accounts—the College takes one-fourth to one-third of the tuition received for the MSW DE courses. This arrangement is unique to the DE program; the campus-based program runs through the central UH Mānoa administrative infrastructure.

Technology

The technology utilized by the program is a course management platform that is funded by the university and thus not seen in the School's budget. (This platform is available to all courses in the UH system, not just DE courses.) Therefore, this technology cost is not included in this analysis. The more advanced technology utilized by the DE MSW program alone is an online synchronous classroom environment (Blackboard Collaborate) that is paid for through a contract with the UH College of Education on a yearly basis based on usage and includes tech support. Last, for many DE courses, interactive television is utilized (Hawai'i Interactive Video Services–HITS), and the cost of this service is 25% of tuition revenue generated by the courses conducted in HITS studios.

Sources of funds

The SSW, as part of a land grant public university, is primarily funded through state-appropriated funds. However, the SSW also has an active program of grants and contracts. The DE program was financed from 2007 to 2011 through appropriations and tuition as well as significant state support through Title IVE training funds. Many other universities have also paired with state agencies to improve the child welfare workforce (Zlotnik, 2003:

Zlotnik & Cornelius, 2000), and in 1996, 29 states were utilizing Title IVE funds for social work education and training (National Association of Social Workers [NASW], 2004).

METHOD

Data in this study are from three state fiscal years: 2008–2009, 2009–2010, and 2010–2011. As a baseline for the costs of the campus-based program offered on O'ahu, we first examined the process that the UH budget office implements on a yearly basis for each campus in the UH system to measure expenditures. The budget office calculates:

1. *Total Direct Expenditures (TDE)*: total expenditures minus unattributable and indirect costs.
2. *Student Semester Hours (SSH)*: the total number of credits offered times the number of students enrolled (for example, a standard 3-credit course that has 20 enrolled students would be a total of 60 student semester hours).
3. *Course Full-Time Enrolled Students (CFTE)*: Total SSH divided by 24 (the number of credits per year to be considered full-time) for graduate students. Essentially, the number of full-time equivalent students served, not the number of discreet individual persons enrolled in the program. For example, if eight students take 20 credits each in one year, CFTE would equal 6.67.
4. *Direct Expenditures per SSH*: Total direct expenditures divided by SSH (TDE/SSH) to reflect the direct expenditure for each student semester hour delivered.
5. *Direct Expenditures per CFTE*: Total direct expenditures divided by CFTE (TDE/CFTE) to reflect the direct expenditures per full time equivalent student (not actual individual students).

SSH and CFTE provide related measures that are utilized in different ways by university communities. As described above, costs for SSH reflect the amount spent to deliver each credit hour of coursework. In contrast, costs per CFTE allow schools to estimate their direct costs per student. Data on SSH and CFTE for the campus-based program are reported each year by UH budget office reports while data on the DE MSW are available from Outreach College reports. Costs associated with DE that *do* appear in UH budget office reports (such as tenure-track faculty salaries) were broken out separately to isolate campus-based expenditures alone. Last, those DE-specific expenses that were broken out were then combined with Outreach reports and other expenditures that were not included in the University reports (e.g.,

Title IVE expenditures) in order to determine the discrete costs associated with the DE MSW program.

Modifications of Reported Expenditures

Rumble (2001b) recommends that, whenever possible in creating cost comparisons, the included cost categories should be as similar as possible to ensure that one is not comparing "apples and oranges." Given that some indirect costs are shared (e.g., electricity for the campus in Mānoa from which courses are delivered), we focused exclusively on *direct* costs that were attributable to the programs. This strategy meant excluding four staff from the analysis (two fiscal personnel, two administrative personnel) who assisted both DE and the campus-based programs in the school as well as the dean's salary. In addition, costs such as rent, phones, facilities, shared technology expenses, and other indirect costs were excluded. Last, costs associated with projects, contracts, or centers were not included.

Expenditures clearly attributed to the campus-based MSW-program and the DE program were computed separately for fiscal years 2008–2009 through 2010–2011. Although the program started in fiscal year 2007–2008, this year it was dropped from the analysis because only one cohort was admitted, and the program is designed to run two cohorts simultaneously. Every year since 2008, there have been two cohorts progressing through the program during each fiscal year, allowing for appropriate comparative calculations.

RESULTS

As can be seen from Table 1, the primary expenses for the DE program were related to personnel, including both salaries and fringe benefits. Although nearly 80% of DE expenditures is a significant proportion of the total, for the campus-based program, just over 90% of direct program costs were personnel costs. In this case study, the additional administrative costs associated with running the DE program through Outreach College were the second largest category of expenditures, followed by technology costs. Although prior cost research has focused predominantly on technology costs, the additional personnel hired to implement the DE program (and related administrative costs) were the most significant portion of the DE MSW program's direct expenditures.

Table 2 outlines the SSH, CFTE, and expenditures for the campus-based and distance MSW programs for fiscal years 2009–2011. Given the national economic turmoil of 2008 through 2010, one can see fluctuations in expenditures from year to year as well as changes in student enrollment. The difference between DE and campus-based expenditures consistently showed

TABLE 1 Proportion of DE Expenditures by Type and Fiscal Year

Type of DE Expenditure	2008–2009	2009–2010	2010–2011
Personnel	82.7%	75.9%	78.5%
Outreach College Fees (Administrative Costs)	8.9%	12.0%	9.5%
Technology	3.6%	2.8%	3.7%
Travel	2.8%	4.3%	2.9%
Materials/Supplies	0.4%	3.5%	2.8%
Other	1.5%	1.4%	2.6%

TABLE 2 Expenditures by Student Semester Hours of Full-Time Equivalent Students by Fiscal Year for Distance Education

Fiscal Year	Modality	Total Direct Expenditures (TDE)	Student Semester Hours (SSH)	Direct Expenditures per SSH	Course Full-Time Enrolled Students (CFTE)	Direct Expenditures per CFTE
2008–2009	Campus	$1,420,944	4,677	$304	195	$7,287
	DE	$737,540	894	$825	37	$19,934
2009–2010	Campus	$1,052,237	4,330	$243	180	$5,846
	DE	$709,150	928	$764	39	$18,183
2010–2011	Campus	$1,195,566	4,575	$261	191	$6,259
	DE	$851,054	882	$965	37	$23,001
3 Year Total	Campus	$3,668,747	13,582	$270	566	$6,482
	DE	$2,297,744	2,704	$850	113	$20,334

that delivering DE courses costs more per student. In year 1, DE delivery expenses were 2.7 times higher than campus-based costs per student. In year 2, DE delivery was 3.6 times higher and, in year 3, it was 3.3 times higher than campus-based delivery per student. Overall, the 3-year totals reflect direct costs of DE that are an average of 3.2 times higher than campus-based costs. Given that the 2010–2011 year reflected the DE team at full capacity (highest enrollments of students as well as being fully staffed), the DE model described above is anticipated to remain three times more costly than the campus-based program.

DISCUSSION

Consistent with prior research, which hypothesized that maintaining high-quality, low-enrollment, interaction-focused DE in social work would not be revenue-generating, this analysis found the DE MSW program at UHSSW was 3.2 times more expensive than the campus-based MSW program. Despite prior concerns about technology costs being the most prohibitive element of DE delivery, this analysis found that the largest expenditure for the

DE program in fact was for the additional personnel needed to provide instruction, administration, and student support.

It is critical to remember this research describes costs but does not address program efficacy or quality. As cautioned by Inglis (2007):

> the question that managers now want answered is not "Which method of delivery is less costly?" but "How can the costs of delivery best be managed?" In other words, given that the decision has been taken to go online, it is important to determine how the quality of courses and programs can be maintained or increased, without at the same time escalating costs. (p. 447)

Most schools of social work do not choose to venture into DE delivery in order to generate revenue but instead make the move to increase equitable access to education (Raymond, 2005). Hence, the higher costs associated with DE delivery should not necessarily be a deterrent, given the prior success of models to address such issues as rural/urban disparities in the availability of trained social workers (e.g., Daley & Avant, 1999; Haga & Heitkamp, 2000; Stotzer, 2012). These preliminary studies have all suggested that DE is just as effective in attaining learning outcomes equivalent to face-to-face programs, but the question remains "at what cost?"

Although this study represents the first to attempt to demonstrate the relative costs of DE and campus-based programs, future studies should measure both costs *and* benefits of DE to students, schools, universities, and their communities. Given that many professional programs struggle to quantify their value and the benefits of their program, the need for such measurement certainly is not an issue unique to DE program delivery. However, research should explore more deeply how different models predict different costs and whether those different models generate differential outcomes (i.e., graduation rates, employment, licensure, etc.).

There are significant limitations to our analysis that should be noted. First, this analysis is based on a very specific model of DE delivery. Although it does offer important documentation to aid programs in their consideration of adopting a fully DE-based graduate degree, more study of the costs of other program models is needed to paint a fuller picture of the range of expenses associated with DE delivery. In particular, the UHSSW's specific (multi-island) geographic limitation, the purposeful limiting of cohort and class size, and the focus on interactivity by increasing tenure-track personnel committed to the DE program are all particular policy and pedagogical choices that lead to a significant pattern of expenditures. Other schools that may choose not to limit class size, decide to invest in a more resource-based asynchronous delivery model, or heavily utilize adjunct lecturers to deliver a large portion of their curriculum will clearly have a different rate and distribution of expenditures. This case study should serve as just one cost model, and further research should explore different DE models to determine their associated costs, so that schools can make more informed decisions about adopting DE options.

Another limitation of this case study is the nature of this comparison of direct costs rather than total costs. This decision was governed by University spending patterns and the range of unattributable costs incurred by all programs. Therefore, it was not possible to compare the total costs of DE delivery, only the comparability of direct costs with the school's more traditional face-to-face delivery model. This case study also provides only a 3-year snapshot of a DE delivery model, while the costs of DE are likely to change over time. In this particular case, the majority of instructional faculty affiliated with the DE project were tenure track assistant professors. Those professors actively seek grants (and possible course buyouts and the need to find lecturers to cover courses) and are pursuing tenure and promotion (leading to increased costs if tenure/promotion is achieved). These personnel changes will result in different expenditures. Other changes in expenditures have been associated with turnover of personnel, shifts in university policy regarding the use of tuition funds, and changes in sources of funds for the DE program. These realities suggest that the costs of DE delivery have a high probability of fluctuating substantially from year to year and that fixed costs are likely to be low compared to variable ones. Again, additional cost analysis is needed with different program models.

Despite these limitations, this cost analysis is the first to compare the direct costs associated with a social work DE degree option to its partner campus-based degree program. Results suggest that DE program delivery is more costly than for face-to-face degree programs and that schools of social work should prioritize locating reliable sources of funds when considering moving toward a DE degree option.

REFERENCES

Bernard, R. M., Abrami, P. C., Lou, Y., Borokhovski, E., Wade, A., Wozney, L., & Huang, B. (2004). How does distance education compare with classroom instruction? A meta-analysis of the empirical literature. *Review of Educational Research, 74*, 379–439.

Bledsoe, C. A. (2008). *Distance education financial expenditures in North Carolina community colleges.* (Unpublished doctoral dissertation). University of North Carolina at Greensboro.

Bray, N. J., Harris, M. S., & Major, C. (2007). New verse of the same old chorus? Looking holistically at distance education research. *Research in Higher Education, 48*, 889–908.

Coe Regan, J. R., & Youn, E. (2008). Past, present, and future trends in teaching clinical skills through web-based learning environments. *Journal of Social Work Education, 44*, 95–115.

Csiernik, R., Furze, P., Dromgole, L., & Rishchynski, G. M. (2006). Information technology and social work—The dark side or light side? *Journal of Evidence-Based Social Work, 3*, 9–25.

Daley, M. R., & Avant, F. L. (1999). Attracting and retaining professionals for social work practice in rural areas: An example from east Texas. In I. B. Carlton-Laney, R. Edwards, & P. N. Reid (Eds.), *Preserving and strengthening small towns and rural communities* (pp. 335–345). Washington, DC: NASW Press.

Forster, M., & Washington, E. (2000). A model for developing and managing distance education programs using interactive video technology. *Journal of Social Work Education, 36*, 147–158.

Haga, M., & Heitkamp, T. (2000). Bringing social work education to the prairie. *Journal of Social Work Education, 36*, 309–324.

Inglis, A. (2007). *Comparing costs of alternative delivery methods.* In *Moore's Handbook of distance education* (2nd ed., pp. 437–450). Mahwah, NJ: Lawrence Erlbaum Associates, Inc.

Inglis, A., Ling, P. & Joosten, V. (2002). *Delivering digitally: Managing the transition to the knowledge media* (2nd ed.). London, UK: Kogan Page.

Kreuger, L. W., & Stretch, J. J. (2000). How hypermodern technology in social work education bites back. *Journal of Social Work Education, 36*, 103–114.

Mason, J. A., Helton, L. R., & Dziegielewski, S. (2010). Psychosocial environmental relationships among MSW students in distance learning and traditional classrooms. *Journal of Social Service Research, 36*, 230–247.

McCormack, T. (1996). Understanding the true cost of distance learning. *The Journal of Academic Media Librarianship, 4*(1) (online). Retrieved from http://wings.buffalo.edu/publications/mcjrnl/v4n1/watch3.html

National Association of Social Workers. (2004). *Fact sheet: Title IV-E child welfare training program.* Washington, DC: Author.

Office of Institutional Research, North Virginia Community College. (2002). *Postsecondary distance education: Issues of student outcomes, access, cost, and quality assurance.* Research Report No. 01–01. Retrieved from http://www.nvcc.edu/oir/reports/distanceeducationreport.pdf.

Office of Institutional Research, Northern Virginia Community College. (2002). *Postsecondary distance education: Issues of student outcomes, access, cost, and quality assurance.* Research Report No. 01–02. Annandale, VA: Author.

Potashnik, M. (1998). Distance education: Growth and diversity. *Finance & Development, 35*, 42–46.

Raymond, F. B. III. (2005). The history of distance education in social work and the evolution of distance education modalities. In P. Abels (Ed.), *Distance education in social work: Planning, teaching, and learning* (pp. 23–42). New York, NY: Springer.

Rumble, G. (2001a). The costs and costing of networked learning. *Journal of Asynchronous Learning Networks, 5*, 75–96.

Rumble, G. (2001b). Analysing costs/benefits for distances education programmes. In *The knowledge series.* The Commonwealth of Learning. Retrieved from http://www.col.org/resources/publications/trainingresources/knowledge/Pages/costBenefit.aspx

Stotzer, R. L. (2012). Serving rural communities with distance education degree programs. *Journal of Technology in Human Services, 30*, 109–117.

Taylor, T. H., Parker, G. D., & Tebeaux, E. (2001). Confronting cost and pricing issues in distance education. *Educause Quarterly*, *3*, 16–23.

Turoff, M. (1996). Costs of the development of a virtual university. *Journal of Asynchronous Learning Networks*, *1*, 17–27.

United States Department of Education, National Center for Education Statistics. (2008). *Distance education at degree-granting post-secondary institutions, 2006–07* [NCES 2009-044]. Washington, DC: Author.

University Budget Office, University of Hawai'i. (2010). Expenditure studies, University of Hawai'i fiscal year 2009–2010. Retrieved from http://www.hawaii.edu/budget/pdfs/Actual%20Expenditures%20by%20Campus%202009-10%20%282%29.pdf

Van Dusen, G. (2000). Digital dilemma: Issues of access, cost, and quality in media-enhanced and distance education. ASHE-ERIC Higher Education Report 27.5. In *Introduction* (p. 5). San Francisco, CA: Jossey-Bass Publishers.

Vernon, R., Vakalahi, H., Pierce, D., Pittman-Munke, P., & Adkins, L. (2009). Distance education programs in social work: Current and emerging trends. *Journal of Social Work Education*, *45*, 263–276.

Wilson, (1999). Distance education and accreditation. *Journal of Social Work Education*, *35*, 326–330.

York, R. O. (2008). Comparing three modes of instruction in a graduate social work program. *Journal of Social Work Education*, *44*, 157–172.

Zlotnik, J. L. (2003). The use of Title IV-E training funds for social work education: An historical perspective. *Journal of Human Behavior in the Social Environment*, *7*, 5–20.

Zlotnik, J. L., & Cornelius, L. (2000). Preparing social work students for child welfare careers: The use of Title IV-E training funds in social work education. *Journal of Baccalaureate Social Work Education*, *51*.

Distance and Online Social Work Education: Novel Ethical Challenges

FREDERIC G. REAMER

School of Social Work, Rhode Island College, Providence, Rhode Island, USA

Digital technology has transformed social work education. Today's students can take individual courses and earn an entire degree without ever meeting their faculty members in person. Technological innovations such as videoconferencing, live online chat, asynchronous podcasts, and webinars enable social work educators to reach students whose personal circumstances and geographical locations make it difficult for them to attend school in person. This paper highlights complex ethical issues associated with the proliferation of digital and online social work education. Key ethical issues concern student access; course and degree program quality and integrity; academic honesty and gatekeeping; and privacy and surveillance.

The digital world has created remarkable opportunities for creative social work education. Videoconferencing, online chat rooms, webinars, podcasts: The electronic options seem endless. And, simultaneously, online and distance social work education have unleashed a staggering array of ethical concerns and challenges for which the profession has few existing guidelines.

In 1994, the Code of Ethics Revision Committee began drafting the current National Association of Social Workers (NASW) *Code of Ethics*. Committee members spent considerable time discussing the ethical implications of social workers' use of electronic communications. At the time, electronic communications primarily included electronic mail (e-mail), fax machines, and telephones. Online social networking and social media as we know them today (for example, Facebook, LinkedIn, Twitter) did not yet exist. In 1994, no social workers provided counseling services using e-mail, Skype, or live chat rooms. No social work educators taught courses using synchronous (real-time) digital tools, webinars, or other web-based platforms.

Fast forward: Both social work practice and social work education have been transformed by the digital era. Social workers entering the profession today now have the option to communicate with clients on social networking sites, provide online and video counseling services to people they have never met in person and who live thousands of miles away, save electronic records in the virtual "cloud," and exchange e-mail and text messages with clients using their respective smartphones. Social work educators now teach clinical courses online using videoconferencing. Indeed, social work students now can earn their degree without setting foot in a traditional classroom or meeting in person with a professor.

THE EMERGENCE OF DISTANCE AND ONLINE SOCIAL WORK

Social work and other mental health services emerged on the Internet as early as 1982 in the form of online self-help support groups (Kanani & Regehr, 2003). The first known fee-based Internet mental health service was established by Sommers in 1995; by the late 1990s, groups of clinicians were forming companies and e-clinics that offered online counseling services to the public using secure websites (Skinner & Zack, 2004). In social work, the earliest discussions of electronic tools focused on practitioners' and educators' use of information technology (IT; Schoech, 1999) and the ways in which social workers could use Internet resources such as online chat rooms and listservs, joined by colleagues, professional networking sites, news groups, and e-mail (Grant & Grobman, 1998; Martinez & Clark, 2000).

Today's social work services include a much wider range of digital and electronic options, including a large number of tools for the delivery of services to clients (Chester & Glass, 2006; Kanani & Regehr, 2003; Lamendola, 2010; Menon & Miller-Cribbs, 2002; Reamer, 2012a; Wells, Mitchell, Finkelhor, & Becker-Blease, 2007; Zur, 2012). These include e-mail counseling, live chat counseling, video counseling, cybertherapy, avatar therapy, self-guided web-based interventions, and the use of social networking and text messaging for therapeutic purposes.

Serious efforts to teach social work courses online using distance technology are more recent. However, the idea of distance education itself is not new, with the correspondence course representing its earliest form. The first such course was the Pitman Shorthand training program that brought cutting edge stenographic practices to the United States in 1852. Using the U.S. Postal Service, self-taught secretaries mailed their exercises to the Phonographic Institute in Cincinnati, Ohio and, after completing the required coursework, received a certificate of expertise in stenographic shorthand skills (Casey, 2008). In 1892, the University of Chicago created the first college-level distance education program for students who lived far from campus; students used the U.S. Postal Service to send their professors completed assignments and lessons (Hansen, 2001). In 1934, the University of Iowa began broadcasting courses by television; in 1963, the FCC created the Instructional Television Fixed Service (ITFS), a band of 20 television channels available to educational institutions to provide distance education. Also in 1963, the California State University system was the first to apply for ITFS licensing (Casey, 2008).

Coastline Community College in California was the first college without an actual campus, and by 1972, colleges in Miami-Dade, Florida; Costa Mesa, California; and Dallas, Texas became pioneers in telecourse offerings. Ten years later, the National University Teleconferencing Network used satellites to transmit programs to its 40 institutional members. In 1985, the National Technological University, located in Fort Collins, Colorado, began to offer online degree courses (in both continuing and graduate education) using satellite transmission to access course materials from other universities which then were downloaded and redistributed by satellite. All instruction was either real-time broadcast or video (Casey, 2008; Matthews, 1999). As Rumble (2008, p. 167) notes:

> Distance education developed significantly in the 1960s and 1970s because it provided a cheaper option of meeting demand, and because it was able to reach people in their homes, thus meeting the needs of those who had not gone to or could not attend regular face-to-face classes. The 1960s' and 1970s' growth in educational provision, including distance education, occurred because governments saw it as both a duty (arising from egalitarian arguments) and a need (arising from thinking on human capital and modernization) to meet the costs of educational provision.

In the early 1990s, the advent of high-speed broadband transmission introduced the Internet as the next distance education frontier. The creation of online course management systems, such as WebCT and Blackboard, transformed colleges' and universities' opportunities to reach off-campus students throughout the world. Today, increasing numbers of social work educators are teaching hybrid (combined in-person and online) and exclusively online courses using web-based platforms. Faculty members offer synchronous (simultaneous interaction in real time) and asynchronous (the absence of simultaneous interaction in real time) instruction; simulcast classes using ITV online; live interactive video technologies and related programmed instruction; and Skype-based seminars and faculty advising via video conferencing. Students now can earn their MSW degrees completely online.

Distance education has brought with it complex ethical challenges, especially when it is online (Reamer, 2012b). As Anderson and Simpson (2008, p. 129) observe:

> Teaching at a distance raises ethical issues particular to the distance context. When distance teaching is also online teaching, the situation is even more complex. Online teaching environments amplify the ethical issues faced by instructors and students. Online sites support complex discourses and multiple relationships; they cross physical, cultural and linguistic boundaries. Data of various kinds are automatically recorded in a relatively permanent form.

As social work educators expand their use of distance instruction, it is essential that they address a wide range of ethical issues. Key ethical questions pertain to student access; course and degree program quality and integrity; gatekeeping and academic honesty; and privacy and surveillance.

Student Access

As a profession, social work is deeply committed to enhancing access to resources. The concepts of fair access and equal opportunity are deeply rooted in the profession's values. According to the NASW *Code of Ethics* (2008), social workers seek "to ensure that all people have equal access to the resources, services, and opportunities they require to meet their basic human needs and to develop fully" (Standard 6.04[a]). Consistent with this widely embraced ethical standard, distance education enhances opportunities for prospective social workers to obtain professional education. Distance education may be particularly appealing to people whose life circumstances (for example, work schedules, family responsibilities, financial status) make it difficult, if not impossible, for them to enroll in bricks-and-mortar social work education programs. Being able to complete coursework (for example, watching online video lectures, listening to podcasts, and reading Internet-based literature) at any time, day or night, is particularly appealing to students who would have difficulty attending classes in person. In addition, distance education options enable students who live in remote locations to complete courses and degrees without the time and financial burden of traveling long distances to attend classes.

Distance education also may appeal to students who prefer learning in nontraditional ways (Kolb, 1984). Several studies have demonstrated correlations between students' learning styles (for example, visual, verbal, nonverbal, auditory, tactile, kinesthetic) and their preference for online versus traditional education (Buerk, Malmstrom, & Peppers, 2003; Federico, 2000; Lippert, Radhakrishnam, Plank, & Mitchell, 2001; Terrell & Dringus, 2000; Zacharis, 2010). Thus, distance and online options may serve to enhance access among students whose learning styles mesh with these modalities of delivery. As Sankey and St. Hill (2008, p. 344) note in their discussion of distance education,

> importantly, as these students learn in different ways, so they may also represent knowledge in different ways, and as performance can be related to how they learn, it may be seen that people can learn more effectively when taught by their preferred approach to learning.

However, the current structure of many social work distance education programs may limit student access as well. Some students may have unique learning needs and styles that make distance and online education difficult. Those who have problems, for example, processing information that is presented in written form online or through online podcasts or have difficulty completing reading and written assignments without the guidance of an in-person instructor may find distance and online education inaccessible and unrealistic (Zacharis, 2010).

Further, several widely publicized online MSW programs charge tuitions that are significantly higher than those charged for their in-residence programs; these tuitions may be out of reach for students of modest financial means and whose prospects for paying off significant loans may be dimmed by moderate-wage social work jobs. For example, the University of Southern California tuition for its 2-year MSW online program (2013–2014) is $87,074. Brey (2006, p. 130) poses a compelling question about access in his discussion of the ethical and social justice implications of distance education: "Does a reliance on computer networks in higher education foster equality and equity for students and does it promote diversity, or does it disadvantage certain social classes . . .?"

Hence, distance and online MSW programs can, simultaneously, enhance access for some students and limit access for others. Kelly and Mills (2008, p. 149) note this contrast in their assessment of the fit between students' learning styles and distance education:

> Open, distance and e-learning institutions of higher education often face ethical issues relating to their distinctive mission, especially where the core role is to open educational opportunities to under-represented groups while maintaining academic standards. Openness is surely a "good thing"; and yet there are often tensions relating to government policies, recruitment, access to technology, curriculum, teaching and student support that sometimes involve uncomfortable trade-offs.

Quality Control and Integrity

Social workers are morally obligated to provide services in a competent manner. Such a commitment is particularly important when social workers offer services that are considered novel and innovative (for example, online graduate education). According to the NASW *Code of Ethics*, "when generally recognized standards do not exist with respect to an emerging area of practice, social workers should exercise careful judgment and take responsible steps (including appropriate education, research, training, consultation, and supervision) to ensure the competence of their work . . ." (Standard 1.0[c]).

Several scholars who have investigated distance and online learning have raised troubling questions about the quality of instruction and the lack of empirical evidence of its effectiveness (Casey, 2008; Leh & Jobin, 2002; Rinear, 2003). Common concerns include unevenness in instructor competence and training, curriculum quality and rigor, use and implementation of online and distance teaching tools, and student monitoring and assessment.

In an unsolicited e-mail communication sent to this author, a seasoned instructor in an online MSW program sponsored by a prominent school of social work expressed his grave concerns about quality control (J. Kanter, personal communication, October 4, 2012). Although this instructor's views are not necessarily representative of the universe of experienced online social work educators, they do offer an unusually detailed, thoughtful, and thought-provoking perspective.

> I began teaching the beginning Social Work Practice with Individuals class in the university's "virtual" MSW program in January 2011. After viewing an advertisement seeking faculty, I submitted my resume and received an e-mail response in December 2010 inviting me to interview for the position. The interview was virtual. There were 10 video questions from a faculty member and I had 3 minutes to respond to each one with a video feed from my personal computer. This was non-interactive. About two weeks later, I received an e-mail inviting me to teach two sections of the introductory Social Work Practice class and offering me a choice of dates and times . . .
>
> Apart from a minority of classes which had lengthy, and rather compelling videos (which the students could essentially watch or not watch), most of the material in the asynchronous classes could be completed in 15–30 minutes. On average, these asynchronous assignments never seemed much more than 1/3 of the 75 minutes of "class time" that they were supposed to occupy and the degree of intellectual challenge seemed extremely low . . . .

Kanter shared a number of concerns about his ability in an online social work practice course to monitor and assess students' interpersonal skills, focus on online course activity, and nonverbal behaviors.

> The technical limitations of the "virtual classroom" are omnipresent. Depending to some extent on the speed of each student's internet connection (wireless, cable, DSL, etc.), the visual acuity of each person's image varies greatly. Of course, the "box" on one's computer screen for each participant is relatively small and facial gestures can be difficult to discern even when internet speeds are high and the images are responsive. However, for the majority of students, their facial images were minimally responsive and it was not possible to observe gestural nuances. Eye contact is not possible with online communication and it was almost impossible to establish non-verbal communication with students when they were silent. Most boxes would evidence a blank stare and it was not possible to differentiate whether students were concentrating on the classroom experience or drifting off thinking about other matters. Of course, other visual cues concerning each student (grooming, posture, etc.) were extremely limited as only faces dominated the visual field . . . .
>
> In all of my four sections, I had one or two students who largely monopolized the discussion. These students were commonly those with more self-confidence and professional experience, and their comments and questions were mostly worthwhile. Yet it was difficult to connect with the "silent" members in the 75 minutes we had allotted. I should note here that it took a minimum of 5 minutes in each class to get everyone "signed in" to the virtual classroom. And, as in any graduate class, there was often 10 minutes of "housekeeping," discussing upcoming assignments and so on. Thus, the time available to discuss each week's course content was frequently 60 minutes or less . . . .
>
> Overall, I don't think there is any question that all online communications, whether student-teacher, patient-therapist, and even friend-to-friend, suffer from the implicit technical limitations of talking to each other via computer networks and monitors. Non-verbal communication is severely curtailed. One cannot see the twinkle in the other's eyes, a look of rapt attention, a bored expression or a quizzical expression of disbelief. One cannot judge well how one's humor is being received. Or if a student's quiet behavior is simply shyness, profound depression, or even emergent psychosis . . . .

Kanter also conveyed his strong concerns about the quality and competence of a number of the students enrolled in his online courses, compared with students he has taught in traditional classroom settings.

> It was my impression that the admission requirements for the online program were not as rigorous as for the traditional MSW program, one of the most selective MSW programs in the nation. This seemed odd as the syllabus had a demanding reading list and 90% of the grade was

> based on a lengthy written midterm and final assignment each semester. Several of the students were barely literate and perhaps at least one-third did not have the intellectual background to digest the complex reading assignments.
>
> Also, half the students had severely limited skills in written communication. By "severely limited," I refer to papers with numerous spelling and grammatical errors, sentences that required multiple readings to decipher the author's intent, and an inability to construct coherent paragraphs. With these students, I often wondered if they would be able to appropriately write an agency report or letter that described a client problem . . . .
>
> It also became apparent that overzealous admissions counselors "oversold" the ease and convenience of the online MSW program. While the time commitments involved in the online MSW program were obviously less than in a conventional MSW program . . . they still were significant and some students were disappointed to learn mid-semester that they could not work full time and matriculate full time. Given the cost of tuition, this was a very expensive lesson for some, leaving them with expensive debts which should have been prevented with appropriate pre-admission counseling. In other situations, clearly unqualified students dropped out of the program leaving them with costly loans . . . .

Kanter shared a number of compelling observations pertaining to the cornerstone of MSW education, field work.

> The field work experience is perhaps the centerpiece of MSW education. However, unlike conventional MSW programs which have an array of ongoing relationships with community agencies and field supervisors, the online program staff were required to develop new relationships with agencies that had to be formed across the U.S. for every student in our sections. As I learned halfway through my first term, this agency "recruitment" was not handled by university staff, but rather by employees from the Utor Corporation (now known as 2U, Inc.) who a lacked knowledge of the communities which the students lived in, and b) were unfamiliar with the learning objectives of MSW-level field internships.
>
> Our faculty cohort (teaching the initial Social Work Practice course) was told upfront that students would not have field placements until Week 7 of the semester. This created problems as the first part of the semester's curriculum focused on basic interviewing and relationship skills that the students would not be able to practice in vivo. Also, the midterm writing assignment (due Week 8) was supposed to be a discussion of a client the students worked with in their placement. Instead, they had to write about a character or situation in a Hollywood movie.

> As the semester evolved, only one student in my sections was in placement by Week 7, only half by Week 11, and all but two by Week 14. My faculty colleagues teaching other sections reported similar delays. Students reported an array of problems including a placement that required a two-hour commute from one student's home (when she lived near a large city with dozens of agencies), a placement that simply asked the student to compile a resource directory (with no client contact), and many that seemed to have no good idea how to deploy an MSW student. As one might imagine, the quality of field supervision seemed universally mediocre as agency supervisors had neither knowledge of the university nor were personally screened by School of Social Work faculty . . . .

Of course, in traditional social work education, it is common for some students to struggle with various aspects of the educational process; this is not unique to online programs. However, the problems are more complicated to address when there is no in-person contact and when adjunct faculty across the continent (or globe) are very loosely supported by the educational institution. Kanter further highlighted a number of novel challenges he encountered managing students who struggled with the academic work and the logistics of online education:

- a student who was literally homeless and without cell phone and Internet hookup for several weeks;
- a student who e-mailed him confidential agency files about a client in preparation for a case presentation (the student had been asked to prepare a brief outline of the case);
- a student who plagiarized a number of passages in her midterm;
- a student who was "absent" without cause for several classes and e-mailed a midterm two weeks late, claiming—without evidence—that a computer problem had caused the delay;
- a student paper, describing a case of a child physically abused by a sibling, with no awareness of any duty to report; and
- two students who were unable to write more than two pages of an 8- to 10-page midterm assignment.

There was a much higher proportion of such problems than when I taught social work practice in a conventional classroom-based program . . .

Gatekeeping and Academic Honesty

Social work educators are deeply committed to upholding high standards of academic honesty, consistent with the NASW *Code of Ethics:* "Social workers should not participate in, condone, or be associated with dishonesty, fraud, or deception" (Standard 4.04). Of course, academic dishonesty, primarily in the form of plagiarism, is possible in any educational setting, including face-to-face social work education programs. Students can "lift" passages from other publications and insert them in their written assignments, hire ghost writers, and cheat on exams. However, distance education poses additional and unique risks because of the absence of in-person contact between instructor and student. Unscrupulous students can arrange to have a knowledgeable acquaintance take an online exam or consult with a friend surreptitiously via text message or e-mail. According to Casey (2008, p. 49),

> the essential nature of distance learning, with teacher and student being separated by both space and time, creates an environment that could threaten the quality of learning that is supposed to take place. The educational institutions, the learners, and the teachers are all subject to the honor system. However, many educators question if the honor system is enough to guarantee an education.

These sentiments are echoed by Olt (2002):

> In considering the issue of ethics and distance education . . . the "age-old concerns about ethical practices in assessment . . . take on new twists in the distance-learning environment" (Abbott, Siskivic, Nogues, & Williams 2000). Students are no longer in close proximity. In fact, they may be separated by thousands of miles. Distance, however, does not diminish the possibility of students cheating, with or without an accomplice, on online assessments; instead of developing codes or passing erasers, students pass private e-mails, which instructors have no means of intercepting. In some cases, students can also download an assessment, look up the answers before actually taking it, and share those answers with classmates. Instead of using crib notes or writing answers within the margins of the textbook or on the desktop, students simply use the verboten sources during the assessment. Instructors can no longer depend on different handwriting, a change in ink color, or the detection of eraser marks on an assessment as evidence that a student has changed answers after having taken the assessment. Under such circumstances, it would seem that ensuring the integrity of online assessment is almost an impossibility, or is it?

Digital Surveillance and Privacy

Respecting privacy and confidentiality is a time-honored value in social work. Since the formal inauguration of the profession in the late nineteenth century, social workers have understood how important it is to respect people's judgment about what information they choose to share about themselves and not to pry intrusively into people's lives (see NASW *Code of Ethics*, Section 1.07).

Online social work education is raising new questions and introducing unprecedented challenges pertaining to student privacy. Many online courses feature electronic chat rooms that provide students with an opportunity to share their opinions about course-related issues; as in face-to-face classes, students sometimes choose to share personal information, for example, related to past trauma or their mental health challenges. Such disclosure can be valuable educationally. However, unlike traditional classroom settings, online learning creates a permanent, written record of such disclosures. Although course management software is typically secure, students who choose to disclose personal details online run the risk of electronic breaches or hacking. Further, an unscrupulous or insensitive classmate might choose to print out a confidential message and share it with a third party. As Anderson and Simpson (2008, p. 135) observe, students often are more relaxed about self-disclosure when they communicate with each other online and do not have to face each other in person:

> In online classes students gradually establish a presence and identity through interaction, becoming known in some way to other members of the class. In fact, Joinson (2001, p. 188) has shown "people disclose more information about themselves during CMC [computer mediated communication] compared to FtF [face to face]." Entering a new course, students bring with them sets of expectations. When the course anticipates or requires interaction with other students, they might realistically expect that only basic information such as their name is provided to other class members, expect that interactions will be constructive and primarily course-focused, expect that students will work together when required, and expect that class discussions are for the class, not for a general audience. Over time, often reflecting practices set by the instructor and beliefs about the nature of teaching and learning, students come to know each other's online persona, beliefs and ideals. At times students reveal other contact information to enable ongoing interaction. The trust that underpins the free exchange of ideas and the flourishing of debate ensures this. Personal details are inevitably recorded—in reasonably permanent text.

Instructors and educational administrators must make earnest and proactive attempts to protect student privacy and confidentiality in online learning situations. This is an extension of the longstanding principle in social work practice to discuss confidentiality guidelines and exceptions at the very beginning of practitioners' work with clients. Instructors similarly should share their expectations with students about their obligation to respect classmates' privacy, consistent with social work values, and obtain students' agreement to honor these expectations.

Further, instructors and administrators must hold themselves to high standards as well by respecting student privacy and ensuring that the course management software provides adequate encryption and protection of electronic communications. Anderson and Simpson (2008) highlight the need for new and strict norms pertaining to electronic surveillance of students' online communications, informed consent, and related privacy protections. They note:

> How can we assess the kind of surveillance that occurs in online courses and make ethical judgments about the use of such data? For used it will be . . . . The large amount of data about students being collected in most learning management systems is usually collected automatically. Lecturers or tutors do not typically make active decisions to collect information about how often or when students are online, reading or posting messages, or working through course content in a particular order. Messages themselves remain as data. The usual safeguards offered to students are guarantees of privacy and of data protection. But, while important, are these safeguards addressing the right issue when an even more fundamental issue, informed consent for data gathering, is overlooked? It is possible that some students are not aware that data about their actions are being recorded. How often do instructors pause to think about whether that recording requires informed consent or at least awareness on the part of the student of the nature and extent of the data gathering? The question of safeguards highlights the possibilities for control, and of judgments about students on the basis of the collected data. Privacy and data protection safeguards do nothing to protect against those aspects of surveillance. (Anderson & Simpson, 2008, p. 134)

CONCLUSIONS AND RECOMMENDATIONS

Online and distance education in social work are coming of age. The bell has been rung, and it is not possible to "unring" it. Clearly, there is much to be said in favor of online and distance education. As noted, students who live in remote areas, have a disability, or have work schedules or family obligations that make traditional, face-to-face instruction difficult or impractical can acquire new knowledge and skills. Online and distance education offer opportunities to tailor instructional tools and media to suit students' unique learning styles. Social work students can access creative and instructive videos, websites, and podcasts at convenient times and develop digital relationships with colleagues around the globe.

Accompanying these benefits and advantages, however, are numerous and serious ethical concerns. Chief among them are troubling issues that must be addressed pertaining to student access; course and degree program quality and integrity; gatekeeping and academic honesty; and privacy and surveillance.

At this relatively early stage in the development of distance and online MSW education, social work educators, therefore, should address several compelling questions. First, what are the overarching motives for promotion of distance and online MSW education? Are educators paying sufficient attention to the quality of the product and student learning outcomes, or are these efforts driven to a significant extent by the revenue that these programs may generate? Decisions about whether to mount profitable distance and online MSW programs must be a matter of conscience, not revenue.

Second, social work educators must ask whether there is sufficient evidence that essential social work knowledge and skills can be taught and learned in distance formats—especially clinical skills. To what extent have schools relaxed admissions standards in order to enroll large numbers of tuition-paying students? Are we satisfied that the distance courses being offered measure up to the high standards associated with rigorous social work education? Does currently available technology enable instructors to truly assess the quality of students' professional demeanor, interpersonal skills, and clinical acumen? To what extent are social work education programs arranging and supervising field placements in ways that ensure close and careful scrutiny of students' performance and field instructor quality? Are program administrators able to develop close working relationships with course and field instructors they have never met in person? Do programs have adequate protocols and mechanisms in place to address instructors' concerns about students' academic performance, field work performance, or impairment?

Third, have programs developed and implemented mechanisms to promote and enhance student honesty and prevent forms of plagiarism and cheating that may be unique to distance and online education? Finally, have distance and online social work educators paid sufficient attention to the unique challenges associated with student privacy, confidentiality, and surveillance? The task here is twofold. First, the education programs must use course management software that truly protects digital communications and avoids any untoward surveillance or misuse of students' electronic data. Second, and more broadly, social work educators must cultivate and promote a new set of norms regarding students' moral obligations to respect and protect classmates' privacy and confidentiality. The concept itself is not new; what is novel are the ways in which students' privacy and confidentiality can be compromised due to the permanent record created by digital communication.

As with so many innovations, the digital revolution is a mixed blessing. In social work education, earnest and principled academicians are now able to share knowledge with vast numbers of students who, but for this technology, would not be reached and served. Further, currently available audio, video, and digital technology is remarkably versatile and enables one to communicate with students in a wide variety of engaging ways. That's the good news. The less-than-good news is that there are troubling signs of ethical problems and compromises associated with the rush toward distance and online social work education. Our moral duty, at this stage of development, is to acknowledge these challenges honestly, wrestle with thoughtful options, and develop principled guidelines and safeguards to ensure that social work education fulfills its principal duty: to educate the next generation of social workers who will carry out the profession's mission to, in the words of the NASW, "enhance human well-being and help meet the basic human needs of all people, with particular attention to the needs and empowerment of people who are vulnerable, oppressed, and living in poverty."

REFERENCES

Abbott, L., Siskovic, H., Nogues, V., & Williams, J. G. (2002). Student assessment in multimedia instruction: Considerations for the instructional designer. Retrieved from Eric on-line database (ED 444 516): http://newfirstsearch.oclc.org

Anderson, B., & Simpson, M. (2008). Ethical issues in online education. *Open Learning: The Journal of Open, Distance and e-Learning, 22*(2), 129–138.

Brey, P. (2006). Social and ethical dimensions of computer-mediated education. *Journal of Information, Communication and Ethics in Society, 4*(2), 91–101.

Buerk, J. P., Malmstrom, T., & Peppers, E. (2003). Learning environments and learning styles: Non-traditional student enrollment and success in an Internet-based versus a lecture-based computer science course. *Learning Environments Research, 6*(2), 137–155.

Carey, K. (2012, December 9). Who will hold colleges accountable? *New York Times*. Retrieved at http://www.nytimes.com/2012/12/10/opinion/who-will-hold-colleges-accountable.html?_r=0

Casey, D. M. (2008). A journey to legitimacy: The historical development of distance education through technology. *TechTrends: Linking Research & Practice to Improve Learning, 52*(2), 45–51.

Chester, A., & Glass, C. A. (2006). Online counseling: A descriptive analysis of therapy services on the Internet. *British Journal of Guidance & Counselling, 34*, 145–160.

Federico, P. (2000). Learning styles and student attitudes toward various aspects of network-based instruction, *Computers in Human Behavior, 76*(4), 359–379.

Gearhart, D. (2001). Ethics in distance education: Developing ethical policies. *Online Journal of Distance Learning Administration, 4*(1). Retrieved from http://www.westga.edu/~distance/ojdla/spring41/gearhart41.html

Grant, G. B., & Grobman, L. M. (1998). *The social worker's Internet handbook.* Harrisburg, PA: White Hat Communications.

Hansen, B. (2001). Distance learning. *CQ Researcher, 11*(42), 1–24.

Haughey, D. (2008). Ethical relationships between instructor, learning, and institution. *Open Learning: The Journal of Open, Distance and e-Learning, 22*(2), 139–147.

Heberling, M. (2002). Maintaining academic integrity in on-line education. *Online Journal of Distance Learning Administration, 5*(2). Retrieved from http://www.westga.edu/%7Edistance/ojdla/spring51/spring51.html

Hinman, L. M. (2000). Academic integrity and the World Wide Web. Retrieved from http://ethics.acusd.edu/presentations/cai2000/index_files/frame.htm

Illinois Online Network. (2001). Strategies to minimize cheating online. Retrieved from http://illinois.online.uillinois.edu/pointer/IONresources/assessment/cheating.html

Joinson, A. N. (2001). Self-disclosure in computer-mediated communication: The role of self-awareness and visual anonymity. *European Journal of Social Psychology, 31*(2), 177–192.

Kanani, K., & Regehr, C. (2003). Clinical, ethical, and legal issues in e-therapy. *Families in Society, 84*, 155–162.

Kanter, J. Personal communication, October 4, 2012.

Kelly, P., & Mills, R. (2008). The ethical dimensions of learner support. *Open Learning: The Journal of Open, Distance and e-Learning, 22*(2), 149–157.

Kolb, D. (1984). *Experiential learning: Experience as the source of learning and development*. Englewood Cliffs, NJ: Prentice-Hall.

Leh, A., & Jobin, A. (2002). Striving for quality in distance education. *Computers in the Schools, 19*(3/4), 87–101.

Lamendola, W. (2010). Social work and social presence in an online world. *Journal of Technology in the Human Services, 28*, 108–119.

Lippert, R., Radhakrishnam R., Plank, O., & Mitchell, C. (2001). Using different evaluation tools to assess a regional internet in service training. *International Journal of Instructional Media, 28*(3), 237–248.

Lyon, D. (2001). Facing the future: Seeking ethics for everyday surveillance, *Ethics and Information Technology, 3(3)*, 171–180.

Martinez, R. C., & Clark, C. L. (2000). *The social worker's guide to the Internet*. Boston, MA: Allyn & Bacon.

Matthews, D. (1999). The origins of distance education and its use in the United States. *T.H.E. Journal, 27*(2), 54–59.

Menon, G. M., & Miller-Cribbs, J. (2002). Online social work practice: Issues and guidelines for the profession. *Advances in Social Work, 3*, 104–116.

National Association of Social Workers. (2008). *NASW Code of Ethics*. Washington, DC: Author.

Olt, M. (2002). Ethics and distance education: Strategies for minimizing academic dishonesty in online assessment. *Online Journal of Distance Learning Administration, 5*(3). Retrieved from http://www.westga.edu/~distance/ojdla/fall53/olt53.html

Reamer, F. G. (2012a). The digital and electronic revolution in social work: Rethinking the meaning of ethical practice. *Ethics and Social Welfare*. Retrieved from http://www.tandfonline.com/doi/abs/10.1080/17496535.2012.738694]

Reamer, F. G. (2012b). The elephant in the (virtual) classroom: The ethical implications of online social work education. *Social Work Today*. Retrieved from http://www.socialworktoday.com/news/eoe_080312.shtml

Rinear, K. (2003). Maintaining a successful distance program: What administrators need to know. *Distance Education Report, 7*(13), 1–2,7.

Rumble, G. (2008). Social justice, economics, and distance education. *Open Learning: The Journal of Open, Distance, and e-Learning, 22*(2), 167–176.

Sankey, M., & St. Hill, R. (2008). Ethical considerations in providing distance education in the light of massification. *Lifelong Learning Conference*. Retrieved from http://eprints.usq.edu.au/4169/1/Sankey_St_Hill_5th_Lifelong_Learning_Conf.pdf

Schoech, D. (1999). *Human services technology: Understanding, designing, and implementing computer and Internet applications in social services*. Binghamton, NY: Haworth Press.

Skinner, A., & Zack, J. S. (2004). Counseling and the Internet. *American Behavioral Scientist*, *48*, 434–446.

Terrell, R., & Dringus, L. (2000). An investigation of the effect of learning style on student success in an online learning environment. *Journal of Educational Technology Systems*, *28*(3), 231–238.

Wells, M., Mitchell, K. J., Finkelhor, D., & Becker-Blease, K. A. (2007). Online mental health treatment: Concerns and considerations. *CyberPsychology & Behavior*, *10*, 453–459.

Zacharis, N. Z. (2010). The impact of learning styles on student achievement in a Web–based versus an equivalent face-to-face course. *College Student Journal*, *44*(3), 591–597.

Zur, O. (2012). TelePsychology or TeleMentalHealth in the digital age: The future is Here. *California Psychologist*, *45*, 13–15.

A Response to 'Distance and Online Social Work Education: Novel Ethical Challenges'

DONI WHITSETT and WENDY SMITH

As faculty members of the USC School of Social Work, with experience teaching in both the onground and online programs, we feel compelled to respond to Dr. Frederic G. Reamer's otherwise very interesting chapter. Comments relating to our program depended almost entirely on the opinions of a single adjunct instructor involved in our online program early on, who is unfamiliar with many changes that have since taken place.

The hiring process now permits greater depth, with an initial virtual interview to rule out unqualified candidates, followed by interviews with lead instructors. The large pool of interested applicants permits much greater selectivity.

"Quality of instruction is uneven" is a comment that might be made about any program. Our innovative and unique Office of Faculty Development provides individual consultation, webinars on instruction, and oversight of student evaluation data. In addition, our new Virtual Field Placement program, in which students role play with actor "clients" from the very first week, allows for immediate introduction to field placement.

Space does not permit a full response to comments regarding quality of students. The School shared the concerns stated about the quality of the students admitted in the beginning, who often were over committed and had misperceptions about the rigor of our program. Currently, students who are working full-time may not enroll as full-time students. It is inevitable also that some students will lack the academic skills necessary to succeed in our program. Nonetheless, some of our best students graduate from the online program and some of our weakest students graduate from the onground program.

Finally, our tuition is high, but it is identical to our onground tuition, and 65-75% of our students receive a scholarship or stipend.

Doni Whitsett, Ph.D., LCSW
Clinical Professor of Social Work
Associate Director of Faculty Development
USC School of Social Work

Wendy Smith, Ph.D., LCSW
Clinical Associate Professor of Social Work
Associate Dean of Faculty Development
USC School of Social Work

Distance Guest Speakers in Online Synchronous Classrooms: Practical and Legal Considerations

MELANIE SAGE
Department of Social Work, University of North Dakota, Grand Forks, North Dakota, USA

Social work students increasingly are served by distance education, which necessitates the use of creative and innovative online teaching methods. An instructor embarking upon online teaching should consider interpersonal and technical issues, be familiar with the Family Education Rights and Privacy Act of 1974, and understand other legal implications related to recording a guest speaker. This paper offers an illustrative example and recommendations regarding the use of guest speakers who visit from a distance in a synchronous classroom.

Social work students increasingly are served by distance education and technology that necessitates exploration of innovative online teaching methods (Vernon, Pittman-Munke, Vakalahi, Adkins, & Pierce, 2009). Improvements in distance learning technologies and synchronous education options make it possible to move past pedagogical barriers of asynchronous learning, such as an inability to see the teacher and students, the difficulty of small-group collaboration, or inability to speak to the teacher after class. Fortunately, many studies have compared distance education methodologies to in-class learning and have found learning outcomes are similar whether students are in the classroom or an Internet-based setting (Schoech & Helton, 2001; Webber, Currin, Groves, Hay, & Fernando, 2010; Wilke & Vinton, 2006; York, 2008).

Distance learning offers opportunities to improve education availability to individuals who may not have geographic access to a campus-based degree (Oliaro & Trotter, 2010; Rafferty & Waldman, 2006). However, distance education may offer some benefits beyond geographical access. Synchronous online educational delivery, in which the class meets at a specific time and interacts "live" through presentation, chat, and collaboration, mirrors the experience of an in-person classroom in many ways, even though participants may be accessing the class from different time zones. One way to capitalize upon the benefit of the synchronous distance classroom is to utilize the expertise of guest speakers who are also at a distance and thus offer presentations that normally are not available to campus-based students.

Guest speakers, of course, frequently are utilized in social work classrooms to offer students the perspective of a practitioner or of a consumer in the social service field (Colvin-Burque, Davis-Maye, & Zugazaga, 2007; Yee Lee & Green, 2008; Scheyette & Diehl, 2004). However, whereas an on-campus program is most likely to draw upon local speakers, technology opens options to invite national and international experts to the synchronous classroom. An instructor might extend invitations to textbook authors, subject experts, leaders of advocacy groups, and prominent individuals across the globe; the opportunities are vast. Nevertheless, several considerations are required before inviting a distant speaker to participate in a live online classroom. An instructor should consider interpersonal and technical issues, have familiarity with the Family Education Rights and Privacy Act (FERPA), and understand further legal implications related to recording a guest speaker in class.

This paper offers an illustrative example of the use of such a guest speaker, along with recommendations for using guest lecturers in a distance synchronous class setting. The specific technology used in this example is Adobe Connect, which is one type of Internet Video Virtual Classroom product that allows video, audio, text between participants and instructor, file sharing, and break-out rooms for small group work (Quinn, Regan, & Schoech, 2008). Although some of the same concepts apply to the use of guest speakers in an asynchronous classroom or on-campus classroom, these examples are based on synchronous learning.

MSW students from Arizona to Canada attend the social work program described in this illustration. Because of the high demand for distance education at this institution, the students who are admitted to the program typically come with significant pre-professional practice experience, which necessitates learning opportunities that will build upon what they already know. Indeed, research suggests that MSW distance education students tend to be older and have more work experience (Wilke & Vinton, 2006). Because they are geographically dispersed, the benefit of inviting a speaker from a "local program" that would acquaint students with regional community services is replaced by the goal of finding the best speaker to stimulate the topical interest and needs of the students.

The speaker in this case is a professional helper who speaks regularly to university students about his young adult daughter's suicide and his family's difficult experience with help seeking. His advocacy interests converge around the complexities of confidentiality, informed consent, continuum of care, and policy change. He speaks about the challenges he faced with coordinating care for his daughter because providers frequently were unwilling to speak to him about services because his daughter was 18 years old. Through his story, students learn about core issues to our profession and its code of ethics related to confidentiality, advocacy, informed consent, and self-determination (National Association of Social Workers [NASW], 1999).

ILLUSTRATIVE EXAMPLE

A former colleague on the West Coast introduced this author to Mr. Smith after he spoke in her class about his daughter's suicide. As a professional in the helping field, Mr. Smith speaks in his local community to school groups and social workers about his personal experience and his policy advocacy work. (Although recommended as a speaker, he had never before spoken online and I had no knowledge of his experience with technology.) By e-mail, I extended Mr. Smith an invitation to speak to the class. He would need a microphone and webcam. When he confirmed interest, we arranged a time for a preparatory session together so we could discuss the class and test out his technology.

Orienting the Guest Speaker

In an entirely synchronous distance program, students are well-oriented to the live online method of learning. However, guests may need an orientation as well as technical assistance. Their computers may require software updates, and cameras and microphones may have to be set as default devices. Cameras with built-in microphones often create an echo in the classroom; therefore, a headset is ideal, but a USB microphone can also be used. Adobe Connect software is utilized at this university, and the program is supported by computer service staff should additional help become necessary.

During the pre-meeting with Mr. Smith, we were able to navigate software and hardware issues. This also was an opportunity to explain to the speaker how students generally interact, the classroom use of voice chat, typing, raising hands, and cameras. Explaining the classroom technology options provided him with knowledge about alternatives he could utilize during his presentation, such as inviting students to use a computerized "show of hands" if they ever had a particular experience (students use an icon that appears next to their name when they click it). I offered him the option to e-mail me documents for student review which I could upload to the shared space in the online classroom, and explained that the lecture would be video-recorded so that students could review it later. (As this was his first online lecture, he also requested a copy of the recorded video.) A few days before our scheduled class, I sent him an e-mail that outlined our discussion goals and a reminder about our class meeting time.

Preparing the Students

It is useful to prepare students to view their classroom from the lens of an outsider and on how to make the speaker as comfortable as possible. In regular online classrooms, students sometimes offer friendly and conversational comments during the class discussion. This might be akin to passing a note or offering casual feedback during a class discussion. Out of respect for the guest speaker, who was not acclimated to the culture of our online classroom, students were asked to refrain from possibly distracting chat during the speaking portion of our class. Further preparation for students included a preview of the topic (and the speaker's experience), with an acknowledgement that some might feel emotionally triggered by the discussion. Students were reminded to use self-care.

Cameras and Microphones

Due perhaps to limited exposure to online speaking, guest speakers may experience interpersonal challenges related to presenting remotely at a distance. They tend to be more accustomed to a particular way of seeing and interacting with their audiences in a typical classroom. When all the students, however, turn on their microphones and speakers at once in a synchronous session, it is quite distracting, limits the viewing area for the principal speaker, and may cause trouble with Internet performance due to bandwidth use. For that reason, students in this course are asked to turn on their microphones only when speaking and use their cameras only when asked to present to the class. The instructor's microphone and camera are turned on while interacting with the group and then turned off when a student is speaking.

Using our cameras and microphones, Mr. Smith and I "met" in the online classroom before his class presentation so that we would recognize each other. However, he did not get the opportunity to view any of the students until he opened up the floor for questions near the end of the online class period. At this time, students raised their hands and turned on their cameras and microphones when talking, a procedure to which they are accustomed (and to which our guest had been oriented during our pre-meeting). Although he saw the list of names of attendees during his presentation, he said later that it felt like he was simply talking to a camera, and it was hard to imagine who else was listening. Therefore, it would have been preferable to have students briefly turn on their cameras at the beginning of class during introductions to help orient the speaker to the students in the classroom at the outset.

FERPA in the Online Classroom

The Family Educational Rights and Privacy Act (FERPA) is a federal law (often called the Buckley Amendment) that limits the ways in which student information may be disclosed. In this case, a recording that is distributed later and includes content about students in attendance could violate FERPA regulations.

In traditional classrooms, a guest lecture typically is not recorded. By way of contrast, in the online environment, technology makes it easy to record the class, so a recording often is maintained for students' future review, and is utilized by students who are absent. While the recording contains a list of student names, the document typically is stored on a password-protected online course management site, which limits information sharing. If it is a clear assumption of the learning environment that videos are to be recorded and stored, and students have forewarning that presentations will be taped. However, because our guest wanted a copy of the video to share outside of our institution, students were offered the option of logging in as "guests" themselves, using their first name or pseudonym, since the recording (and roster) might be shared outside of class by the speaker. Students were so informed by e-mail prior to class and again at the beginning of class, and they gave permission for external use. Although FERPA does not mandate an IRB review, instructors who are concerned about FERPA requirements could include a signed release from students, providing permission to appear on a video that may be shared beyond the classroom.

Other Legal Issues

This author's university legal counsel confirmed that it was acceptable to give a copy of the recording to the guest speaker; in fact, speakers have ownership of their performance in the class. To demonstrate diligence regarding permission to record the video, an instructor can request a signed consent to record the class from the guest speaker, which would include information about how long the lecture is to be stored and who will have access. However, an instructor should consider other copyright issues. For instance, third-party material sometimes is presented during guest lectures, such as a copyrighted mental health inventory, a proprietary video clip, or a case study from an agency. In cases where it is entirely acceptable to share this information in a classroom, it may in fact be a copyright violation to make a stored recording of the same information.

The Technology Education and Copyright Harmonization (TEACH) Act of 2002 is legislation that specifically addresses the use of copyrighted material in the online classroom and provides additional guidance for distance education instructors (Copyright Clearance Center, 2005). Even when works fall under the fair use doctrine, it may be necessary to attach copyright notices; fair use may no longer apply if the video later is used in another setting, such as a paid speaking engagement. Because these laws are open to interpretations, instructors should consult their university's copyright officer for further instruction (Crews, 1994).

When a video broadcast may be kept online for perpetuity, implications of verbal miscues are more important than they might be during a unrecorded one-time presentation in a traditional classroom. Practical ethical considerations of video-taped lectures include the problem of a slip of the tongue, in which either the speaker, student, or instructor offers inaccurate information, makes an inappropriate statement, breaches confidentiality, offers excessive personal disclosure, or has some other error or slip in conduct that one would not want recorded indefinitely. The instructor also should consider whether the technology offers the ability to edit out these mistakes, so that they do not cause future embarrassment to the university, speakers, or students.

Some classroom recordings require students to log in to a system (such as Blackboard) for access, while others generate a URL or create a widely accessible copy. In reality, any recorded classroom material potentially could be copied and re-shared, and therefore the instructor should evaluate the content of a classroom recording with this in mind and make the guest speaker aware of how information will be accessed and stored.

Student Feedback

The next time the students met as a class, they offered informal reflection about the guest presentation. Because they are quite accustomed to online presentations as students in an online degree program, the methodologies used in bringing a distance speaker "to campus" were not entirely novel for them. Nonetheless, several students described how they were impacted by the speaker's story and social action, which increased their awareness of the complexities inherent in decision making in direct practice and helped them understand connections between policy and practice. The students offered overwhelmingly positive feedback regarding the guest presentation, and one student, impressed by the presentation, forwarded a thank-you card via the instructor to the presenter.

DISTANCE SPEAKERS IN TRADITIONAL CLASSROOMS

As we become more connected in virtual synchronous classroom settings (and in our personal lives) to those at a distance, there will be more opportunities to connect speakers to their audiences. Next semester, we plan to use a guest speaker who lives many states away through the use of Skype, a free voice- and video-conferencing software program, for an on-campus class. Our video camera will point toward the classroom so our guest speaker can see the students, and she will use a headset for voice projection. Video projection will allow her to be seen clearly by the entire class and permit the faculty member to introduce the guest expert to the students.

DISCUSSION

Fast-moving technologies make it difficult to imagine how classroom visitors might inhabit both our online and real-life classrooms in the future. Our access to far-away expertise now offers us opportunities to create global classrooms to enrich the social work education experience. Next-generation learners expect that professional education will be technology-savvy and, as they emerge, we should make the best use of the new tools at our disposal. Although an excited professor should not delve prematurely into using a guest speaker, using video technology to support social work learning offers many benefits in both the real and virtual classroom. Students consistently report satisfaction with having access to online video recordings and options for synchronous learning and generally rate their interactive experiences very favorably (Stocks & Freddolino, 2000).

As our expertise in technology increases, it is important to explore ways in which technology can enhance the learning experiences of our students. With respect to the use of distance guest speakers, further research should explore best practices for preparing speakers, students, and instructors, as well as ethical guidelines for selecting, preparing, and recording guest speakers. These admonitions regarding ethical practice may be relevant with the use of potentially vulnerable guest speakers, such as women who are victims of abuse, people with developmental disabilities, or young adults aging out of the foster care system.

REFERENCES

Colvin-Burque, A., Davis-Maye, D., & Zugazaga, C. B. (2007). Can cultural competence be taught? Evaluating the impact of the SOAP model. *Journal of Social Work Education, 43*(2), 223–241.

Copyright Clearance Center. (2005). The TEACH Act: New roles, rules and responsibilities for academic institutions. Retrieved from http://www.copyright.com/media/pdfs/CR-Teach-Act.pdf

Crews, K. D. (1994). *Copyright, fair use, and the challenge for universities, promoting the progress of higher education*. Chicago, IL: University of Chicago Press.

National Association of Social Workers. (1999). *Code of ethics of the National Association of Social Workers*. Washington, DC: NASW Press.

Oliaro, L., & Trotter, C. (2010). A comparison of on-campus and off-campus (or distance) social work education. *Australian Social Work, 63*(3), 329–344.

Quinn, A. S., Coe Regan, J., Ann, R., & Schoech, D. (2008). Online synchronous audio and video environments for education, training, and human service delivery: A review of three products. *Journal of Technology in Human Services, 26*(1), 89–104.

Rafferty, J., & Waldman, J. (2006). Fit for virtual social work practice? *Journal of Technology in Human Services, 24*(2-3), 1–22.

Scheyett, A., & Diehl, M. J. (2004). Walking our talk in social work education: Partnering with consumers of mental health services. *Social Work Education, 23*(4), 435–450.

Schoech, D., & Helton, D. (2001). Qualitative and quantitative analysis of a course taught via classroom and Internet chatroom. *Qualitative Social Work, 1*(1), 111–112.

Stocks, J. T., & Freddolino, P. P. (2000). Enhancing computer-mediated teaching through interactivity: The second iteration of a world wide web-based graduate social work course. *Research on Social Work Practice, 10*(4), 505–518.

Vernon, R., Pittman-Munke, P., Vakalahi, H., Adkins, L. F., & Pierce, D. (2009). Distance education programs in social work: Current and emerging trends. *Journal of Social Work Education, 45*(2), 263–276.

Webber, M., Currin, L., Groves, N., Hay, D., & Fernando, N. (2010). Social workers can e-learn: Evaluation of a pilot post-qualifying e-learning course in research methods and critical appraisal skills for social workers. *Social Work Education, 29*(1), 48–66.

Wilke, D., & Vinton, L. (2006). Evaluation of the first web-based advanced standing MSW program. *Journal of Social Work Education, 42*, 607–620.

Yee Lee, M., & Green, G. (2008). A teaching framework for transformative multicultural social work education. *Journal of Ethnic and Cultural Diversity in Social Work, 12*(3), 1–28.

York, R. O. (2008). Comparing three modes of instruction in a graduate social work program. *Journal of Social Work Education, 44*(2), 157–172.

Current Challenges in Social Work Distance Education: Responses from the Elluminati

WILLIAM PELECH, DAN WULFF, ELLEN PERRAULT,
JESSICA AYALA, MYRA BAYNTON, MARGARET WILLIAMS,
RACHAEL CROWDER, and JANKI SHANKAR
Faculty of Social Work, University of Calgary, Calgary, Alberta, Canada

One of the first tasks of the Social Work Distance Education Network at the Faculty of Social Work at the University of Calgary was to review the literature and address three research questions to inform policy making and planning relating to distance social work education programming. This paper is intended to disseminate responses to these questions from a small group of dedicated and experienced distance educators who have adopted the moniker Elluminati. (The Elluminati adapted their name from a popular online audio-conferencing program.) These questions include: (1) What is the optimal class size for a distance delivery offering? (2) What supports does an online course require for development and effective delivery? (3) What types of courses are suitable/unsuitable for online learning?

> *At no time in history has it been more important to invest in higher education as a major force in building an inclusive and diverse knowledge society and to advance research, innovation and creativity.* (UNESCO, 2009)

For many, the idea of being educated in anything but the traditional face-to-face instructional milieu seems to conflict with the very purpose of social work education. As Vernon, Vakalahi, Pierce, Pittman-Munke, and

Adkins (2009) have noted, "Social work educators and practitioners often describe themselves as 'people persons' who value human encounters. This is an understandable ethos given the nature of our profession" (p. 269); however, such a position may limit the scope and creativity that can be brought to social work education. For, if we teach social work only in a conventional classroom environment, only those who have access to the classroom can benefit. Moreover, the notion that social work education can be conducted *only* in a traditional classroom may be becoming a confining and antiquated notion.

BACKGROUND AND CONTEXT

In a recent American survey, the Commission on Accreditation of the Council on Social Work Education (CSWE) found that "more than a third of the BSW programs and a quarter of the MSW programs did not require a face-to-face experience as an integral component of coursework. Instead, these programs offered courses that were entirely online, without direct human contact" (Vernon et al., 2009, p. 269). From this survey of 137 social work programs, it was found that 61% of BSW and 83% of MSW programs were delivering, developing, or contemplating distance education and were "open" to using technology to provide courses for their students. As the authors of the 2009 CSWE report noted, "it is readily apparent that distance education has expanded exponentially in only a decade" (p. 274).

In addition to technological change, two factors may be driving this transformation. First, there is student demand. Students are voting with their feet, or perhaps more accurately, with their browsers. The 2010 Sloan Survey of Online Learning in the United States reveals that nearly 30% of students take at least one online course in their degree programs, with enrollment having risen by almost 1 million to 5.6 million students from a prior year. This is the largest ever year-to-year increase in the number of students studying online (Allen & Seaman, 2010). One may ask if this increase arises from greater accessibility offered by online courses, or student preference, or both?

The second factor driving the transformation is institutional pressure. According to Vernon and colleagues (2009), nearly two-thirds of social work program respondents reported being pressured from within institutions to develop online courses. There may be several reasons for such pressure, not the least of which are the substantial investments in distance education infrastructure and technology and the perceived profits associated with online classes (Vernon, et al., 2009). Another reason, according to Simonson (2004), may be the result of one of the misconceptions in distance education that posits that online classes are scalable. That is, given that online classes are not limited by the constraints of a physical classroom, it does not matter how many students are enrolled in a class so long as the course is properly organized.

On the other hand, Simonson (2004) identifies an opposing myth that suggests that, due to the additional time demands of teaching online, smaller classes are more equitable in relation to faculty workload. Ironically, concluding what is likely the most often cited one-page op-ed in the annals of distance education, Simonson (2004) asks:

> And finally, traditional education has answered questions about class size and work load, if not by research, at least by common practice. Any professor or teacher can tell you how many students should be in class, and they know within limits what constitutes a fair workload. Where are the distance education researchers to help us develop our own answers? (p. 56)

THE ELLUMINATI

In 2011, the Faculty of Social Work at the University of Calgary created a network of social work educators under the name of the Social Work Distance Education Network (SWDEN). One of the first tasks of the SWDEN was to review the literature and to respond to three questions: (1) What is the optimal class size for our distance delivery offerings? (2) What supports does an online course require for its development and effective delivery? (3) What types of courses are suitable/unsuitable for online learning?

The name Elluminati was created by a SWDEN member to convey the collective wisdom and skill possessed by Network members in distance education. The *Elluminati* bring years of experience in various forms of distance and traditional social work education. The Elluminati include the director of e-learning and distance education, who has been involved in the delivery of various forms of distance education since 1989; another member who completed a dissertation focused on distance education; and other members who bring years of experience with various forms of distance education. The name, Elluminati, is an adaptation of the brand of the online audio-conferencing software, *Elluminate Live*, that is currently in use by the University of Calgary. More sophisticated than other commonly used online audio-conferencing programs (such as *Skype* and *Google Talk*), Elluminate Live enables students to participate in a virtual classroom and real-time class discussions. Indeed, one of the ways that distance education has improved over the years has come from the increased interactivity afforded both students and instructors through the use of synchronous audio-conferencing. In this paper, we will offer a brief survey of the literature, followed by a summary of discussions among the Elluminati.

DOES CLASS SIZE MATTER?

Many have commented on how administrators, perhaps in response to both diminishing resources and an increasing demand for online courses, have been challenged to find a balance between budgetary considerations and faculty workloads (Orellana, 2006; Simonson & Schlosser, 2004; Tomei, 2006). As Tomei observed:

> It is not uncommon for higher education administrators in particular to view online, distance learning-based courses as the "mother lode" for sizeable tuition revenue increases. After all, to the uninitiated, the argument can be made that if a traditional classroom teacher can accommodate a class of 25 students with the demands of face-to-face instruction, scheduled office hours, and individualized assessment, why shouldn't an online instructor be capable of handling 50 students? Why not 100? (p. 533)

For this reason, considerable attention has been given to addressing Simonson's (2004) question of whether online course development and delivery require considerably more time than traditional instruction. For example, when comparing the time required in a course delivered to 22 technology and education students, half of whom learned online and the other half in a traditional classroom setting, Tomei (2006) found that approximately 14% more hours were required to teach the same number of students online than in the traditional classroom (and this calculation did not take into account the time required for curriculum development). He also found that delivering instructional content online necessitated 43.5% more time than classroom-based teaching. He added that advising required an additional 16.3% more hours for online, with traditional assessment requiring 7.6% less time than online assessments. Based on these results, he concluded that the ideal class size for traditional classes was 17 students and for online courses was 12.

A now somewhat dated case study by Visser (2000) concluded that online courses seem to take more teaching and development time than traditional courses. However, it was noteworthy that, as corroborated by others (Anderson, 2003; Hislop & Ellis, 2004), delivery time and effort may be mediated by instructor experience with the technology as well as by the level of institutional support. Similarly, Orellana (2006), in a survey of 154 faculty members and researchers at the 2004 National Convention of the Association for Educational Communications and Technology, found that on average, a perceived optimal class size for online courses (averaging 18.9) as recommended by respondents was smaller than their actual reported class sizes (averaging 22.8).

In perhaps the most cited comparative study, Cavanaugh (2005) found that course preparation and student contact required considerably more time for an online course than a traditional one. However, these conclusions are challenged by earlier studies (DiBiase, 2000; Hislop & Ellis, 2004), which found that teaching time per student in online courses was not greater than in their traditional versions.

In addition to instructor familiarity with educational technologies and levels of institutional support, there are other variables to consider when determining optimal class size. These factors include andragogical issues such as the desired level of interaction and the role and function of the instructor. Traditionally, interaction has been viewed as an essential ingredient in higher education. For this reason, three of seven of Chickering and Gamson's (1987) *Principles of Good Practice in Undergraduate Education* focus on peer and instructor-student interaction. This view is shared by eight regional accrediting commissions in the United States that developed the *Statement of Commitment for the Evaluation of Electronically Offered Degree and Certificate Programs*. The *Statement* declares "that learning is dynamic and interactive, regardless of the setting in which it occurs" (Eaton, 2001, p. ii). In subsequent research relating to activity and exchange in online learning, student interaction with peers and instructors has been associated with improved outcomes (Bender, 2003; Wilson, Pollock, & Hamann, 2007) and higher perceived course quality (Taylor & Ku, 2011). Moreover, in a profession where the relationship is the key element in professional practice, one might be prone to recognize the value of interactions in social work distance education.

In a review of the literature, Orellana (2006) found that the size of the class dramatically affects the types of learning activities that can be introduced as well as the nature of interaction. As Simonson and Schlosser (2004) have noted, there are three forms of interaction available in any classroom: student-to-content, student-to-instructor, and student-to-student. The class size choices that faculties make will clearly impact such interactions. For example, larger classes may be more conducive to student-to-student interactions in the form of group learning activities (Orellana) and online community building (Vrasidas & McIsaac, 1999). They can obviously reduce the extent of instructor-student interaction (Dykman & Davis, 2008; Simonson, 2004).

Simonson, Schlosser, and Orellana (2011), summarizing what is known, have observed that the early research in the field assumed that fostering all forms of interaction was essential to quality online education. Perhaps illustrative of this assumption in terms of the importance of student-instructor interaction would be the comments of Dykman and Davis (2008) on the impact of larger class sizes:

> In a conventional setting, delivering lectures to a group of fifty instead of twenty is mostly a matter of getting a bigger lecture hall. But in an online setting, these are very different situations. There would be considerably

> more work needed with the larger class to maintain quality at acceptable levels. For example, there would be much more posting and dialoging, many more relationships to maintain, etc. A typical professor probably could not allocate that much time to one class. So, how would more students change the content in an online class? Clearly, there is much less time to discuss issues in the online environment with many students. So, the content would have to be limited to only the most important points, theories, or whatever. The fullness of the curriculum would be limited. Fewer deliverables, much less feedback for students, much more of the 'sink or swim' mentality would be necessary. Quality of the online teaching and learning experience would suffer dramatically. (p. 278)

Implicit in this statement of course is an assumption of the importance of instructor-student interaction to the quality of online education. Clearly, with the ongoing enhancement of distance learning technologies from manualized correspondence programs, to interactive television and, most recently, to online course management systems with audio/video-conferencing capabilities, the opportunities for interaction in distance learning have greatly expanded. While the importance of interaction has been viewed as a vital element to high-quality education, Simonson et al. (2011) question whether instructor-student interaction is as essential as Dykman and Davis would have us believe. Moreover, we wonder if a largely teacher-to-student dialogue would be desirable in *any* classroom setting. Dykman and Davis (2008) offer an important caution in relation to class size. They argue that the size of the class *determines* the learning objectives and course design. An online course designed for 15 to 20 students is necessarily a different kind of course from one designed for 35 or 50. It is unwise to take a class designed for 20 students and enroll 40 or 50 in it (p. 278). While Dykman and Davis's view here is noteworthy, to be more proactive one could restate this point by noting that one needs to be purposeful in instructional design and generate learning objectives that are appropriate to the needs and numbers of students. For larger classes, one simply must organize the course to accommodate interaction among a larger number of students.

Just such an accommodation occurs in an online undergraduate program offered by the University of Calgary, known as the BSW Virtual Learning Circle. This Virtual Learning Circle (VLC) offers predominantly online modularized social work courses annually to approximately 60 students across Canada.[1] In the VLC, additional discussion areas and audio-conference

[1] As Canada has two official languages, French and English, bilingual services are required for programs offered by federal government agencies. In Canada, there are many social work education programs available in either French or English, and a few of them offer social work education programming in both official languages. The Faculty of Social Work follows the mandate of the University of Calgary, which is to offer courses in English. Cost constraints limit our ability to also offer coursework in French. Students seeking instruction in French therefore would be referred to a Canadian university offering such courses.

groups were created in several courses to accommodate larger numbers of students. Additional supports also were offered in the form of teaching assistants and graders to reduce the workload faced by instructors. However, contrary to Dykman and Davis (2008), learning objectives here were not appreciably altered to accommodate the doubling of class size. These purposeful adaptations are supported by the literature, where the recommended number of students participating in discussions would range between 10 and 20 students (Boettcher, 2006; Colwell & Jenks, 2004; Frey & Wojnar, 2004; Reonieri, 2006; Schellens & Valcke, 2006). Generally in higher education, as Gilbert (1995) has noted:

> The research clearly indicated that quality education occurs in certain circumstances and these conditions are not exclusive to small classes. In fact, size per se and what it necessitates appears to be a small component of quality education. Small class sizes are neither necessary nor sufficient to ensure high quality student learning, growth and development. What matters is not the size of the class but what goes on in the class. (p. 5)

A RESPONSE FROM THE ELLUMINATI

Perhaps due to their relative comfort with online learning, discussions among the Elluminati identified higher optimal class sizes than did some of the above-cited researchers. Such class sizes ranged from 25 to 35 students. Some Elluminati indicated that they had instructed classes as large as 300 students supported by five teaching assistants. In that case, the delivery largely was focused on content, with limited student interaction. Others noted that class sizes could increase substantially depending upon the nature and purpose of the class and the availability of support from teaching assistants. Our discussions deepened to note that groupings of different sizes would be appropriate for different types of technologies. Larger classes would require additional discussion forums. Similarly, depending on the purpose and amount of interaction desired, online audio-conference sessions could range up to 25 students, including small group discussions to support greater interaction. Our discussions similarly focused on the andragogy and goals of instruction. Questions were raised as to whether we come from a banking approach, which King (1993) called the "sage on the stage," or a liberatory one? While a banking approach would support simple content delivery by an expert instructor, it would not be an approach congruent with our client-centered approaches to practice. To sum up our discussions, the available supports and the technologies utilized, as well as the instructional purpose, substantive content, and professional values, will help to determine optimal class size.

Supports for Online Learning

Largely absent from much of the debate and comparative studies pertaining to appropriate class sizes is a discussion of the resources and preparation necessary to support large online classes. As Dykman and Davis (2008) have noted, there are consequences to anticipate when one increases the number of students in an online course. Clearly, some outcomes may arise regardless of the delivery strategy. The time required for the grading of assignments naturally will increase proportionally if one increases the number of students in a course without changing the assignments. Also, as Dykman and Davis point out, if an instructor wishes to respond to every student posting, a larger number of students will proportionally increase this workload demand. Thus, larger online classes may demand changes in the way one teaches online, calls for additional supports, and suggests reduced workload consideration. One may ask whether larger classes, without additional supports, will result in fewer or shorter assignments, the need for more objective assessment measures (such as multiple choice exams), and less feedback to students. Are such changes consistent with the objectives of social work education which emphasize critical reflection and thinking?

The American Association of University Professors (AAUP; cited by Orellana, 2006) has posted sample policies for distance education programs, including one that states that class size should be based on andragogical considerations and that large sections should be compensated by additional credit in load assignment as they would for traditional classes. In addition, the AAUP recommended that workload allocations should take into consideration that high-quality distance education course development takes two to three times as long as comparable course development (for delivery in a traditional format) and that additional time will be required to answer student inquiries and provide support at a distance (Orellana, 2006). While the AAUP's recommendations are helpful, they are very broad in their conceptualization, spanning across the disciplines.

There are supports that are specifically associated with teaching online. First, instructors will need the support of ongoing technical assistance and peer mentorship. As Vitale (2010) notes, instructors who proceed to course development without an introduction to the technologies, technical assistance, and peer mentorship are destined to struggle.

Second, along with larger classes comes increased interaction. Nevertheless, the instructors can choose to reduce their centrality by shifting some of the responsibility for responding to students. This approach suggests having students play a greater role in responding to one another and having a class member monitor and facilitate discussions. The use of small group discussions, a technique commonly deployed in traditional classes to promote student-to-student interaction, can be utilized in formatting online discussion groups (Berry, 2008). Finally, as in any large traditional class, teaching assistants and graders may play an important role in reducing the workload demands experienced by instructors of large classes.

A Response from the Elluminati

These strategies have been used widely by the Faculty of Social Work at the University of Calgary. In discussions among the Elluminati, members recognized a need to differentiate the roles of teaching assistant and grader. The Elluminati believed that, since all of our teaching assistants were doctoral students who would one day become social work educators, teaching assistants should be freed from the limited and mundane role of simply attending class and grading assignments. Their role needed to have far less involvement in grading and a greater focus on enhancing their own teaching skills by direct engagement with students. Consequently, graders, who normally are MSW students, would be needed to focus on grading, under the direct supervision of the instructor. The instructor would be expected to orient graders and provide them with clear rubrics for student assessment.

The Elluminati advised that a teaching assistant be added when classes exceed 35 students. Also recommended was a grader for each increment of 25 students. Hence, when a class exceeded 35 students, a teaching assistant and grader would be needed. (A class that exceeded 50, of course, would require a teaching assistant and two graders.) These numbers might change if the course were a practice skills class where smaller sections and/or blended delivery would be advisable. Differing views were given regarding workload and remuneration for online classes, depending on the supports provided, ranging from a 1-to-1 ratio to a ratio of 1 to 1.5.

The literature also offers a number of strategies to work "smarter rather than harder" in larger online classes. For example, in addition to training and support in structuring online discussions, Berry (2008) affirms the importance of assessment of discussion board postings including the use of rubrics to evaluate online discussions. Instructors also need to be purposeful with respect to how and when they interact in online discussions. Rather than responding to individual postings, the instructor (or a teaching assistant or student) may elect to post a response to the themes emerging from groups of student postings. In addition, Ko (2007) has proposed a number of strategies that may be considered in working with larger classes. Many of them involve rebalancing the interaction from student/instructor, to student/student, and instructor to group. First, Ko suggests organizing students into discussion groups of up to 10 members and then having them post a summary of their discussions to a class discussion board. Instructors in larger classes could respond to multiple posts at one time and encourage students to respond to their fellow classmates. According to Ko, students also can play a role in assessments, including utilizing a rubric for the peer review of class postings.

Courses Suitable for Online Learning

While the Faculty of Social work was one of the early adopters of distance education at the University of Calgary, the early literature has been divided with respect to the appropriate social work courses to offer. While some have argued that a broad range of courses may be delivered online (Miller, Walker, & Ayala, 2003), others have noted that social work programs that offer distance education often may be appropriately reluctant to offer distance-based methods and practice courses because of their emphasis on learning through face-to-face interaction (Petracchi, Mallinger, Engel, Rishel, & Washburn, 2005; Siebert, Siebert, & Spaulding-Givens, 2006). This caution is curious since online learning has been associated with increased interaction when compared to traditional classroom settings (Thurmond & Wambach, 2004).

Indeed, a growing body of evidence indicates that a wide variety of social work courses can be offered effectively online. MacFadden, Dumbrill, and Maiter (2000) found positive results for an online graduate social work course designed to improve multi-cultural competencies and skills. Stocks and Freddolino (1998) compared an Internet-based class using computer mediated communication with a traditional face-to-face version of the same class. Their course was a research methods class. Students in the Internet course reported that they were not as bored, did not feel talked down to, did not feel the instructor dominated the course, and were pleased that they could learn at their own pace. The results in course achievement showed no significant difference between the two modes of delivery. However, students overwhelmingly noted that it was the computer-mediated communication that made the class successful, in addition to the flexibility and self-pacing and the ease with which they could ask questions and revisit course materials. Moreover, over a decade of research comparing online and traditional instruction appears to have found no differences in academic achievement across a wide array of disciplines (Hylton, 2006; Petracchi et al., 2005; Woehle & Quinn, 2009; York, 2008).

Perhaps indicative of a shift in perception over the past decade relating to the appropriateness of online practice courses, Vernon and colleagues (2009) found that the majority of online courses were elective in nature, 35% for BSW and 39% for MSW programs. They observed that, "In rank order, practice courses were the most prevalent in core curriculum offerings for both MSW and BSW courses" (p. 268). Indeed, a greater proportion of BSW and MSW programs offered practice courses (14.5% and 20%, respectively) than policy courses (14% and 13%, respectively). While the evaluative literature in this area is quite limited and with generally small sample sizes, among the three studies that were found, two involved online instruction only (Seabury, 2005; Siebert et al., 2006); and one, involving a hybrid approach, reported no significant differences between the two delivery methods in relation to student academic achievement (Petracchi et al., 2005).

A Response from the Elluminati

Given these more recent trends, the Elluminati chose to reframe this question from "What courses are most suitable to teach online?" to "How do we teach online courses well?"

Discussion focused on what makes a good course, whether it is online or traditionally delivered. Here, as with many of the issues and questions addressed in this paper, the boundaries between traditional and online teaching blur. As Madoc-Jones and Parrott (2005) have noted,

> Good practice in education and learning are the same whether this takes place in the classroom, at a distance through correspondence or in the virtual world of the World Wide Web. Online learning is not inherently any more capable of providing good educational experiences and developing criticality than classroom based or distance learning based courses. Much depends on how the learning medium is exploited. (p. 758)

To this end, Graham, Cagiltay, Lim, Craner, and Duffy (2001) adapted *Seven Principles of Good Practice in Undergraduate Education* (Chickering & Gamson, 1987) for online education. First, they note that instructors should encourage student-to-teacher contact by setting clear expectations regarding timelines and the preferred form for communication. In this way, clarity regarding how to communicate (and how quickly the instructor will respond to student inquiries) promotes confidence in students that they will not be ignored and makes the instructor's workload more manageable. Second, the instructor can promote interaction and cooperation among students by creating well-designed discussions that promote meaningful and focused student discourse. As with the first principle, clear expectations, relating to the form and the nature of postings, need to be established. Third, good practice engages students in active learning through the use of student projects. In the BSW VLC, student engagement and interaction are promoted via integrative projects. Students from across the country utilize audio-conferencing and discussion forums to collaborate on group projects. Fourth, consistent with many of our student evaluations, good online practice teaching involves providing prompt feedback. Indeed, in an online environment, where student access to an instructor often is limited by distance, a responsive instructor who provides immediate feedback will be valued. Graham and colleagues (2001) further specify that this feedback needs to include both information and acknowledgement. Fifth, while one of the many advantages of online learning is the flexibility that it offers to busy students, explicit deadlines (that are realistically scheduled) can add useful structure. Sixth, Graham et al. observe that an instructor needs to promote high expectations in student academic work, including the posing of challenging tasks, relevant case studies, and offering public praise for high-quality work. Of course, as with all of these principles, accountability goes both ways so that instructors need to practice what they teach in terms of modeling the types of interactions expected in discussion forums. Finally, good teaching encourages the expression of diverse views and respects different learning styles. Two of the hallmarks of social work education are critical thinking and respect for diversity. In most social work classes, students are expected to critically appraise prevailing theories. In the VLC, however, students are encouraged to explore their own interests and passions through integrative projects and portfolios that incorporate their diverse points-of-view (Siebert & Spaulding-Givens, 2006).

While the implications of our responses appear to counter the current global trends in distance education—where dedicated virtual institutions such as Coursera, the University of Phoenix, and Open University are turning to automated massive open online courses to feed higher education courses to a mass market—one question that emerges is whether social work is ready and appropriate for instruction by *Professor Robot* (Carr, 2012). Certainly, distance education is well-suited for a spread-out and relatively sparsely populated nation like Canada, particularly in rural areas where there seldom are sufficient students to sustain local delivery of courses. However, just as Abraham Flexner questioned the rigor of mail-ordered correspondence courses in 1928 (Carr, 2012), our discussions certainly question the maxim of "bigger is better."

CONCLUSION

In conclusion, we have addressed three questions relating to online education in social work. While there are diverse opinions relating to optimal class size, the complex array of factors that mediate the issue make this question difficult to answer in a simple or uniform manner. However, providing mentoring and training can enable instructors to work smarter in terms of how they design their courses for larger numbers of students. Supports would include release time for course development, workload consideration, and the deployment of teaching assistants and graders. Finally, we have noted that the range of courses deemed suitable for online delivery has broadened over the past decade, leading us to reframe the question to ask: "How can we more effectively teach *across the curriculum*?" In sum, we need to ask how we can teach more effectively to larger classes across the curriculum and what supports will we need in order to do so.

REFERENCES

Allen, I. E., & Seaman, J. (2010). *Class differences: Online education in the United States, 2010*. Wellesley, MA: Babson College.

Anderson, T. (2003). Modes of interaction in distance education: Recent developments and research questions. In M. G. Moore & W. G. Anderson (Eds.), *Handbook of distance education* (pp. 129–144). Mahwah, NJ: Erlbaum.

Bender, T. (2003). *Discussion-based online teaching to enhance student-learning*. Sterling, VA: Stylus.

Berry, G. (2008). *Asynchronous discussions: Best practices*. Paper presented at the 24th Annual Conference on Distance Teaching & Learning, Madison, Wisconsin. Retrieved from http://www.uwex.edu/disted/conference/resource_library/proceedings/08_12701.pdf

Boettcher, J. V. (2006). How many students are just right in a web course? Design for learning. Retrieved from http://www.designingforlearning.info/services/writing/number.htm website:

Carr, N. (2012, September). The crisis in higher education. *MIT Technology Review*. Retrieved from http://www.technologyreview.com/featuredstory/429376/the-crisis-in-higher-education/

Cavanaugh, J. (2005). Teaching online—A time comparison. *Online Journal of Distance Learning Administration*, *8*(1), 1–11. Retrieved from http://www.immagic.com/eLibrary/ARCHIVES/GENERAL/U_WGA_US/J050300C.pdf

Chickering, A., & Gamson, Z. (1987). Seven principles of good practice in undergraduate education. *AAHE Bulletin*, *39*, 3–7.

Colwell, J. L., & Jenks, C. F. (2004). The upper limit: The issues for faculty in setting class size in online courses. Retrieved from http://www.ipfw.edu/tohe/Papers/Nov%2010/015__the%20upper%20limit.pdf.

DiBiase, D. (2000). Is distance teaching more work or less? *American Journal of Distance Education*, *14*(3), 6–20.

Dykman, C. A., & Davis, C. K. (2008). Online education forum—Part 3: A quality online educational experience. *Journal of Information Systems Education*, *19*(3), 281–289.

Eaton, J. S. (2001). *Maintaining the delicate balance: Distance learning, higher education accreditation, and the politics of self-regulation* (Council for Higher Education Accreditation Monograph Series, 2001, No. 1). Retrieved from http://www.chea.org/pdf/mono_1_dist_learning_2001.pdf

Frey, B. A., & Wojnar, L. C. (2004). Successful synchronous and asynchronous discussions: Plan, implement, and evaluate. Retrieved from http://www.educause.edu/ir/library/pdf/MAC0426.pdf website:

Gilbert, S. (1995). Quality education: Does class size matter? *CSSHE Professional File*, *14*, 1–7.

Graham, C., Cagiltay, K., Lim, B.-R., Craner, J., & Duffy, T. M. (2001). Seven principles of effective teaching: A practical lens for evaluating online courses. *The Technology Source*, (March/April). Retrieved from http://technologysource.org/article/seven_principles_of_effective_teaching/

Hislop, G., & Ellis, H. (2004). A study of faculty effort in online teaching: *Internet and Higher Education*, *7*(1), 15–31.

Hylton, M. E. (2006). Online versus classroom-based instruction: A comparative study of learning outcomes in a diversity course. *The Journal of Baccalaureate Social Work*, *11*(2), 102–114

King, A. (1993). From sage on the stage to guide on the side. *College Teaching*, *41*(1), 30–35.

Ko, S. (2007). Tips for managing larger online classes. *DE Oracle @ UMUC*. Retrieved from http://deoracle.org/online-pedagogy/classroom-management/tips-for-managing-larger-online-classes.html

MacFadden, R., Dumbrill, S., & Maiter, S. (2000). Web-based education in a graduate faculty of social work: Crossing the new frontier. *New Technology in The Human Services, 13*(1/2), 27–38.

Madoc-Jones, I., & Parrott, L. (2005). Virtual social work education-theory and experience. *Social Work Education, 24*(7), 755–768.

Miller, P. A., Walker, J., & Ayala, J. (2003). Technology integration as a transformative catalyst and tool. *International Journal of Learning, 10*, Retrieved from http://ijl.cgpublisher.com/product/pub.2037/prod.2230.

Orellana, A. (2006). Class size and interaction in online courses. *The Quarterly Review of Distance Education, 7*(3), 229–248.

Petracchi, H., Mallinger, G., Engel, R., Rishel, C. W., & Washburn, C. (2005). Evaluating the efficacy of traditional and web-assisted instruction in an undergraduate social work practice class. *Journal of Technology in Human Services, 23*(3/4), 299–310.

Reonieri, D. C. (2006). *Optimizing the number of students for an effective online discussion board learning experience.* (Unpublished master's thesis). Thomas Edison State College, Trenton, N.J.

Schellens, T., & Valcke, M. (2006). Fostering knowledge construction in university students through asynchronous discussion groups. *Computers and Education, 46*, 349–370.

Seabury, B. A. (2005). An evaluation of on-line, interactive tutorials designed to teach practice concepts. *Journal of Teaching in Social Work, 25*(1–2), 103–115.

Siebert, D. C., Siebert, C. F., & Spaulding-Givens, J. (2006). Teaching clinical social work skills primarily online: An evaluation. *Journal of Social Work Education, 42*(2), 325–336.

Siebert, D. C., & Spaulding-Givens, J. (2006). Teaching clinical social work skills entirely online: A case example. *Social Work Education, 25*(1), 78–91. doi:10.1080/02615470500477953

Simonson, M. (2004). Class size: Where is the research? *Distance Learning, 1*(4), 56.

Simonson, M., & Schlosser, C. (2004). We need a plan: an instructional design approach for distance education courses. *Distance Learning, 1*(4), 29–38.

Simonson, M., Schlosser, C., & Orellana, A. (2011). Distance education research: A review of the literature. *Journal of Computing in Higher Education, 23*, 124–142.

Stocks, J., & Freddolino, P. (1998). Evaluation of a world wide web–based graduate social work research methods course. *Computers in Human Services, 15*, 51–69.

Taylor, J. E., & Ku, H. (2011). Measuring active learning to predict course quality. *Performance Improvement Quarterly, 24*, 31–48.

Thurman, V., & Wambach, K. (2004). Understanding interactions in distance education: A review of the literature. *International Journal of Instructional Technology and Distance Learning, 1*(1), 9–26.

Tomei, L. A. (2006). The impact of online teaching on faculty load: Computing the ideal class size for online courses. *Journal of Technology and Teacher Education, 14*(3), 531–541.

UNESCO. (2009, July 5-8). *Communique*. Paper presented at the 2009 World Conference on Higher Education: The Dynamics of Higher Education and Research for Societal Change and Development, Paris.

Vernon, R., Vakalahi, H., Pierce, D., Pittman-Munke, P., & Adkins, L. F. (2009). Distance education programs in social work: Current and emerging trends. *Journal of Social Work Education*, *45*(2), 263–275.

Visser, J. (2000). Faculty work in developing and teaching web-based distance courses: A case study of time and effort. *The American Journal of Distance Education*, *14*(3), 21–32.

Vitale, A. T. (2010). Faculty development and mentorship using selected online asynchronous teaching strategies. *Journal of Continuing Education in Nursing*, *41*(12), 549–556.

Vrasidas, C., & McIsaac, M. S. (1999). Factors influencing interaction in an online course. *American Journal of Distance Education*, *13*(3), 22–36.

Wilson, B. M., Pollock, P. H., & Hamann, K. (2007). Does active learning enhance learner outcomes? Evidence from discussion participation in online classes. *Journal of Political Science Education*, *3*(2), 131–142. doi:10.1080/15512160701338304

Woehle, R., & Quinn, A. (2009). An experiment comparing HBSE graduate social work classes: Face-to-face and at a distance. *Journal of Teaching in Social Work*, *29*(4), 418–430.

York, R. O. (2008). Comparing three modes of instruction in a graduate social work program. *Journal of Social Work Education*, *44*(2), 157–172.

Part 2: Teaching and Simulating Practice

Teaching MSW Social Work Practice in a Blended Online Learning Environment

SHELLEY LEVIN and DONI WHITSETT
School of Social Work, University of Southern California, Los Angeles, California, USA

GARY WOOD
Social Work Curriculum and Faculty Relations, 2U, Inc., Los Angeles, California, USA

Blended learning is a newly emerging trend in higher education and is defined as the purposeful integration of synchronous and asynchronous learning to provide educational activities that maximize the benefits of each. This paper describes the development of a graduate social work foundation-year practice class in a blended online environment in which both asynchronous and synchronous activities transpire online. The course's underlying pedagogical principles are illustrated, and the perceptions of instructional faculty are reported in key areas, including engagement and participation, activities, and the challenges of technology, socialization, etiquette, and nonverbal cues.

Computers have been used in the education of social workers for more than three decades. Methodologies have included computer-assisted instruction, interactive videodiscs (Seabury & Maple, 1993), computer-based expert systems (Kelly, 1994), computer simulation (Wodarsky & Kelly, 1987), and virtual classrooms (Ouelette, 2000).

Although the use of computer-mediated technology as an instructional medium has been rapidly increasing in the field of social work education (Shibusawa, VanEsselstyn, & Oppenheim, 2006), social work has lagged behind in incorporating technology in the teaching of practice under the assumption that practice should be taught in person (McNutt & Menon, 2002). In a national study that examined the perceptions of social work faculty concerning the effectiveness of web-based instruction, practice courses received the lowest scores (Moore, 2005). Despite these oft-mentioned concerns, a 2001 survey by the Council on Social Work Education (CSWE) of 137 MSW and BSW programs found that 23 BSW programs and 38 MSW programs were teaching practice online; in the intervening decade, those figures are likely to have increased.

In October 2010, the University of Southern California School of Social Work expanded access to its MSW degree program by developing a web-based, distance-education version of its on-campus MSW degree. This program is offered through the school's new Virtual Academic Center (VAC), which parallels the school's four existing geographically defined academic centers. Students may enroll in the MSW program full- or part-time and, in their advanced year, currently may complete any of the school's five concentrations and the Military and Veteran Services sub-concentration (although the first two cohorts of VAC students were restricted to the Mental Health and Families and Children concentrations and the Military sub-concentration). The gradual introduction of concentrations online was based on pragmatic reasons and student demand; converting all concentration courses simultaneously was not deemed feasible, so concentrations were developed based on student preference. (None of the school's dual-degree programs, such as MSW/JD, is currently offered as an option for online students, although this remains a future possibility.) The VAC offers coursework and degree requirements identical to those of the campus-based program and consists of a blended synchronous–asynchronous curriculum in conjunction with a traditional (although geographically dispersed) field internship. This paper describes the development of the foundation-year practice course of the VAC program.

Online blended learning is a newly emerging trend in higher education and is defined as the purposeful integration of synchronous and asynchronous learning to provide educational activities that maximize the benefits of each (Ayala, 2009). All curricular content—syllabi, readings, supporting materials (e.g., videos, handouts) and assignments—is identical to the content of the campus-based program. By using blended learning methods, the faculty was able to combine the best of synchronous and asynchronous learning approaches to meet specific educational goals.

THE LEARNING MANAGEMENT SYSTEM

Crucial to any online education is the delivery of curricular content, which is accomplished through a learning management system (LMS). LMSs (such as Blackboard) frequently have been adopted by faculty and are ancillary in many traditional campus-based courses for purposes of class management—posting grades, course documents, or Internet links.

The LMS designed for USC's VAC consists of three primary and integrated components: (1) a system for students to engage with asynchronous (or pre-produced) curriculum content; (2) an access portal to enter synchronous classes, meetings with peers, and office hours with professors; and (3) social network devices (walls, profiles, student affinity groups, etc.) that promote student interaction outside of class time. Of primary importance to this paper are the first two components, which will be discussed in greater detail. As noted, students also attended a traditional field placement in their geographic locale.

An important early decision of school leaders was that courses would be conducted such that 50% of the students' class time would be in synchronous meetings with instructors and other students and the remaining time spent working through asynchronous learning activities. This 50–50 split fostered the benefits of asynchronous content (such as access flexibility, standardization of content) while also promoting traditional small-group learning that is a hallmark of most social work programs, especially for practice classes. Such classes require an environment of mutual trust among students and with instructors, because discussions and role-playing often necessitate a degree of risk on the part of students.

The Asynchronous Component

The asynchronous component of the course work is composed of learning activities that faculty members design for students to complete each week *prior* to attending the synchronous portion of the class. By definition, asynchronous material is reviewed individually by students. In addition to the didactic material embedded in the LMS, a range of learning activities can be planned, including viewing faculty presentations, watching case vignettes and standard videos that would typically be shown in campus classrooms, participating in threaded forum discussions (sometimes called *discussion boards*), and taking self-check quizzes. Each week's asynchronous content provides the foundation for that week's synchronous session. For instance, a filmed vignette might prompt discussion about how best to approach a situation similar to the one depicted or might lead to role-playing various approaches.

The Synchronous Component

Each week, students have a synchronous class meeting for each class they are taking. Class times are scheduled as they would be on campus, and each student adjusts for time zone. The class sessions are conducted via the Internet and feature real-time audio and video connections. Classes are composed of a maximum of 12 students and an instructor. All students and the instructor can see and hear one another. Instructors and students report that these synchronous classes can feel more intimate than a campus-based class, everyone has a front-row seat, and everyone can see one another. *Social presence* is the term used in the online literature to refer to students' sense of community or connection to others in their classes and has been an elusive quality in many online courses (Tu & McIsaac, 2002). Because of the use of real-time audio and video, students and instructor are able to hear and see emotional expression, vocal inflection, and a full range of verbal and nonverbal communication. Social presence has been greatly increased as a result.

At present, synchronous sessions are enabled through the use of commercially available software (Adobe Connect Pro). This provides the instructors with a robust set of tools for conducting class sessions. They can create PowerPoint presentations, display documents, use a white board, assign students to smaller breakout sessions for role-playing or small group discussion, utilize a polling tool to quickly assess class opinion on an issue, or use the chat box to send messages to the whole class or individual students. Generally, synchronous class sessions involve an application or elaboration of concepts presented in the learning activities of the asynchronous components.

Underlying Theoretical Principles

The underlying principle of the course design was the concept of pedagogy with respect to adult learning. In 1833, German educator Alexander Knapp coined the term *androgogik*, or andragogy, when referring to adult learners as opposed to *pedagogy*, which seemed more specific to children (Knowles, 1968). However, today the terms are often used interchangeably. Knowles (1980) identified six principles of adult learning:

1. Need to Know: Adults need to know the reason for learning something.
2. Foundation: Experience (including error) provides the basis for learning activities.
3. Self-Concept: Adults need to be responsible for their decisions regarding education and involved in the planning and evaluation of their instruction.
4. Readiness: Adults are most interested in learning about subjects that have immediate relevance to their work, personal lives, or both.
5. Orientation: Adult learning is problem-centered rather than content-oriented.
6. Motivation: Adults respond better to internal than to external motivation.

Knowles's assumptions are incorporated into both the asynchronous and synchronous portions of the course in a variety of ways. The *Need to Know* principle is built into the material by continuously demonstrating to students how particular information is important in helping them understand client behavior and situations. The material is continuously linked and applied to clinical practice. For example, during the synchronous portion of the class, instructors might present a clinical vignette to the students and ask them to apply material from the asynchronous portion. This standard is also embedded in the synchronous portion of the course through the discussion of issues students are encountering with current clients, as well as in written assignments.

Foundation is included in the asynchronous content through the use of "test yourself quizzes." In the synchronous portion of the course, students experience the material through role-playing and discussion of case vignettes.

Self-Concept, the principle that adults need to be responsible for their decisions regarding education and involved in the planning and evaluation of their instruction, is featured in the asynchronous portions of the course by having materials accessible at the convenience of each student; offering the option to partially complete the materials and return later when time permits; and providing the opportunity for students to review course materials any time during the semester.

Forum questions are an additional example of the application of the *Self-Concept* principle. They are queries posed throughout the asynchronous material that result in student responses and subsequent discussion, similar to a blog. Finally, additional readings, assessment instruments, and Internet links are posted by the instructor and available at any time to the students. The *Self-Concept* principle is also applied in the synchronous sessions through discussion of the forum postings and elements presented in the asynchronous section.

The concept of *Readiness* is included in the asynchronous material through embedded videos and media-rich slide presentations produced by USC faculty. In the synchronous portion of the course, *Readiness* is met through the use of case discussions, vignettes, and role-playing. Students also are able to introduce current issues from their field placements for discussion, just as they do in campus-based courses.

Orientation, the principle that adult learning is problem-centered rather than content- oriented, is operationalized in the asynchronous portion of the course through case studies and journal articles with accompanying questions. In the synchronous portion of the class, student responses to the questions are reviewed.

Finally, the principle of *Motivation* is asynchronously addressed via self-checks at the end of each unit. In the synchronous portion of the class, electronic polling is used in response to instructor-generated questions.

PERCEPTIONS OF FACULTY

VAC instructors represent a very similar configuration as campus-based faculty members teaching foundation practice courses (i.e., relatively few tenure-track faculty and mostly full-time non-tenure-track clinical and adjunct faculty, including many with a long history of teaching at the school).

The following information was collected from an informal survey sent to the foundation practice faculty members, who taught virtually, as well as gleaned from discussions at curriculum meetings. The purpose of the survey was to obtain feedback regarding how the program was perceived by faculty and to ensure that the quality of the online practice courses was seen as equivalent to campus-based courses. Although more formal evaluation methods have since been instituted at the school, with a focus on student outcomes, the following themes reflect the experiences of the instructors; many have also taught in the classroom and are in a position to make those comparisons.

The Relationship

Forming a relationship with students online seems to have a different trajectory than when on campus. Many of the instructors felt that it took longer to form such a relationship, partly because they spent less time with the students (75 minutes in each weekly synchronous session versus 2.5 hours in the campus-based classroom) and partly because of the medium. However, once developed, the relationship was perceived as stronger. Faculty members became more creative and assertive in reaching out to students, such as connecting with them via e-mail between classes and posting discussion questions on the LMS to which all students had to respond. One instructor noted the following: "I greet each student as they arrive in the classroom and before class begins. If a student is absent, I send an email to 'check in' and this small exchange helps to get to know them." A key to building the relationship appears to be between-class contact. Instructors used both Skype and the LMS for private meetings and office hours with their students.

Although many instructors noted a lag time in building a relationship for several reasons, they felt that the relationship often was more intimate than those in campus classrooms. First, the number of students in each section was approximately half of those on campus (10–12 versus 18–20, respectively). Second, some instructors noted that because most students joined the class from their homes, the setting was more personal and informal, and they had the feeling of being invited into the students' lives. However, an unanticipated consequence of this informality was that some students came to class in their pajamas or spent class lying in bed; the issue of decorum, therefore, will be discussed below.

Engagement and Participation

Engaging students virtually seemed to take more effort, and instructors felt they needed to be more creative and active than they were in campus settings. In addition to the strategies mentioned above, instructors used the private chat box for this purpose. This feature allowed them to encourage quieter students to participate in class discussions without having to call on them publicly and risk embarrassing them. An instructor could ask privately whether a student was not feeling well that day if he or she were acting contrary to their usual demeanor. Additionally, the Adobe program came equipped with several features that facilitated engagement, such as polling (which is equivalent to the interactive classroom response system) and other features described in the next section.

Moreover, unprepared students could not hide behind others in a back row. Shy students frequently felt more encouraged to participate in this more intimate setting. As one student in the first graduating cohort stated in an e-mail:

> There's a certain amount of personal courage that goes into speaking in front of a webcam. It's not like in a physical classroom where a small comment can be just that. In the VAC any comment you make is show stopping, for everyone in the class has eyes on you. There is no hiding in the back of class. Wimps need not apply and if they do they will no longer be wimps. You HAVE to participate. You HAVE to be brave.

Activities

Classroom exercises had to be modified to accommodate the virtual platform. Instructors initially had been concerned about the ability of students to role-play client situations. To the contrary, role playing was easily conducted; the program, in fact, allowed instructors to put students in separate "rooms" for this purpose. The instructor then could enter individual rooms, observe the role-playing exercise, and use the private chat box to give suggestions to the student playing the therapist. In this respect, the virtual program proved to have an advantage over the campus-based program, where students generally are limited to one classroom, the noise level can be distracting, and the instructor may have difficulty moving around the room to help students individually.

Instructors could also replicate many campus-based activities in the virtual environment, such as provide PowerPoint presentations, handouts, and case vignettes. Assignments consisted of papers submitted via the LMS, which could be read and corrected online, and grades could be entered electronically.

Challenges

Technology

Although not unique to practice courses, initially the challenge of the technology itself must be noted. As the technology improved with upgraded versions of the program, such issues of course diminished. Nevertheless, there were situations beyond faculty control, such as poor weather in different parts of the country that sometimes compromised Internet connections. Through our partnership agreement with 2U, Inc., a technology support group helped manage these issues by assisting students and faculty with technological glitches. Having a third party mediate these issues proved extremely important to ensuring that student and faculty time would be focused solely on teaching.

Socialization

There was a clear learning curve in terms of socializing students to the program. Two components were integrally related. The first, decorum, was unanticipated, although in retrospect probably should have been foreseen. The second, the reputation of online programs, led to the first. Online programs historically have been viewed by some as less rigorous than programs in traditional schools—specifically, the quality of education and the demands of the program. Although most students choose online programs for the convenience of location and scheduling and often had families and careers, in the early days of the innovation, some students appeared to have expected a less rigorous program. We were adamant that the USC reputation and brand not be compromised, so we ensured that the program's quality, delivery, rigor, and expectations were fully equivalent to those on campus. This level of rigor was unsettling for many initial students who expected otherwise; many dropped to part-time status, and others dropped out altogether. At the time of this writing, there is a lower attrition rate than in previous years, as the program's reputation has "gone viral," and incoming students appear to be more knowledgeable about expectations.

Etiquette

Part of the socialization process was the issue of decorum. Perhaps ingenuously, we expected that students would come to class dressed appropriately, as they would on campus. When some students showed up in pajamas or drinking beer, with children present in the room or with partners visible in their underwear, we had to take a more proactive stance. Norms for behavior were discussed in each classroom, and the director of the program, Dr. June Wiley, compiled a document (in collaboration with the faculty) that she posted on the virtual bulletin board and was discussed during orientation (see the Appendix).

In terms of the actual practice course, there is no question that the virtual environment presents certain challenges to a faculty accustomed to teaching in a brick-and-mortar setting. However, the challenges spurred us to be more creative in course delivery. For example, one of the challenges involved the use of videos, which often are shown during class time in campus-based classes. One of the solutions was to embed the video into the asynchronous portion of the course and use it for discussion during the synchronous sessions. In addition, some used case vignettes that were filmed with professional actors, frankly providing a more engaging and real-life client situation than possible with paper-based sketches.

Nonverbal cues

The most prevalent concern with respect to the practice courses was whether facial expressions and body language would be visible on the screen. The answer to this question was mixed. Some felt that, because the class was small and everyone is facing front, facial expressions could easily be picked up. However, some instructors noted that if computer resolution was not good or lighting in the room was poor, facial expressions were hard to discern. With experience, instructors learned to advise students how to properly light their faces, and students were encouraged to use adequate broadband connections. Likewise, body language was limited to the upper half of a student's body. Nonetheless, most faculty members felt that these limitations were compensated for in the field, where students have an in vivo experience and where facial expressions and body language can be more accurately addressed.

Ethical Issues

As with any new venture, we encountered some challenges that might fall under the rubric of ethics. As previously noted, issues of decorum, and who should be present in the virtual classroom, arose very quickly. With input from the VAC instructors, a policy statement was developed, posted, and then discussed with all students. The guidelines state that no one other than the student should be present during the synchronous sessions. This requirement presented logistical difficulties for some students who were parents of young children. When their children were home from school, such as during spring break, and there was no one to supervise them in another room, the student had to miss class that day. Because sensitive clinical material was discussed and confidentiality had to be maintained, we did not feel comfortable allowing children to be privy to the synchronous discussions.

The most troubling ethical issue was that several students disclosed (or manifested) mental health issues, especially when other assignments came due and stress was high. Although these disclosures of course are not uncommon in campus-based programs as well, instructors felt they had fewer resources available to help manage these situations and ensure a good outcome. Although field faculty members intervened when they could, often making appropriate referrals to the students' local social service agencies, class instructors felt more was needed. This dilemma has been addressed and hopefully resolved. At the time of this writing, school administrators have hired a full-time mental health counselor who is solely responsible for assisting VAC students with personal and emotional issues.

Another issue that was raised concerned reporting laws. What would happen if an instructor became aware of an abuse situation during the synchronous class time that needed to be reported to the police or child protective services? Because each state has its own laws and protocols, for example, regarding the reporting of child and elder abuse or neglect, what is reportable and to whom may differ, depending on the locus of the program (Schulman, 2009). Practice instructors noted these differences and asked each student to find out what the reporting laws were in his or her particular state.

CONCLUSION

Our experience at the University of Southern California School of Social Work demonstrates that, despite the trepidations of many clinicians and our own faculty, it is possible to successfully teach practice in an online environment, with several important caveats. The first is that a blended learning model should be considered because it allows for a wide variety of learning experiences, in the most effective medium (synchronous or asynchronous). The blended environment counters many of the concerns that faculty contemplating online programs have expressed, such as the lack of interpersonal contact, which is essential to social work practice. Of major concern here was the application of didactic material, which is mostly provided by each week's synchronous class sessions

Second, it is vitally important to have a learning management system that supports the faculty's choice of the placement of learning activities. Pedagogically, some activities are more theoretically suited to an asynchronous modality, whereas others require the interaction imbedded in the synchronous portion of the class.

Third, careful student preparation for learning in this type of environment is essential. Students who choose a web-based program must have a strong, reliable Internet connection, a web cam, and a well-lit, private room. (A coffee shop is not an appropriate venue!)

Finally, faculty must approach teaching online in a thoughtful manner, recognizing the differences in teaching online versus a campus setting. Our experience is consistent with Wolf's (2006) findings that faculty must be highly motivated to teach in an online environment and be open to new experiences, such as reaching out to students between scheduled classes to help build a supportive relationship.

Taking all the concerns fully into account, we conclude that there is great promise for the future of social work practice education in a blended online learning environment.

REFERENCES

Ayala, J. S. (2009). Blended learning as a new approach to social work education. *Journal of Social Work Education, 45*, 277–288. doi:10.5175/JSWE.2009.200700112

Council on Social Work Education. (2008). *Educational policy and accreditation standards*. Alexandria, VA: Author.

Kelly, M. J. (1994). Teaching applications of expert systems. *Journal of Teaching in Social Work, 9*, 37–47. doi:10.1300/J067v09n01_04

Knowles, M.S. (1968). Andragogy, not pedagogy. *Adult Leadership, 16*(10), 350–352, 386.

Knowles, M. S. (1980). *The modern practice of adult learning: From pedagogy to andragogy* (rev. ed.). Englewood Cliffs, NJ: Cambridge.

McNutt, J., & Menon, G. (2002). Teaching Internet-based social work advocacy practice in cyberspace: A course example and conceptual framework. *Electronic Journal of Social Work, 1*(1), 1–6.

Moore, B. (2005). Faculty perceptions of the effectiveness of web-based instruction in social work education: A national study. *Journal of Technology in Human Services, 23*(1–2), 53–66. doi:10.1300/J017v23n01_04

Ouelette, P. M. (2000). Moving toward technology-supported instruction in human service practice: The "virtual classroom." *Journal of Technology in Human Services, 16*(2–3), 97–111. doi:10.1300/J017v16n02_08

Schulman, L. (2009). *The skills of helping individuals, families, groups, and* communities (6th ed.). Belmont, CA: Brooks/Cole.

Seabury, B. A., & Maple, F. F. Jr. (1993). Using computers to teach practice skills. *Social Work, 38*, 430–439. doi:10.1093/sw/38.4.430

Shibusawa, T., VanEsselstyn, D., & Oppenheim, S. (2006). Third space: A web-based learning environment for teaching advanced clinical practice skills. *Journal of Technology in Human Services, 24*(4), 21–33. doi:10.1300/J017v24n04_02

Tu, C.-H., & McIsaac, M. (2002). The relationship of social presence and interaction in online classes. *American Journal of Distance Education, 16*, 131–150. doi:10.1207/S15389286AJDE1603_2

Wodarsky, J. S., & Kelly, T. B. (1987). Simulation technology in social work education. *Arête, 12*(2), 12–20.

Wolf, P. D. (2006). Best practices in the training of faculty to teach online. *Journal of Computing in Higher Education, 17*(2), 47–78. doi:10.1007/BF03032698

APPENDIX

VAC Classroom Decorum

Expectations

- It is expected/required that students complete the asynchronous portion of each unit prior to attending the synchronous session as it provides a significant portion of class lecture and activities. This will also enhance our discussions and promote advanced learning.
- As you engage in the asynchronous portion of the class, please take time to fully and thoughtfully reflect on and think about the questions posed throughout the units. These questions are meant to enhance self-awareness and promote further discussion.
- Please take notes of any questions/comments/thoughts/feelings you have while engaging in the asynchronous units and please be prepared to share those questions/comments/thoughts/feelings during the synchronous session.

The Virtual Environment

- Although we are not in a physical classroom, we need to still treat the virtual environment with respect as a learning environment and try to keep external distractions to a minimum. Please do your best to find a quiet, well-lit space prior to logging onto the synchronous session.
- Here are some additional tips for maintaining a safe virtual environment.
  - When posting written communication, you may want to avoid typing in ALL CAPS or all bold, as this is often seen as equivalent to yelling in most online communities.
  - Please remember to use a salutation (e.g., Dear Ms./Mr./Professor) when sending e-mails to your professors, administrators, and field liaisons/instructors. Using a salutation conveys courtesy and respect for the individual rather than just jumping into the body of the e-mail.
  - Use emoticons and other symbols to indicate tone. When posting on an Internet discussion forum, there is an absence of indicators that help one to decipher tone and the forum poster's intention.
  - Take time to critically think about the messages posted and how you want to formulate your response. Think about whether it accurately reflects what you are truly trying to say. Remember that we are all in the process of learning, and our thoughts do not have to be perfectly formulated; however, what we type needs to remain respectful.

Classroom Decorum

It is important to be cognizant of the following:

- Appropriate use of the chat box
  - Classroom attire: dress code (proper dress attire is always important).
- Learning Environment
  - Children: Children should not be on the student's lap or in the vicinity of the camera's view in respect to other students
  - Pets: Pets should not be in the same room to respect the learning environment of the other students in the classroom
  - Media distractions: Both television and music should not be on during class time nor should music be listened to on your computer; your classmates and instructor are able to hear what you are hearing and can view any distraction in the background
  - Sitting upright at computer desk: Unless for medical reasons or with permission from the instructor, students should be sitting upright at a table or desk as they would in a physical classroom
  - Quiet space: Not in a coffee shop or loud public space. You and your computer should be in a place where you can hear the instructor and other classmates without distractions
- Conduct
  - The following items are not allowed and will not be tolerated in the classroom: alcohol and smoking.
- Classroom Etiquette
  - Language: Academic discourse is encouraged at all times, whether it is through speech, chat room, or e-mail.
  - Camera-ability to see student in well-lit room: In respect for your instructor and other students, your learning space should be a well-lit, quiet room, and your camera should give full view of your face in order to engage with the others in the classroom.
  - Cell phone use in front of camera: Unless used for class, your cell phone should be in the off or silent position during class time. It is inappropriate to answer phone calls during class time and especially in view of the camera. Certain instances occur when it is necessary; however, for most cases, use of a cell phone during class time is prohibited.
  - Behavior: As in any academic setting, appropriate behavior is expected at all times. Third-party distractions take away from the classroom setting and disrupt the learning environment.
  - Auditing class: When auditing a class, it is important to notify the instructor as well as be respectful to the other students enrolled.
  - Timeliness: Students should attend class in a timely manner as well as in completing the class; students should not attempt to leave early unless the instructor is notified or an emergency has taken place.

Although virtual, it is still a classroom and should be respected as such, in compliance with the USC student conduct code.

Teaching Direct Practice Skills Using Web-Based Simulations: Home Visiting in the Virtual World

AMY BLANK WILSON
Mandel School of Applied Social Sciences, Case Western Reserve University, Cleveland, Ohio, USA

SUZANNE BROWN
Wayne State University School of Social Work, Detroit, Michigan, USA

ZOE BREEN WOOD and KATHLEEN J. FARKAS
Mandel School of Applied Social Sciences, Case Western Reserve University, Cleveland, Ohio, USA

Social work programs increasingly are engaged in deploying distance education models, yet questions remain about how to teach direct practice skills within this context. As field agency changes have limited practice opportunities for social work students, methods for helping interns develop direct practice skills in diverse field practicum settings also are needed. This paper describes a direct practice course initiative in which a virtual simulation of a home visit was developed in Second Life. Descriptions of the steps that were involved in developing and implementing this initiative, feedback from the students and instructors, and resources necessary to launch such an initiative are discussed.

The authors thank Sue Shick, instructional designer working in the Department of Instructional Technology and Academic Computing at Case Western Reserve University for her dedication and invaluable assistance in developing and implementing the project described in this paper. This project was funded in part by a curriculum innovation grant from the Mandel School of Applied Social Sciences, Case Western Reserve University.

Traditionally, classrooms and field settings have been the major venue for social work education, but advances in technology and distance education capabilities have created additional opportunities and challenges for teaching social work content and practice skills (Abels, 2005). Distance education has been a part of social work education since the nineteenth century (Regan & Youn, 2008). Online education, which is the most popular form of distance learning in use today, and computer-mediated learning technologies associated with this educational format currently are becoming an increasingly common educational platform in social work (Vernon, Vakalaha, Pierce, Pittman-Munke, & Adkins, 2009).

Social work educators have been seen by some as late adopters of the online education format (Siebert, Siebert, & Spaulding-Givens, 2006). Yet, despite this perception, a recent survey found that half of the MSW programs and 4 of 10 BSW programs surveyed were actively engaged in distance education. In this study, distance learning was defined as

> delivering part or all of a course or courses through the Web, or through television or other media where students neither meet physically in the traditional classroom setting, nor meet simultaneously via one of the aforementioned forms of distance education. (Vernon et al., 2009, p. 265)

When programs that were in the process of developing (or were actively considering developing distance education programs) were included, 61% of BSW programs and 83% of MSW programs were found to be in the process of engaging distance education formats to provide at least some courses for their students (Vernon et al., 2009).

Research has found that the education outcomes for face-to-face and online classrooms generally are equivalent (Russell, 1999; Young, 2000), even in clinical courses taught in a number of disciplines (Fieldhaus & Fox, 2004; Siebert et al., 2006; Yucha & Princen, 2000). In a comparison of field instructor ratings of social work students' practice skills, few if any differences were found between distance education versus on-campus students (Kleinpeter & Potts, 2000). However, despite these positive findings, many concerns remain among social work educators about the ability to effectively teach practice skills, especially clinical skills, in an online environment (Moore, 2005; Siebert et al., 2006; Siegel, Jennings, Conklin, & Flynn 1998). These worries were clearly expressed in the most recent survey of online education in social work, where a number of respondents expressed the opinion that direct practice classes should not be offered in an online format.

This opinion finds some support in the evaluation of a skills-based clinical course that was taught in the first entirely online master's program accredited by the Council on Social Work Education (Siebert et al., 2006). The quantitative portion of this evaluation found that students in the online program had perceptions of the course that were similar to those in the face-to-face class and reported feeling better prepared to provide the services after they completed the online course. However, results from the qualitative portion of the evaluation found that online students felt they were disadvantaged due to the lack of hands-on teaching of skills in their online course (Siebert et al., 2006). The concerns voiced by students in this evaluation echo those frequently expressed by social work educators regarding the teaching of direct practice courses in an online setting. Indeed, instructors have expressed doubts about their ability to teach clinical skills effectively in an online environment in part because online classrooms have traditionally lacked the educational technology needed to support face-to-face interactions, such as role plays, live supervision, and simulated counseling sessions (Vernon et al., 2009; Wilke & Vinton, 2006).

Nonetheless, despite these widely held concerns about teaching direct practice skills online, the most recent survey of distance education programs in social work found that social work was in fact the most common foundation year course being offered through the medium of distance education (Vernon et al., 2009). The significance of this finding can best be understood by comparing it to an earlier survey of distance programs (Siegel et al., 1998), which found that most schools of social work were limiting their online programs to courses in policy and research. Thus, the present prevalence of direct practice courses being offered in distance formats represents a more recent, yet substantial, shift in the types of classes that social work programs are willing to offer in this format. The trend also brings to the forefront a need to develop educational technologies that can support the face-to-face instructional methods that are perceived by faculty and students as being essential components of the educational experience in such courses.

THE USE OF INTERACTIVE WEB-BASED TECHNOLOGY IN DIRECT PRACTICE CLASSES

From an instructional standpoint, direct practice classes need to engage instructional opportunities that will allow students to practice the skills that they are learning in the classroom before using them in the field. These practice exercises can take many forms—as group activities, role plays, or practice simulations—but a central feature of each of these activities involves the opportunity for students to interact with one another face-to-face (Regan & Youn, 2008). Such interactions are critical components professional training because they provide opportunities for students to practice new skills before using them with real clients (Cook et al., 2011).

The problem with translating these learning opportunities to online programs is finding web-based technology that can offer all three different types of educational interactions (student to content, student to teacher, and student to student) required to support students' efforts to practice the skills they are learning in the classroom (Moore, 2005). This challenge stems from the fact that, until recently, web-based educational technology focused mainly on supporting the first two forms of interaction (student to content and student to teacher) because there still were limited options available to support student to student learning (Gorini, Gaggioli, Vigna, & Riva, 2008).

The challenges associated with developing web-based technology capable of supporting real-time interactions between students could not have come at a better time. First, the literature suggests that social work educators are being encouraged to use a variety of electronic media in their face-to-face and online programs (Regan & Youn, 2008). This emphasis comes at a time when a number of new interactive web-based technologies have become available. They include podcasts, blogs, wikis, video conferencing, and 3-D virtual worlds (Regan & Youn, 2008), and all of these technologies have potential applications for direct practice online classrooms. Emerging 3-D virtual worlds, which are computer-based, simulated multi-media environments where users can interact via graphical self-representations (referred to as avatars), have opened up as-yet-unexplored avenues for creative peer-to-peer interactions in online education (Boulos, Hetherington, & Wheeler, 2007; Gorini et al., 2008). Some of the purported benefits of using virtual world tools in educational settings include providing opportunities for students to become immersed in a physical setting, where they can interact with and manipulate objects; role playing; case simulation; and real time one-to-one verbal interaction (Boulos et al., 2007).

3-D Virtual Worlds

3-D virtual worlds are web-based virtual environments that became available with the advent of Web 2.0 and the increased capacity of the Internet to support these resource intensive programs (Petrakou, 2010). Virtual worlds provide a 3-D platform where multiple users can interact at the same time, through avatars—virtual representations of individual users projected into the 3-D world. Some have pointed to the fact that the openness of these virtual worlds (and the high degree of user control associated with them) creates a wide range of teaching and learning opportunities that we have only just begun to explore (Mayrath, Traphagan, Jarmon, Trived, & Resta, 2010).

Second Life is the most popular 3-D virtual world in use today in higher educational settings (Baker, Wentz, & Woods, 2009). It was originally launched in 2003 by Linden Lab and is reported to have several million users from around the world. It is a free, computer-simulated, multi-media environment that supports its own day/night cycle, weather, its own economy with its own currency, and land that can be privately owned and developed for economic and/or educational gain (Boulos et. al., 2007).

Second Life has been used in a number of different capacities in higher education. For example, this technology is being deployed in classrooms throughout the country as a means to facilitate activities as routine as office hours and lectures as well as simulcast of special events, exhibitions of student work, and providing web-based simulations in both face-to-face and online classrooms (Baker et al., 2009). These web-based simulations are being used in educational settings as diverse as Stanford University's virtual emergency rooms, the U.S. National Oceanic and Atmospheric Administration's isle, and the U.S. Centers for Disease Control and Prevention's Genome Island (Mayrath et al., 2010).

The preceding description of 3-D virtual worlds and how they are being used in educational settings highlights the potential this technology has to provide solutions to some of the problems associated with teaching direct practice skills online, but the simulations and virtual practice exercises that can be developed also have potential applications for teaching direct practice skills in face-to-face classroom settings as well (Regan & Youn, 2008). There is a substantial body of literature in the medical and health-related fields that documents how this technology is being used to create computer simulations and virtual practice exercises that offer opportunities for students to practice skills in face-to-face classrooms (Boulos et al., 2007). In these sister disciplines, virtual worlds have been found to be especially useful in teaching skills that cannot be simulated realistically or ethically in field settings or in face-to-face role plays (Rockinson-Szapkim & Walker, 2009). However, very little has been published related to how social work educators are using this technology in their face-to-face or distance education programs.

The aim of this paper is to begin to fill this gap in knowledge by providing a description of a recent initiative that was launched in a face-to-face foundation direct practice course in an MSW program accredited by the Council on Social Work Education. In this course, the virtual simulation of a home visit was developed in Second Life in order to provide students with the opportunity to practice the engagement and assessment skills associated with the generalist practice model. Our discussion of this initiative will include an overview of the simulation that was developed, descriptions of the steps that were involved in its development and implementation, and resources needed to deploy this educational tool. We also will include discussion and feedback that was systematically collected from the students and instructors related to their learning experiences with this simulation as part of a formative assessment of ongoing efforts to improve the delivery of the course content. This project was reviewed by the university's IRB, and since it would be part of ongoing classroom improvement activities, was granted exempt status.

Project Description

As noted, the web-based home visiting simulation described in this paper was used in a foundation MSW direct practice course that teaches the generalist practice model and the direct practice skills needed to work with individuals and families. This course is divided into several sections each year, each of which meets once a week for 3 hours. This web-based simulation was implemented in three sections of this course in the fall of 2011. A total of 41 students participated in this Second Life web-based home visiting simulation, 35 women and 6 men.

All sections of this class included both a weekly lecture and a lab component. The lab used structured role plays designed to provide students with an opportunity to practice the skills they were learning from their readings, classroom lectures, and discussions each week. During the first 6 weeks of lab, students work with each other in dyads, using structured role plays to practice the skills needed to work with individuals during the five stages of the generalist practice model. These role plays are based on six pre-set client scenarios. The labs were structured so that each student in the dyad took a turn acting as the social worker practicing the skills associated with the lesson that week, and the other played the client. The students then switched roles and repeated the process using a different scenario so that each member of the dyad had a chance to play the role of the social worker in each lab session. At the end of this 6-week lab module, students produced and handed in a "client file" that included a bio-psychosocial assessment and case plan (among other items) based on the information that the student obtained during the lab sessions. Both teacher feedback and student evaluations indicated this format had been effective in teaching direct practice skills.

One skill set, home visiting skills, had been missing from the course. From a pedagogical standpoint, home visiting skills traditionally have been taught in the field; however, the delivery of social work services has changed so that not all students currently are able to learn this skill in their field settings (Jarman-Rohde, McFall, Kolar & Strom, 1997; Wayne, Bogo & Raskin, 2006; Wayne, Bogo & Raskin, 2010). The faculty therefore decided to add a module on home visiting to this course in order to help students develop the skills necessary to engage practice in this setting because working with clients in their own homes has long been deemed a distinguishing feature of social work practice (Allen & Tracy, 2009). However, the face-to-face role-play techniques used in the course lab could not provide students with the opportunity to develop the engagement and assessment skills needed for home visiting. Hence, in order to provide students with a hands-on opportunity to practice home visiting skills, a web-based home visiting simulation was developed.

Simulation Development

After the decision was made to develop such a simulation, the two full-time faculty members, an assistant professor and an instructor who both teach in the direct practice concentration, assembled an instructional team to support this initiative. This team included the chair of the Direct Practice Concentration, a project manager (who was a graduate student with substantial teaching and practice experience), and an instructional designer who was designated by the university to work on all Second Life educational projects. Since none of the faculty involved in this project had prior experience in virtual environments, as a first step, members of the instructional team worked with the university instructional design specialist to learn how to access and negotiate Second Life themselves. This process sensitized members of the instructional team to the activities that would be needed to support students' orientation to this web environment while also providing them with the opportunity to work.

The university where this initiative took place was a medium-size, private urban university in the midwest that had a pre-established presence in Second Life. This presence included investment in resources, such as private university-owned land in Second Life, and instructional design staff with experience building educational simulations in this environment. (Table 1 illustrates both the personnel and non-personnel resources required to implement this project.) Yet despite the presence of this considerable support, the instructional team realized it would need additional resources to implement this project in multiple classrooms in the upcoming year. The team, therefore, sought leadership and administrative support from within the social work school in order to secure the additional resources requisite to support the development and implementation of this initiative. This assistance came in the form of a small curriculum innovation grant provided by the dean's office, which was used to pay for a graduate assistant to be the project manager and assist the faculty in carrying out the development, implementation, and assessment of the initiative. Since there was no faculty release time associated with this project, the project manager's role was to provide support with many of the additional tasks that were imbedded in creating this program. For example, she worked with the appropriate information and technology departments in the university to ensure that the necessary computer hardware and software would be available. She also provided office hours (and training sessions outside of regular classroom hours) to ensure that students obtained the support needed to access and interact in Second Life and then assisted in assessing students' experiences with this initiative.

Once the necessary resources were obtained to support this project, the instructional team began in earnest to develop this web-based simulation. This work involved a 2- to 3-month period before the class began where the team endeavored to develop, test, and refine the home visiting simulation. As with the face-to-face role plays, the web-based home visiting simulation involved a structured scenario that was developed based on the practice experience of the faculty and graduate student overseeing the project. The

TABLE 1 Suggested Web Simulation Resources

Resource	Description	Approximate Effort and Cost
PERSONNEL		
Instruction Designer	• Consultation: use of Second Life (S.L.) • Development: scenario	• 80 hours: Consult and Development. Hourly rates vary between 50 and 100 dollars. Hourly rate with experience range between 50 and 100 dollars/hour
	• Training: Access and Skills in S.L. • Support: PRN Instructional Support	• 80 hours: Development of training materials PRN support. Hourly rate varies with experience range between 50 and 100 dollars/hour
Project Manager (graduate assistant)	• Oversee integration of Second Life software and hardware into classrooms • Assist in the development and testing of simulation • Coordinate training for Second Life across classrooms • Office hours • Assist students in completing simulation • Conduct an assessment of students learning experience	• 300 hours: Effort calculated at 10 hours per week for 6 months @ $16/hour = $4,800
NON-PERSONNEL		
Second Life Land and Avatars	• Acquisition and maintenance of S.L. "Private Island" for 50 Avatars	• $1,000 acquisition/set-up; $295 monthly maintenance
	• Development of avatars, smart bots and accessories for the simulations	• Each accessory in Second Life has a specific cost. This project used existing university resources so there was no charge.
Equipment	• Hardware and software to operate S.L.	• $500–$2,000 range
	• Computer specifications to operate S.L.	• Second Life requires cable or DSL internet connection and has specific requirements regarding computer operating system, processor, memory, screen resolution and graphics card in order to run properly. For further information, go to the Second Life website, www.secondlife.com
	• Headphones for each participant session	• $15–$30 per headphone

simulation was designed so that students could carry out some of the role play that they were conducting in the face-to-face portion of the lab sessions in the role of avatars in the home environment, created in Second Life. The goal of this component of the role play was to provide students with an opportunity to practice the engagement and assessment skills that are specific to home visiting, such as gaining entry to the home, observation of the physical environment, and how to deal with distractions or interruptions in the setting. Students then had to integrate what they learned from this simulation into the larger biopsychosocial assessment-focused assignment they were completing as part of this lab assignment. The actual simulation consisted of two avatars (one client and one social worker) that students would use for interaction within the context of an apartment that was designed to have a number of occupants and environmental hazards that social workers may encounter when conducting home visits. A picture of the kitchen developed for the simulation can be seen in Figure 1. In this figure, the client avatar is sitting at the kitchen table and the social worker avatar is standing. Figure 2 shows a portion of the living room in this simulation and contains a picture of the client avatar (female avatar seated on the couch), the social worker avatar seated in the chair, and a scripted avatar who was present in the home when the social worker avatar arrived (seated male avatar). The male avatar was programmed to get up and walk around while the social worker was in the home, and his presence during the home visit would be an unexpected event for the social worker conducting the visit.

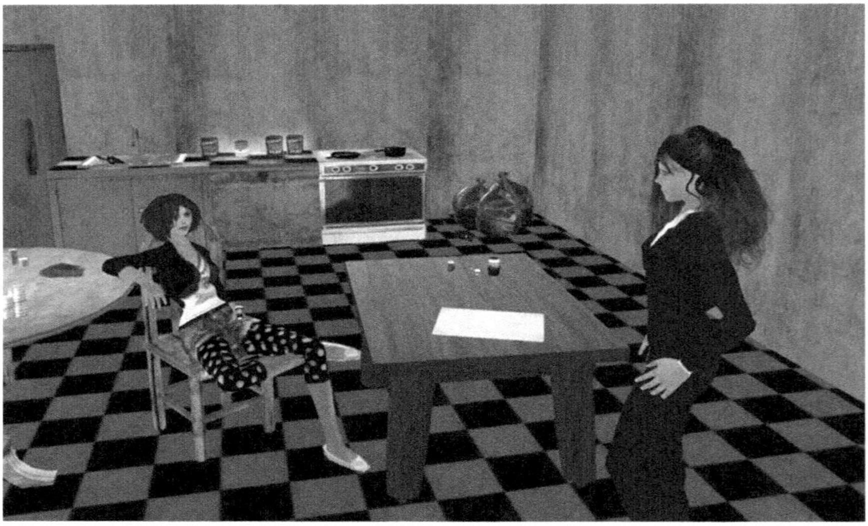

FIGURE 1 Social worker avatar in the kitchen with seated client avatar (color figure available online).

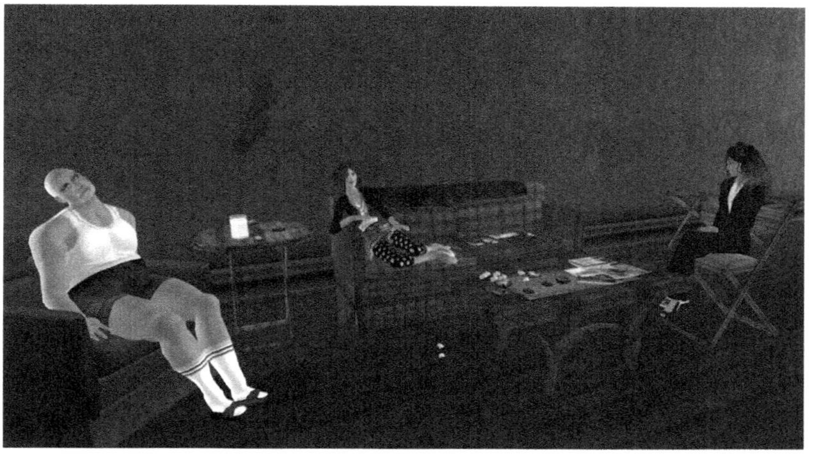

FIGURE 2 Social worker (seated in chair), client (seated on couch), and scripted avatar (seated on lounge chair) in the living room (color figure available online).

(This scripted avatar became one of the issues that students had to address as part of the simulation.)

Simulation Implementation

The implementation phase of this project involved four stages. Instructors introduced the home visiting simulation as part of the larger discussion of the 6-week individual dyad lab sessions. Then the next week students received a live in-class demonstration of Second Life technology using an office-based simulation where the project manager (i.e., graduate assistant) was present in the room operating an avatar (a young man with schizophrenia). The goal of this demonstration was for the students to interact with the avatar as a class. In this demonstration, students themselves did not enter Second Life as avatars. Rather, they worked together to observe the graduate assistant's avatar in the simulated office, projected onto a screen in front of the classroom. The students interacted with the avatar through the graduate assistant, who was always present in the room, listened to their questions and responded to them via the avatar. This demonstration provided students with an introduction to Second Life and the nature of web-based simulated role plays. Using this new medium, it also gave them a chance as a class to practice the engagement skills they were learning in class.

The second stage of implementation involved providing students with an orientation to the mechanics of accessing and interacting in Second Life. This orientation was run by the graduate assistant and offered outside of regular class hours as an optional event which students could attend during lunch hour. (Those who attended received professional development hour credits.) During this orientation, the graduate assistant demonstrated how to access Second Life and offered a tutorial on how to operate the avatar in the Second Life environment. Students were provided also with an opportunity to ask questions and to practice their skills during the session. The graduate assistant held office hours as well during this stage of implementation in order to allow students to obtain individual instruction in the use of Second Life technology if they so desired.

The third stage of implementation involved actually using the home-visiting simulation as part of the lab. The instructors prepared students for this component by giving a lecture on home visiting that provided an overview of the role of home visiting in social work practice, reviewed the mechanics for arranging these visits, and taught the skills needed to ensure safety while engaging clients in their home and conducting an assessment of the environment. A checklist was distributed that was designed to take them through the skills they needed to practice during the simulation exercise. After the lecture, students had a week to complete the home visiting component of their lab. This exercise was scheduled outside of regular class time so that the graduate student could be present, while each dyad engaged in the simulation, in case they found a need for assistance.

The final stage of implementation involved debriefing sessions with the students and faculty who participated in the initiative. Systematic formative feedback was sought related to students' experiences with the simulation and suggestions that they might have on its improvement for use with future classes. The simulation described here was part of ongoing efforts at the school to improve the educational experiences of students in this class. Therefore, all 41 students enrolled in the classes using these role-plays participated in the simulation exercises. All of them then were invited to a voluntary lunchtime meeting after the course was completed to give them an opportunity to provide informal feedback on their experiences with the web-based home visiting simulation. Of the 41 students, 10 attended these sessions, 7 women and 3 men. Faculty feedback was sought as well during the regular end of semester debriefing process associated with this course. The reflections received from both students and faculty were reviewed by the instructional team and found to fall into two categories: issues related to developing the technical skills needed to use Second Life technology and interact in this environment, and, issues related to knowledge construction and applications.

Instructor and Student Feedback

Second Life skill development

Both faculty and students noted that it was essential to have course time and resources devoted to helping both groups develop their proficiency with interacting in Second Life. However, students reported that they would have gotten more from the simulation if they had had additional time to practice interacting with one another as avatars prior to engaging in the assignment. They noted this would have helped them to focus more on the assignment and less on the mechanics of operating their avatar. Students offered several suggestions in this area that included posting a videotaped demonstration of the simulation on Blackboard to watch prior to engaging the simulation exercise, and having them bring their lap tops to class to practice interacting with one another as avatars prior to the simulation exercise.

Knowledge constructions and application

Both students and faculty gave feedback indicating that they thought the simulation provided meaningful learning opportunities with respect to home visiting. Both cohorts felt that the simulation provided students with opportunities to practice their assessment skills in a realistic home environment. They both believed that participation in the simulation exercise accomplished the objective of sensitizing students to the challenges associated with conducting home visits with regard to issues of safety and dealing with personal biases when conducting assessments of peoples' homes. Additional feedback spoke to needing more support in the classroom, after the simulation was completed, aimed at helping students to integrate what they had learned in the home visit into a larger biopsychosocial assessment. Faculty specifically reported that they had not anticipated the amount of difficulty that students would experience trying to integrate the information they had obtained in the home visit with their larger overall assessment. Both groups indicated this task was especially challenging for students when the information they obtained from the home visit contradicted what the client had said during the office sessions.

Students remarked that the simulation helped them to understand the types of skills needed for home visiting and that participating in the simulation helped them to think about the unanticipated situations that can occur in these settings and how they might respond. They also reported that the simulation exercise sensitized them to the fact that they can learn things about clients in their homes that would not be accessible in office settings. They also stated that home visits can change the nature of the relationship with their client and bring up new boundary issues that need to be addressed.

Faculty felt that the simulation helped to expand students' conceptualizations of their clients' circumstances and the resources available to them. They also felt that participation in this simulation gave students more confidence in their home-visiting ability. Finally. faculty reported that the simulation provided a realistic environment that allowed students to practice their skills "without risk" and that gave students an opportunity to process their reactions to what they experienced in the simulation, and identify areas for future learning.

DISCUSSION

The instructors and students who participated in this initiative reported that participation in the web-based home visiting simulation added important learning and skill development opportunities that would not have been possible without access to the virtual simulation. A number of factors were found to be critical to the success of this initiative, many of which can be built upon in future efforts. Before asking them to engage the simulation assignment, it is critical to give students enough time and individual support to master the mechanics of Second Life. Similar to Salmon, Nie, and Edirisingha (2010), we found that the first step in implementing this initiative in the classroom needed to focus on introducing this specific technology to the students. They needed to use it as a part of class so they could develop proficiency in accessing Second Life, operating their avatars, and interacting with one another. However, time alone was not enough; it also was necessary to provide individual support to students developing these skills.

In this initiative, this assistance was provided through live demonstrations during a professional development seminar that was held outside of class time. However, like Salmon et al. (2010), the instructional team decided that in future classes it would be important that this training be provided within Second Life. This type of training would likely better provide the immersion needed to build students' confidence in their skills and gain greater control more quickly.

Second, the instructional team found that this project benefited greatly from having access to private space in Second Life to run the simulation, along with the support of instructional designers experienced with this technology. The fact that our university owned several islands in Second Life allowed the instructional team to control who could access the private space where the simulation was run, thereby protecting the students from some of the hazards that prior educators have found when running simulations in *public* Second Life spaces (Ahern & Wink, 2010). The university's prior investment in this technology also gave the social work faculty access to instructional design staff with the experience necessary to ensure that the simulation would create a realistic home environment. These two resources worked together to create a learning environment where students felt safe to use the skills they were learning in a setting that produced a meaningful and realistic practice opportunity.

Third, the instructional team identified the importance of instructor "buy-in" to the use of distance education in social work generally, and the use of web-based technology to teach direct practice skills specifically. In this initiative, the simulation was used in a number of course sections taught by instructors who had varying degrees of comfort and prior exposure to distance education and the use of web-based simulation in direct practice. The success of future efforts, therefore, would be best supported by the selection of instructors who come with an interest in using these simulations in the classroom and a relative ease with using web-based technology. Such comfort and openness are essential to projects like this for a number of reasons. First, faculty who feel comfortable with the technology can better anticipate and resolve technical problems that may arise. Second, faculty can better transmit their own enthusiasm about the simulation if they have a full understanding of it. Finally, a thorough grounding in the technology can help faculty better envision its potential uses and how to construct a simulation that will best lead to student learning. Developing this knowledge of and grounding in simulation technology may require schools to provide not only training for faculty members but reasonable release time to prepare such simulation exercises.

As a final point, classes that use the home-visiting simulation in the future need to build in more time in class to help students learn how to incorporate information learned from the home visit into a larger biopsychosocial assessment. The instructional team had assumed that students would need assistance learning how to conduct an assessment during a home visit. However, they naively believed that once students learned how to collect this information, they would know how to integrate it into a comprehensive assessment. To our surprise, what was learned was that students across the board struggled with what to do with the information they gained from the home visits. This problem especially was prevalent in instances where students' learned information *from* the home visit contradicted what their clients had told them *before* the home visit.

IMPLICATIONS

The computer-based simulation used in this Second Life initiative was found to provide an important bridge between what was learned in the practice class and in the field. The use of this bridge to teach home-visiting skills was found to be of special value because a number of students were in field placements where they would not have the opportunity to engage in home visits. Opportunities for students to engage clients directly at their field placement continue to shrink due to changes in licensing requirements, insurance reimbursement limits on who can provide billable services to clients, cases that are seen as too complex for students, and limited supervisory resources. It is likely that more of the onus for skill development will fall on learning that takes place in the classroom if such practice trends continue.

As noted, several other practice-related professions, such as medicine, nursing, and dentistry, have been using technology-enhanced simulations to teach practice skills for some time (Decker, Sportsman, Puetz, & Billings, 2008). However, despite the promise this technology offers, much is yet to be learned about its impact on the development of practice skills, especially in the counseling arena where its use is relatively new. The findings associated with this initiative are promising, but research needs to begin to systematically assess the impact that these simulations have on student learning with much larger cohorts, especially in social work educational settings where their use is in the nascent stage.

While much is yet to be learned about the impact that educational activities taking place in virtual reality have on educational outcomes, the virtual simulations used in this initiative (and the 3D web-based technology that provided the pivotal support) have a lot of potential application for teaching practice skills through the medium of online education. The technology used in this simulation offers an instructional platform to support a type of interaction that has been missing from many previous programs: real-time, student-to–student, and student-to-faculty interaction. This special feature of Second Life could be deployed as well to support the development of more informal socialization activities that are important to educational outcomes, but lacking in traditional on-line programs (Petrakou, 2010). Such interactive web-based technology also offers another avenue to carry out a number of routine educational activities that are not easily supported by traditional 2D technologies, such as office hours, breakout sessions, and group learning projects. Moreover, three-dimensional simulations offer one of the only viable ways for students to role-play with one another and with faculty in an online setting. As such, there is a clear need for additional investment in both the development and continuing evaluation of this technology and its impact on teaching practice skills in both face-to-face and online educational formats.

REFERENCES

Abels, P. (Ed.). (2005). *Distance education in social work: Planning, teaching and learning*. New York, NY: Springer Publishing.

Ahern, N., & Wink, D. M. (2010). Virtual learning environments: Second Life. *Nurse Educator*, *35*(6), 225–227.

Allen, S. F., & Tracy, E. M. (Eds.). (2009). *Delivering home-based services: A social work perspective*. New York, NY: Columbia University Press.

Baker, S. C., Wentz, R. K., & Woods, M. M. (2009). Using virtual worlds in education: Second Life as an educational tool. *Teaching of Psychology*, *36*, 59–64.

Boulos, M. N. K., Hetherington, L., & Wheeler, S. (2007). Second Life: An overview of the potential of 3-D virtual worlds in medical and health education. *Health Information and Libraries Journal*, *24*, 233–245.

Cook, D. A., Hatala, R., Brydges, R., Zendejas, B., Szostelt, J. H., Wang, A. T., . . . Hamstra, S. J. (2011). Technology enhanced simulation for health professions education: A systematic review and meta-analysis. *Journal of the American Medical Association*, *306*(9), 978–988.

Decker, S., Sportsman, S., Puetz, L., & Billings, L. (2008). The evolution of simulation and its contribution to competency. *The Journal of Continuing Education in Nursing*, *29*(2), 74–80.

Fieldhaus, C. R., & Fox, P. L. (2004). Effectiveness of an ethics course delivered in traditional and non-traditional formats. *Science and Engineering Ethics*, *10*(2), 389–400.

Gorini, A., Gaggioli, A., Vigna, C., & Riva, G. (2008). A second life for ehealth: Prospects for the use of 3-D virtual worlds in clinical psychology. *Journal of Medical Internet Research*, *10*(3), e21.

Jarman-Rohde, L., McFall, J., Kolar, P., & Strom, G. (1997). The changing context of social work practice: Implications and recommendations for social work education. *Journal of Social Work Education*, *33*, 29–46.

Kleinpeter, C. H. & Potts, M. K. (2000). Distance education: Teaching practice methods using interactive television. *Professional Development: The International Journal of Continuing Social Work Education*, *3*(3), 37–43.

Mayrath, M. C., Traphagan, T., Jarmon, L., Trived, A., & Resta, P. (2010). Teaching with virtual worlds: Factors to consider for instructional use of Second Life. *Journal of Educational Computing Research*, *43*(4), 403–444.

Moore, B. (2005). Faculty perceptions of the effectiveness of web-based instruction in social work education: A national study. *Journal of Technology in Human Services*, *23*(1/2), 53–66.

Petrakou, A. (2010). Interacting through avatars: Virtual worlds as a context for online education. *Computers & Education*, *54*, 1020–1027.

Regan, J. R. C., & Youn, E. J. (2008). Past, present, and future trends in teaching clinical social work skills through web-based learning environments. *Journal of Social Work Education*, *44*(2), 95–115.

Rockinson-Szapkim, A. J., & Walker, V. L. (2009). Web 2.0 technologies: Facilitating interaction in an on-line human services counseling skills course. *Journal of Technology in Human Services*, *27*(3), 175–193.

Russell, T. L. (1999). *The no significant difference phenomenon: A comparative research annotated bibliography on technology for distance education: As reported in 355 research reports, summaries and papers*. Raleigh, NC: North Carolina State University.

Salmon, G., Nie, M., & Edirisingha, P. (2010). Developing a five-stage model of learning in Second Life. *Educational Research*, *52*(2), 169–182.

Siebert, D. C., Siebert, C. F., & Spaulding-Givens, J. (2006). Teaching clinical social work skills primarily online: An evaluation. *Journal of Social Work Education*, *42*(2), 325–336.

Siegel, E., Jennings, J. G., Conklin, J., & Flynn, S. (1998). Distance learning in social work education: Results and implications of a national survey. *Journal of Social Work Education*, *34*(1), 71–80.

Vernon, R., Vakalaha, H., Pierce, D., Pittman-Munke, P., & Adkins, L. F. (2009). Distance education programs in social work: Current and emerging trends. *Journal of Social Work Education*, *45*(2), 263–276.

Wayne, J., Bogo, M., & Raskin, M. (2006). Field notes: The need for radical change in field education. *Journal of Social Work Education*, *42*(1), 161–169.

Wayne, J., Bogo, M., & Raskin, M. (2010). Field education as the signature pedagogy of social work education. *Journal of Social Work Education*, *46*(3), 327–339.

Wilke, D., & Vinton, L. (2006). Evaluation of the first web-based advanced standing MSW program. *Journal of Social Work Education*, *42*(3), 607–620.

Young, J.R. (2000). Faculty report at University of Illinois casts a skeptical eye on distance education. *The Chronicle of Higher Education*, *46*(19), A48.

Yucha, C., & Pricen, T. (2000). Insights learned from teaching pathophysiology on the World Wide Web. *Journal of Nursing Education*, *39*(2), 68–72.

Establishing a Community of Inquiry through Hybrid Courses in Clinical Social Work Education

MARIA FERRERA, NOAM OSTRANDER,
and SONYA CRABTREE-NELSON
Department of Social Work, DePaul University, Chicago, Illinois, USA

Utilizing the conceptual framework of Garrison, Anderson, and Archer for critical inquiry, this paper outlines the importance of the community of inquiry (COI) model and how it may inform online social work education. Integrating the COI model, we discuss how online learning in the classroom with a hybrid approach has been used to facilitate critical reflection and discourse. To illustrate this approach, we provide two case examples from clinical courses taught in an MSW program.

INTRODUCTION

Colleges and universities increasingly have embraced distance learning and online education over the last 20 years (Sandell & Hayes, 2002). In keeping with this trend, social work programs also have moved toward more online course offerings (Maidment, 2005). However, some social work educators hesitate to consider online formats given social work's focus on human interactions and social presence (Burton & Seabury, 1999). Additionally, many social work educators worry about the disparity that can exist between themselves and their students with respect to both knowledge and access to current computer technology (Maidment, 2005).

A compromise between strictly online coursework and the traditional classroom setting is a hybrid approach. Loosely defined, a hybrid stance blends face-to-face teaching with online instruction. Beyond that broad definition, the specifics of a hybrid format vary widely. Such courses have the benefits of (1) reaching students through a medium that they embrace and often prefer; (2) enhancing teaching, social and cognitive presence within the actual or virtual classroom; and (3) teaching and modeling interaction with current social media and information and communication technologies (ICTs) that our students can take to their internships and their future jobs.

To illustrate this hybrid compromise, examples are provided here of the ways face-to-face teaching has been blended with online instruction. For example, some scholars of hybrid courses recommend utilizing face-to-face class sessions in the beginning, middle and end of the academic term (Martyn, 2003). These class sessions then are supplemented with group work, quizzes, and some discussions online. It is worth noting that in general, college students enrolled in hybrid courses have demonstrated similar learning outcomes as students enrolled in traditional face-to-face courses (Ernst, 2008). Nevertheless, within the social work arena, some argue there are few positive outcomes from web-based learning (Kreuger and Stretch, 2000). Other critics simply argue that practice and methods courses should be taught within traditional formats (Siegel, Jennings, Conklin, & Flynn, 1998). However, some claim that it is entirely possible for social work graduate students enrolled in online courses to have equivalent outcomes with those in traditional, face-to-face *clinical* courses (Siebert & Spaulding-Givens, 2006).

CONCEPTUAL FRAMEWORK

As social work educators increase their use of ICTs, so does the need to look at the impact of this approach on student learning. Garrison, Anderson, and Archer (2000) have developed a model that is useful in examining the effectiveness of online learning and the use of ICTs, which highlights the importance of teaching, cognitive, and social presence (Figure 1). "Social Presence" is currently explained in the social work literature as being the numerous ways that people associate with one another (LaMendola, 2010). Garrison and colleagues add that it is the ability of participants to identify with the community (e.g., professional identity or course of study), communicate purposefully in a trusting environment, and develop interpersonal relationships by way of projecting their individual personalities. Such social pressure may include face-to-face interactions, telephone calls, or various types of social media interactions. "Teaching presence" is the design, facilitation, and direction of cognitive and social processes for the purpose of realizing personally meaningful and educationally worthwhile learning outcomes (Anderson, Rourke, Garrison, & Archer, 2001). This involves the actions required to establish an infrastructure for the course, including the integration of appropriate technologies (supported by the teaching

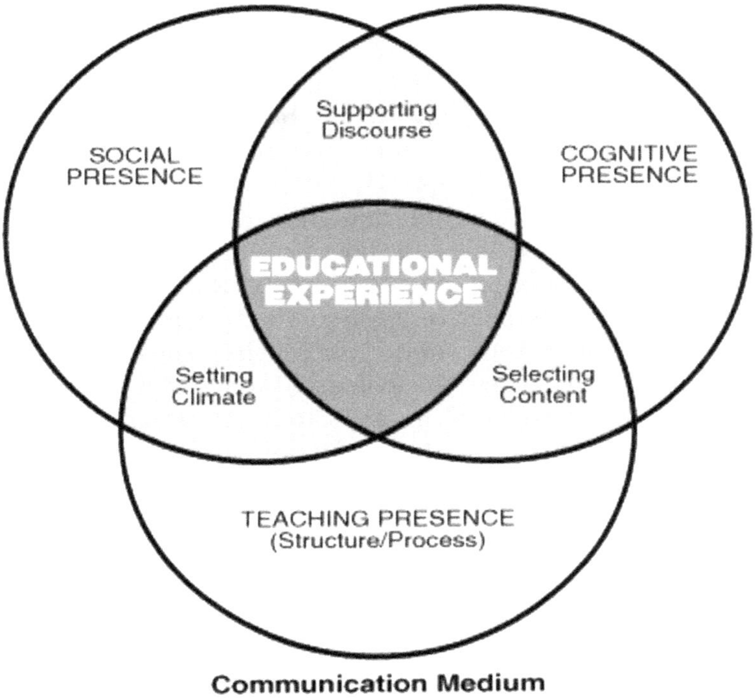

FIGURE 1 The community of inquiry model. *Source:* Garrison, Anderson, & Archer, 2000.

institution), details of assignments, course outcome expectations, and opportunities to relay questions, seek assistance, and receive feedback from the instructor.

"Cognitive presence" is the extent to which learners are able to construct and confirm meaning through sustained reflection and discourse (Garrison et. al., 2000) and involves how the educator facilitates the process of critical thinking. Cognitive presence is indicated among students who exchange information, display a sense of puzzlement, apply new ideas, and make connections between theory and practice. Multiple perspectives and opinions are developed, considered, evaluated, and challenged. Online communication may be tailored to provide opportunities for written communication, which in turn allows time for reflection and critical thinking about complex issues. It is argued that cognitive presence is the most basic element to success in learning. Yet, strong cognitive presence can be facilitated only by an effective teaching presence, both of which are tempered by social presence. Thus, the relationship between these three elements in a community of inquiry is intimate, and the elements are never mutually exclusive of one another. The synthesis of all three elements creates a community of inquiry as the social context and communication medium from which higher order thinking and meaningful educational experiences can occur.

CREATING A SENSE OF COMMUNITY WITHIN THE COMMUNITY OF INQUIRY

Notwithstanding the requisite investment of time and attention to logistics and detail—as well as adjustment in comfort level to utilizing diverse technologies necessary to structure the course online (Siebert & Spaulding-Givens, 2006)—thoughtfulness and time also are required to sustain one's "presence" as a clinical social work educator. The requirements of ethical social work education and practice demand sensitivity to culture and diversity, critical reflection, and self-reflexivity. Social work educators have the responsibility to bring sensitive and controversial issues of oppression, discrimination, and inequality into the dialogue of the social work classroom on a regular basis. In order for meaningful learning to occur, strongly held values and beliefs may be expressed by individual students as well as between peers. How, then, do you respond to students who may have difficulty in this cognitively and emotionally provocative process within an online course? How do you establish a foundation level of trust and sense of safety among students? Mixing face-to-face interaction with online dialogue in a hybrid clinical social work course is possible when the instructor is able to develop a sense of community within the COI in innovative, effective, and creative ways. We now will discuss how this can occur in a hybrid course and how social, cognitive, and teaching presence can be established and sustained.

Ground Rules in Communication

Effective teaching promotes collaborative learning through critical discussion. In networked learning environments, where communication is web-based, there are advantages and disadvantages when promoting collaborative learning. Because debate is inherent within critical discussion, ground rules for communication must be made explicit at the onset to create a safe environment. In a hybrid course, these ground rules may need to be reiterated since the medium of communication is in constant change, switching, for example, from face-to-face to online. Hence, clinical instructors are more challenged to facilitate, steer, and re-direct feedback when students participate in online discussion and debate (Pilkington & Walker, 2003). Since computer-mediated communication can be fragmented, or "interactionally incoherent," the struggle to "see" or "hear" other participants in the process of "speaking" is a barrier to establishing and sustaining meaningful dialogue which the instructor must overcome (Herring, 1999).

A strong teaching presence should provide explicit and detailed guidelines for discussion that promote focus in discussion, expectations for the quality and quantity of "posts" and responses, and recommendations for responding in both a respectful and a critical way. Thus, what is learned in the hybrid classroom will be timely and sensitive to how many individuals, families, and groups have grown accustomed to relating and communicating with one another. As we examine the nuances of this communication among students, we become more acutely aware of the challenges that today's communication mediums bring to family functioning and relationships.

Through the online discussion, students must work together in their efforts to participate in dialogue, listening to each other's opinions, reacting, and interacting. There is social presence here. As educators, we can highlight the strengths of student contributions, and how they build on their arguments and depth of thinking together. Within this collaborative process, there is a potential for thoughts, opinions, and perspectives to be challenged and adjusted.

The Non-Vocal Student May Become Vocal

We often are unsure why certain students may not be vocal within the class. It can be for a myriad of reasons: reserve/shyness, uncertainty, lack of self-confidence, language barriers and, perhaps, culture. As we teach, often to first-generation students, we must recognize that some may come from collectivist or family cultures where it is not always perceived as appropriate to voice one's own individual opinion or to be vocal. Although we want to encourage the practice of being professionally assertive in order to advocate effectively on the behalf of those who often do not have a voice, it may serve us well to be sensitive to the possibilities of why to do so may be counter-cultural. Online discussion often allows those students to weigh their thoughts and opinions and gives them time to articulate those thoughts in a less pressured manner, at their own pace.

Based on these observations and the conceptual framework of COI, we offer two examples from our experiences in the classroom at a private moderate-size urban university located in the Midwest. It is worth mentioning that both of these examples come from the instructors' first experiences incorporating a hybrid model.

CASE EXAMPLE 1: DIRECT PRACTICE COURSEWORK FOR FIRST-YEAR MSW STUDENTS

One of the authors of this study taught a course that serves as the foundation-level direct practice course for our MSW program, spanning direct practice with individuals, families, groups, and communities. Based on her experiences from the previous two quarters with the same student cohort, the instructor learned that she would need to make some adjustments due to the class size (24 students), desired level of engagement via presentations she hoped to have, and the number of speakers scheduled on campus for spring quarter. She realized in the first two quarters that several students had important contributions to the class discussion but did not always get their points heard during class or did not feel comfortable speaking up in the classroom setting and instead used the Desire to Learn (D2L) discussion board. She wanted to build on this pattern, while continuing to allow in-class opportunities for discussion as well. The instructor also did not want to take class time for 24 individual presentations, based on the amount of time the class had spent on presentations during the winter quarter. Thus, she wanted to try something new in the spring quarter. To accommodate, the instructor chose to incorporate more online tools and interface time, utilizing a form of hybrid class design. The course would meet in person 8 of the 10 classes. (Students also were expected to attend presentations by two on-campus speakers and post comments about the content as it related to the course readings and discussion.) The instructor utilized the university's D2L online interface as a place for all students to post their class presentations rather than use class time for 24 individual presentations. The assignment was linked to a large paper due at the end of the quarter. The online presentations allowed students to outline their findings along the way, obtain feedback from their classmates and instructor, and then incorporate that feedback into their final paper. Students were instructed to read and comment on the presentations of their peers. Written, detailed instructions were given for all of these aspects of the course. The expectations also were covered in class and the instructor checked with the students weekly.

Benefit to Students

On reflection, the instructor found that her emerging understanding of hybrid technology as paired with a clinical course highlighted three main areas in which she feels the students benefited. These were an increase in their critical thinking, the creative process brought to assignments, and the level of engagement with the course content.

The instructor learned that the use of hybrid technology in clinical courses can serve to offer more opportunity for critical thinking. In this course, the use of the D2L system for engagement outside of class appeared to deepen and enhance student learning. Students were instructed to utilize reflections and postings during the week in response to course readings, videos shown, and speakers. The instructor found not only that students did this regularly, without prompting, but that the level of thought in the comments often was greater than in class discussions. This may be because students had time to think about their comments prior to posting. One comment on the anonymous course evaluation stated,

> The articles we read for class introduce new ways of thinking about subject matter that turns out to be more complex than it seems at first and we always get to incorporate our own experience into the class and D2L discussion.

The course demonstrated that students were engaging with the material in a thoughtful manner. They were able to have differing opinions in a respectful way and share links to new information for fellow classmates.

Creativity is something the instructor hopes to foster in her students' practice as social workers. This is modeled for them by allowing numerous ways for students to interpret assignments. The instructor found, for example, that when students were instructed to post their presentations on D2L in lieu of in class presentations, and were encouraged to be as creative as they wanted to be, they came up with myriad ways to present information. Examples included the use of Prezi, PowerPoint and various types of videos. A student commented on the anonymous course evaluation,

> The variety of class discussions, activities, lectures, and presentations [were beneficial]. I think that in order to really absorb a concept, it is good for students to learn in a variety of ways. The different activities that were presented in this class were always helpful.

Students were also able to give feedback directly to one another. Moreover, students were required to comment on at least several of their classmates' presentations; most students commented on almost all of them and engaged in ongoing dialogue with one another via D2L. They shared resources and debated points of view in a notably open and respectful manner.

The engagement via D2L often was deeper and more complex than the instructor has ever before experienced in a classroom setting. This could be because students who were normally quiet were able to reflect and engage in this format, which may have felt more comfortable and less intimidating. Students also appeared to take time to think through the various issues and respond from a place of deeper reflection than they were able to "in the moment" during class discussion. One student stated, "I also like the discussion board for people who do not like to talk in class, it seems that a lot of people are getting use out of it." It also appeared that this connection to the course material during the week led to deeper discussion during class sessions. The students were continually engaged in the material as opposed to just revisiting it once per week.

CASE EXAMPLE 2: HYBRID APPROACH TO HUMAN BEHAVIOR IN THE SOCIAL ENVIRONMENT

Like many social work educators, this instructor came to online teaching with doubt and reluctance, given his belief that not only was there something intrinsically valuable about being in a room with students but also because of his conviction that social work education requires face-to-face contact. Despite these hesitations, the instructor enrolled in his home institution's training program for online teaching. In this training program, each faculty member was paired with a technical consultant who would help construct an online or hybrid course. Essentially, this provided a union of someone skilled in content with someone skilled in technology.

For this training process, the instructor selected his upcoming two-course sequence on human behavior and the social environment. With 31 students in the course, he decided on a hybrid framework where class would meet in person for 5 weeks, spread evenly across the 10-week academic term. When class did not meet, students were expected to participate in discussion board threads on the course website and complete assignments based on the readings in order for the instructor to assess comprehension and application of the material.

The students responded positively to this framework, which was evident in their comments on the anonymous course evaluations. One student wrote, "I loved the fact that this was a hybrid course. As students in internships, we are all very busy and it was nice to not have to come to class sometimes and work on the assignments from home." This comment, which echoed numerous others, hints at another benefit the class structure had for social work students: flexibility. Like all graduate social work students, they had to spend 16 to 20 hours a week at their internships. (This requirement often is on top of classwork, any paid employment they may have, and other responsibilities they may have at home. Although every assignment had a specific due date for the weeks when class was online, they had the flexibility to do the work wherever and whenever their schedule allowed.) As an additional benefit, a different student commented on the course evaluation, "I liked the hybrid format. I think that it gives us a chance to express ourselves in a way in which we feel comfortable." This comment echoes the previous case study and hints at literature discussed above in terms of making classes more accessible for students with different learning and communication styles.

Like the students, the instructor also took time to reflect on the experience of teaching a hybrid course. From his perspective, one particular strength stood out. The hybrid and online formats require a greater level of structure than traditional courses. In this sense, the hybrid format improved his teaching presence, which was referenced above in the COI model. The University's training program underscored this need for improved teaching presence and went to great lengths to work through objectives and assessment measures for every learning module. The instructor, who had been teaching social work for 7 years, found this approach particularly helpful because he, like most faculty members, did not necessarily learn how to teach in his doctoral program; rather, teaching was a skill that he, like most social work instructors, was expected pick up along the way. The hybrid framework drove this instructor to develop more structured courses. With that improved structure, which included more frequent and targeted assessment, the instructor also noticed that students were able to develop a stronger grasp of the material and were able to apply what they learned in subsequent class sessions.

The shadow side of the hybrid and online courses, however, is that they require a tremendous amount of preparatory effort before they can be launched. This work is not only extensive but also often concentrated in a compressed amount of time. While this work pays dividends once the course is launched, it can be daunting for faculty who are first entering into the realm of online teaching. The faculty member noted that he also made mistakes that he hopes to learn from with future courses. For example, with the increased number of assessments, the instructor found that he had much more grading to do. The instructor addressed this issue in the second half of the course by having slightly fewer modules, which meant fewer assessments. Additionally, more of the content assessments morphed into quizzes that could automatically be graded through "widgets" that the technology consultant helped create for the course. While this level of support may not be available at all colleges and universities, faculty delving into this area should consider ways to make their grading work manageable given the increased number of assessments that may come with online courses.

Overall, the instructor found teaching these hybrid courses to be rewarding and useful. The format provided him with both greater structure and flexibility. The structure made him a better teacher and improved the students' comprehension of the material. The flexibility allowed interactions with students in formats where they felt more comfortable (in person or online) as well as some respite from being in the classroom every week. Further, it did not appear that the classroom lost any sense of community, despite the fact that the students were not in the same room together every week.

CONCLUSION

Perhaps instinctively, as clinical social work educators we shared our initial reservations about using online learning. This caution stemmed from the responsibility to effectively teach social work students fundamental practice skills that involve "human," face-to-face interaction. However, with institutional support, we were challenged to expand the repertoire of tools within our own pedagogy as well as improve our teaching presence.

At the same time, there are some notable challenges that come with hybrid and online education that instructors should consider prior to and during the development of a course. The case studies already mentioned the extensive time commitment involved in developing an online or hybrid course, the increased time dedicated to responding to discussion board threads, and the additional time spent grading a greater number of assessment measures. Other considerations should include the technological assistance that students may require as they learn new features of online education as well as the reality that students might not have access to computers with up-to-date software and high-speed internet connections at home. This second consideration can be mitigated in the course design process. One can simplify the course design, limit the number of streaming videos, and explore the cost and availability of specialized software. With these considerations in mind, instructors engaging in online and hybrid courses may anticipate conundrums and save themselves and their students challenges that otherwise could be frustrating and affect the learning outcomes.

Nevertheless, the hybrid approach allowed us to reach and engage students in diverse ways, often through mediums to which they were already accustomed. Integrating online learning, however, required a deeper level of consciousness regarding the course structure and, perhaps more important, the incremental, minute processes that contribute to the learning experience as a whole. Throughout the course, week to week, there is an iterative and interactive exchange of information between educator and students (as well as among students) within the context of a collaborative learning environment. Through the use of discussion boards, online presentations, and learning programs that allow faculty to provide infrastructure within the course (such as D2L and Blackboard), educators are able to assess student work, level of understanding of course material, and critical thinking capacity on an ongoing basis. In turn, more opportunities are provided for students to receive feedback that is attuned to where they are at in their individual learning. Students also are empowered to express themselves more reflectively, creatively, and adeptly within the constraints of their often-demanding personal lives and work schedules. The collaborative learning process is encouraged not only in the classroom but also online, providing ample opportunities for students to share ideas and express diverse opinions and for critical discourse to occur. All of these elements contribute to the COI, where teaching, social, and cognitive presence are strengthened, and the student learning experience may be enhanced.

REFERENCES

Anderson, T., Rourke, L., Garrison, R., & Archer, W. (2001). Assessing teaching presence in a computer conference context. *Journal of the Asynchronous Learning Network*, *5*(2), 1–17.

Burton, D., & Seabury, B. (1999). The virtual social work course: Promises and pitfalls. *New Technology in the Human Services*, *12*(3/4), 55–64.

Ernset, J. (2008). A comparison of traditional and hybrid online instructional presentation in communication technology. *Journal of Technology Education*, *19*(2), 40–49.

Garrison, D. R., Anderson, T., & Archer, W. (2000). Critical inquiry in a text-based environment: Computer conferencing in higher education. *The Internet and Higher Education*, *2*(2–3), 87–105

Herring, S. (1999). Interactional coherence in CMC. *Journal of Computer-Mediated Communication, 4*, 4. Retrieved from http://jcmc.indiana.edu/vol4/issue4/herring.html

Kreuger, L W., & Stretch, J. J. (2000). How hypermodern technology in social work education bites back. *Journal of Social Work Education*, *36*(1), 103–114.

LaMendola, W. (2010). Social work and social presence in an online world. *Journal of Technology in Human Services*, *28*, 108–119.

Maidment, J. (2005). Teaching social work online: Dilemmas and debates. *Social Work Education*, *24*(2), 185–195.

Martyn, M. (2003). The hybrid online model: Good practice. *Educause Quarterly*. Retrieved from net.educause.edu/ir/library/pdf/EQM0313.pdf

Pilkington, R. M., & Walker, S. A. (2003). Facilitating debate in networked learning: Reflecting on online synchronous discussion in higher education. *Instructional Science 31*, 41–63.

Sandell, K., & Hayes, S. (2002). The web's impact on social work education: Opportunities, challenges, and future directions. *Journal of Social Work Education*, *28*(1), 85–99.

Siebert, D. C., & Spaulding-Givens, J. (2006). Teaching clinical social work skills entirely online: A case example. *Social Work Education*, *25*(1), 78–91.

Siegel, E., Jennings, J. G., Conklin, J., & Flynn, S. A. N. (1998). Distance learning in social work education: results and implications of a national survey. *Journal of Social Work Education*, *34*(1), 71–80.

Utilizing Video Conferencing to Introduce an International Perspective to Foundation Practice

MARY ANN FORGEY
Graduate School of Social Service, Fordham University, New York, New York, USA

HILDA LOUGHRAN
Department of Social Policy and Social Work, University College Dublin, Dublin, Ireland

JOHNA HANSEN
Graduate School of Social Service, Fordham University, New York, New York, USA

Video conferencing has much potential to enrich international social work education. In this educational initiative, video conferencing was used to deliver a joint foundation social work practice class to students attending an MSW degree program both in the United States and in Ireland. Student feedback indicated that they gained an appreciation of the global nature of social work practice. They reported a deeper understanding of shared theoretical perspectives in relation to client engagement, and of the differences in many fields of practice. Students recommended additional opportunities for international discourse using both synchronous and asynchronous distance education methods.

Over the past two decades, social work education programs throughout the world have attempted to internationalize their curricula (Asamoah, Healy, & Mayadas, 1997; Rotabi, Gammonley, Gamble, & Weil, 2007). Many rationales have been put forth for this direction including the need for students to better understand how domestic social problems are precipitated by international events and forces; to expand students' program and policy development skills by exposing them to alternative approaches and programs used in other cultures; to better prepare students to work with diversity; and to train them for careers in international practice (Nagy & Falk, 2000). Movement toward internationalization also has led to much discussion and debate about what content should be addressed (Midgley, 2001; Powell & Robison, 2007) and how it should be organized within a program's curriculum (e.g. Asamoah, Healy, & Mayadas, 1997; Powell & Robison, 2007). As the field of international social work education continues to grow, attention must also be given to the issue of methodology, that is, what are effective and innovative ways for students to gain an international perspective (Nagy & Falk, 2000).

LITERATURE REVIEW

International Exchanges and Study Abroad Programs

Experiential learning through international exchange programs, study abroad, and international field placements, which allow the student to be immersed in another culture and engage in "international discourse," have been the methods most often acknowledged within the social work literature as the means for development of an international perspective (Carrilio & Mathiesen, 2006; Cincatta, Tokatlian, & Miller, 2006; Gilin & Young, 2009; Midgley, 2001). Those advocating for the internationalization of social work education call for increased opportunities for faculty and students to attend international conferences and participate in international internships and exchanges (Yuen, 2009). Students who participate in such exchanges and immerse themselves in another culture have been found to experience a range of positive learning outcomes including increased cross-cultural competence and understanding, innovative ideas about practice, and deepened identification as a social work professional (Boyle, Nackerud, & Kilpatrick, 1999; Gilin & Young, 2009; Holmes & Mathews, 1993).

While these findings point to the academic advantages of this type of experiential learning, concerns have been raised about the many interorganizational and administrative challenges involved in setting up study abroad programs and international field placements (Carrilio & Mathiesen, 2006; Gilin & Young, 2009). Due to an absence of resources, such as time and money, the goal of participation in this type of learning experience may be unrealistic for many, especially older students who have family responsibilities and other commitments (Powell & Robison, 2007).

Internationalization Using Web-Based Distance Education Technologies

In response, there appears to be a growing interest within social work education in what Hendriks, Kloppenburg, Gevorgianiene, and Jukutiene (2008) term an "internationalization at home" approach, that is, the use of distance education methods to promote communication among social work students across borders. Web-based technologies such as e-mail, discussion boards, chat rooms, and file sharing now are being used in innovative ways in a variety of social work education programs as delivery methods for furthering the internationalization of the curriculum (Bye, Prom, Tsybikdorzhieva, & Boldova, 2006; Carter-Anand & Clark, 2009; Ford & Rotgans-Visser, 2005; Hendriks et al., 2008; Johnson, 1999; Larsen, Sanders, Astray, & Hole, 2008).

Qualitative evaluations of the learning outcomes for students participating in these innovations suggest that they are contributing to the internationalization of social work courses. For example, Hendriks et al. (2008) conducted a pilot study of a cross-national learning experience involving students from four European social work programs. While working in small groups, the students engaged in a cross-national online case analysis of a client with disabilities. The evaluation revealed that the pilot increased the students' identification with social work as an international profession, with a great amount of shared theory, methods, and values. It also revealed that the students' insights into their own country's social policy and national perspectives increased.

In another example involving an electronic student exchange using e-mail and chat rooms, social work students from Trinity College Dublin in Ireland and the California State University at Fresno in the United States participated in similar modules focused on equality studies, diversity, and oppression (Carter-Anand & Clark, 2009). Content analysis of the exchanges found that the interpersonal contact between the students raised consciousness of the diversity of global issues and new awareness of the socio-cultural differences in welfare systems and social structures.

Internationalization Using Video Conferencing Technology

Video conferencing, also known as interactive video or, in its earlier version, interactive television, is another distance education method that has much potential to increase the international perspective of students by facilitating synchronous virtual cross-national exchange. This method differs significantly from the online web-based methods noted above. With video conferencing, the interaction is in real time (synchronous) and includes both video and audio communication, allowing participants to experience both nonverbal and verbal expression as they would in traditional face-to-face communication. While its use has been documented within international social work education as a way to provide supervision to students participating in international field placements (Panos, 2005), there are no published reports to date of its cross-national use in social work education for the purpose of creating a virtual, collaborative classroom learning experience.

Nonetheless, other disciplines have successfully used video conferencing technology to facilitate cross-national student learning. Ekblad et al. (2004) report on a pilot study involving the use of international video conferencing in teaching medical students from Sweden, Australia, and the United States about transcultural psychiatry. In the sessions, students had the opportunity to interview both actual and simulated clients as a way to learn about assessment and intervention with immigrant and refugee populations and to experience the transcultural issues that emerged. Students rated the sessions from good to very good, and the video conferencing was seen as a major strength of the 4-day course. In a second study, university students in the United Sates and South Africa participated in a graduate seminar on globalization and the information society using synchronous (video conferencing) and asynchronous (online) technology. In the evaluation, students indicated a preference for the lectures being delivered synchronously via video conference (Cogburn & Levinson, 2003).

Social work education is well positioned to use such technology for the purpose of creating a cross-national collaborative learning experience. The use of video conferencing (i.e., interactive television) dates back to the 1980s (Raymond, 2005). It is described in the social work literature as part of an earlier generation of distance learning that preceded online web-based technology (Raymond, 2005; Vernon, Vakalahi, Pierce, Pittman-Munke, & Adkins, 2009; York, 2008). The initial impetus for its use was in response to the changing needs and life circumstances of students and the resultant demand for more part-time and satellite campus programs. However, much scepticism was expressed initially about this method due to the distance involved between teacher and learner and social work's traditional preference for face-to-face interaction. Its eventual growth is attributed to the rapid development of new technologies coupled with the reduced implementation costs (Raymond, 2005); the mounting research evidence of comparable or better learning outcomes, compared to traditional face-to-face teaching (Coe & Elliot, 1999; Coe-Regan & Freddolino, 2008; Hollister & McGee, 2000; Petracchi & Patchner, 2000; Wilke & Vinton, 2006); and the growing recognition that distance education fulfilled social work's commitment to social justice and equality by increasing education access to disadvantaged populations (Abels, 2005).

Given the expense of, and limited student access to, the experiential learning provided by traditional international exchange and study-abroad programs, video conferencing represents a viable yet untapped distance learning. Social work education programs have a significant record of experience with this method for the purposes of expanding the national reaches of their individual programs (Vernon et al., 2009) but have not yet used this methodology to enrich the international dimension of social work education.

This paper will describe an educational initiative that used video conferencing to deliver a joint social work foundation practice class to students attending an MSW degree program in the United States and in Ireland. The background and rationale for the project will first be addressed. The developmental tasks completed prior to its delivery will then be described, followed by the results of a content analysis of student feedback. Based on what was learned, the strengths and challenges of using video conferencing as a delivery method in cross-national social work education will be discussed. Future plans for expanding the project will also be noted, including ways that video conferencing technology and web-based learning could be combined to strengthen an international perspective in social work education.

PROJECT BACKGROUND AND RATIONALE

The idea for this project developed during the semester in which the first author, a tenured U.S. faculty member at Fordham University Graduate School of Social Service, was a visiting Fulbright Scholar at the University College Dublin (UCD), Ireland.[1] During her Fulbright semester, she co-taught several courses with Irish faculty. One of the courses was in the foundation practice area that she co-taught with the second author, who was also a tenured professor at UCD. As a result of this experience, both the U.S. and the Irish faculties gained an increased appreciation for the similarities shared between the two programs, particularly in the foundation practice area, as well as differences, which led to discussions of how this international perspective could be shared more fully with their students. Initially, there was some consideration of developing a traditional student exchange program, but concerns were raised about the viability of this option for the majority of students, given the time and financial resources involved. In response to these accessibility concerns, the idea emerged to use distance learning technology to create a joint teaching and learning experience for faculty and students. The overall purpose of the initiative would be to increase awareness of the global nature of social work practice through an understanding of some of the practice similarities and differences between the two countries.

The first joint video conference took place in 2008. Discussion with students indicated that they valued the experience, and faculty were encouraged to continue with the project. The video conference became an annual event and, in 2011, after obtaining IRB approval from each university, formal feedback was gathered from students about their experience and reflections. This paper deals with what was learned from that specific event.

---

[1] Fordham University is a large private Jesuit University with campuses in New York City and Westchester County in New York. University College Dublin (UCD) is Ireland's largest public university.

INTERNATIONAL VIDEOCONFERENCE DESCRIPTION

Development Activities

Prior to implementing this initiative, planning occurred that involved joint decision making about the content and process of delivery. The groundwork also involved coordination with administration and with the Internet technology (IT) departments within each of the universities. Given the importance of this early work to the overall initiative, a more detailed description follows regarding the decisions made and the coordination activities completed.

Content

From the knowledge that both the U.S. and Irish faculty had gained about each other's foundation practice curriculum, a decision was made for the content of the joint learning experience to be infused into an initial foundation practice course required by both programs, and offered at each institution during the fall semester. The preliminary sessions of this course center on the development of basic social work practice skills such as empathic listening and styles of questioning. Later sessions focus on building upon these skills in the teaching of multi-level assessment and intervention.

The topic of "Engaging the Involuntary Client" was selected for the joint session, since this is a population frequently encountered by social workers in most fields of practice in both countries and requires a specialized skill set. Course readings specifically related to social work with involuntary clients (see DeJong & Berg, 2001; Rooney, 1992) and other relevant readings on the stages of change and motivational interviewing (see DiClemente & Velasquez, 2002; Miller & Rollnick, 2002) were selected to be read prior to the class. In earlier class lectures and readings, both sets of students had been introduced to basic interviewing skills and the strengths perspective of social work practice (Saleebey, 2008). The joint session, therefore, was part of a continuum of learning and built upon what had come previously.

Teaching Methods

Role play was selected as the major teaching strategy to be used within the session. Both faculty members had extensive experience with this method for teaching practice skills in the classroom. They also saw role play not only as a way to teach engagement skills but also as an important way to highlight the similarities and differences in social work practice settings. Support exists for the effectiveness of this method in teaching motivational interviewing skills (Mounsey, Bovbjerg, White, & Gazewook, 2006). Ekblad et al. (2004), in the study reviewed earlier, also used role play effectively as a teaching method in the international video conferencing sessions with medical students who were learning transcultural psychiatry.

This decision required each professor to develop a representative case involving an involuntary client. The Irish case was set in the field of probation in Ireland, and the U.S. case was set in a court-mandated treatment program here for perpetrators of domestic violence. Two students from each country volunteered to enact the social worker and client roles. The faculty members spent time with both volunteers to help them prepare for their role. Detailed information about the client characteristics, background, and presenting situation was provided to each student enacting the client role. Only basic referral information was provided to each student enacting the social worker role in order to mirror reality as much as possible during the role play.

Part of the developmental process also included the decision to use a telecommunication-based video conferencing system (Polycom VSX 7000s) as the distance education method to deliver this session, since having a dedicated line and IP address taken off a standard server provided the greatest assurance of a smooth connection throughout the class session. Other systems such as Skype were not considered for the joint class since they might pose difficulties due to the lack of control over interconnectivity when using freeware systems. Although other asynchronous web-based technology options were considered, the decision to use videoconferencing was informed by a number of factors. First, video conferencing would allow the students to see and hear one another in real time. In addition, the wide-angle lens and audio capacity of the cameras in both locations would allow the students to see one another's entire class and had the ability to zoom in on individual students when they spoke. Thus, all the students would be able to observe one another's role plays, including facial expressions and tone of voice. When the role plays were completed, students could share immediate reactions to what they had heard and observed, discuss spontaneous questions that emerged from the interaction, and experience "in the moment" learning together as a team. As such, it provided a more comparable experience to being physically together in a classroom than any other form of distance learning. Second, participation in this method of delivery did not require extensive training on the part of either the faculty or students, beyond gaining some familiarity with how a video conference operates. Prior experience with local video conferencing and participating in a brief test run to get comfortable with the camera were seen as sufficient faculty preparation. Finally, there was no additional expense associated with the connection since both systems were found to be compatible and, therefore, could be connected using a static IP address at no cost.

Coordination Activities

In addition to planning the content and teaching methods for the joint session, both faculty members engaged in coordination activities with university administration in relation to course scheduling and time differences. After some exploration on both sides, a time that would work for the joint session was found, due to the Irish university's ability to move their class time on the day of the video conference to a later time slot, as all of their students were in class together throughout the day. The American university did not have this ability, given its much larger size and the fact that the students were spread out among classes throughout the day.

Each faculty member also coordinated with his or her respective IT departments prior to the session to ensure IT staff and equipment availability on that day. It was also necessary for the two IT departments to be in direct communication with each other well in advance to assess compatibility, exchange IP addresses, and conduct a test run of the connection.

Joint Session Description

Sixteen students from Ireland and 25 students from the United States participated in the 90-minute joint session. (Both sets of graduate students had worked together in their respective foundation practice class for approximately 5 weeks prior to the joint session.) The joint session was co-facilitated by the Irish and U.S. faculty members, one in each location. A member of the IT department set up the conference at each location, was available to address any technical issues, and operated the camera during the session.

At the start of the joint session, students introduced themselves and identified their area of interest in social work. This exercise immediately highlighted some of the similarities and differences in practice contexts and led to questions and discussion about some of the differences. For example, several of the U.S. students had field placements within school systems. This was of particular interest to the Irish students as school social work is not a field of practice in Ireland. Students shared views on the role of social work and the opportunities for preventative and early interventions that arise in this field of practice. Likewise, the U.S. students were curious about the number of Irish students with field placements in probation. The probation service in Ireland employs almost 30% of social work professionals, second only to child protection and welfare services. In fact, probation in Ireland had recently introduced the MSW as the preferred qualification for its probation and welfare officers. The American students also were interested in the fact that almost all of the Irish students complete a field placement in child welfare.

Next, the students were asked to identify the settings in which social workers generally find themselves working with involuntary clients. This discussion also provided the students with knowledge about some of the similarities and differences in practice settings that serve these populations.

After this introductory portion of the session, each professor took turns briefly highlighting what the students had read about the stages of change, beginning motivational interviewing skills and specific strategies for engaging the involuntary client. As part of this overview, each faculty member referred to handouts that had been distributed to both sets of students at the beginning of this class.

The next part of the session involved the two student volunteers from each class, one playing the social worker and one playing the client, enacting their respective role-plays of a first interview, and attempting to use the knowledge and skills learned thus far about engagement. The two Irish students enacted an initial session between a probation social worker and a juvenile in trouble with the law, and the two American students demonstrated a first interview between a social worker and a man mandated by the court for treatment upon conviction for domestic violence. Each role-play lasted approximately 10 minutes. After each role-play, the student who played the social worker was given the opportunity to reflect on his or her performance, followed by the student who played the client. Then the other students from both classes were asked to discuss what they had observed about the client's stage of change and any interviewing skills demonstrated that may have facilitated the engagement process. Given that this was the first (and would be the only) "face-to-face" encounter between the Irish and the U.S. students, they were encouraged to focus their feedback on the strengths observed in each role play. During the discussion, students were also encouraged to ask questions and learn about variations in the role of the social worker in each scenario, the legal framework for social work practice in each case, and the variability in the practice settings within which social workers operated in both countries. The session ended by giving the students the opportunity to ask one another any further questions about social work practice and education that they had as a result of the joint session.

EVALUATION OF STUDENT FEEDBACK

At the end of the joint class session, both sets of students were provided with the same feedback form, which they completed anonymously. The students had been informed about this feedback form during the prior class and on the written informed consent, as required by each university's IRB. Students who voluntarily chose to fill it out were asked to return it (unsigned) to an envelope in each professor's mailbox.

The feedback form asked the students the following questions:

1. What did you learn from this class session?
2. Was there anything that you learned because it was an international joint session?

3. On a scale of 1 to 5, with (1) being not comfortable at all and (5) being very comfortable, can you rate your level of comfort with the technology? Explain your rating.
4. Do you have any recommended changes?

A total of 26 feedback forms were returned, 18 from the U.S. students and 8 from the Irish students. A content analysis of the responses to each of the questions was conducted to identify specific themes. The themes identified for questions 1 and 2 overlapped, and therefore the findings were combined.

Similarities as Social Work Professionals

In response to questions 1 and 2, many of the American and Irish students commented that as a result of the joint session, in which they were required to observe and comment on one another's work, they learned about the similarities in theoretical approaches to client engagement used within each country. Recognizing these similarities increased their understanding of, and appreciation for, the universal aspects of social work practice.

- "I feel that the exchange made me think of social work as international with a cohesive bond and cause." (U.S.)
- "I learned that social work has a consistent theme across international borders. There seems to be a uniformity of social work speak & thought." (Irish)
- "It was very interesting to learn that very little difference appeared between the two countries in theoretical approach to the situations." (U.S.)

Collaborative Learning Process

Within the responses to questions 1 and 2, students also commented about the learning process itself and, in particular, the collaborative learning that occurred within the joint session through the use of the student role-plays, followed by a structured cross-national discussion.

- "I found the class very rewarding in that as a class we worked as a team. It was fascinating to link in with our American counterparts" (Irish)
- "I learned (saw) visually how to use the skills in the first interview that we learned in class. It was very helpful to see how the social work and client interacted, to critique and learn from them." (U.S.)
- "I got to see motivational interviewing in action and how effective it is. It was also good to see other students' views and opinions on it." (Irish)

- "By watching the interviews I gained a better understanding of the skills I read about." (U.S.)

Differences Identified

In response to the initial two questions, the students identified differences with regard to the fields of practice of child welfare, probation and school social work. Many of the U.S. students expressed surprise that the MSW degree was required to work in child protection and probation in Ireland. Many saw this as a standard that the United States should adopt. Irish students found it interesting to learn about the field of school social work in the United States, which does not exist in Ireland.

- "I learned that there are many differences in the field of social work between the U.S. and Ireland. First, Ireland's child welfare workers all have their MSWs, and I think this is an incredibly positive requirement considering the challenges child welfare workers face. Secondly, all of the probation officers have their MSWs. I think this is also a positive example and it may help to increase the success of parolees. Since our country has so many in the criminal justice system and our system does not seem to be that effective, it could be a good model of change." (U.S.)
- "It raised my awareness as to the different types of social work functions available in America, for example, school social work." (Irish)
- "I was extremely interested to hear that many [Irish] social work students had interests in going into child protective services, as this is not viewed in the US as one of the major areas that attracts MSW students." (U.S.)
- "I also learned about the different roles of social work in the states in schools." (Irish)

Comfort Level with the Video Conferencing Technology

Among those who responded, the majority of American students (15 of 18) and half of the Irish students (4 of 8) rated their comfort level to be high (either at 4 or 5). Two American students and three Irish students rated it a mid-point of 3, with the remaining one American and one Irish student rating it below mid-point at 2. (The transmission was interrupted and had to be reconnected during the U.S. student role-play, which may explain the lower comfort ratings given by a few of the students.)

Student Recommendations

In response to Question 4, students made comments related to how opportunities for international discourse with their social work peers could be increased in the future by adding another video conferencing session and employing other forms of distance education technology.

- "Possibly a second session. I found the role plays and feedback extremely helpful in seeing the techniques of motivational interviewing utilized effectively by my peers." (U.S.)
- 'Perhaps, if possible, do it in two sessions—get more out of it." (Irish)
- "It would be nice to have more interaction with the Irish students, not just a one time video conferencing. Maybe we could have extra credit or guided instruction by communicating via e-mail or other ways to continue to contact. Student to student contact would be great." (U.S.)

Last, in response to Question 4, some students also made comments about their overall experience of the joint session.

- "It was very eye-opening to connect and communicate with students from a school in Ireland. I believe that this is the shape of things to come and that there will be more opportunities for this type of communication as well as more advanced and sophisticated technology to facilitate it in the future." (U.S.)
- "Enjoyed the experience–loved the idea of the link and being part of [the U.S. University's] day as we finished and they started." (Irish)

DISCUSSION

The results of the student feedback about the joint session indicate that overall the students did gain an appreciation of the global nature of social work practice and some of the shared theoretical perspectives between the two programs as well as some of the differences that exist in relation to fields of practice. The findings also suggest that the teaching methods chosen for the session, namely the use of telecommunication-based video conferencing technology, role play, and discussion, were an effective means for learning this content. Some of the major strengths of the joint session optimized the value of the single-session, and cross-national interaction resulted from the extensive planning that occurred prior to its delivery. Other professions that have used video conferencing to teach students cross-nationally also have highlighted the importance of planning. For example, Bontempi, Runyan, and Heath (1999) reported a detailed and extensive planning process prior to a telecast video conference designed to teach medical students from different countries about community-based injury and violence prevention programs.

The planning that occurred also ensured that the content and teaching methods for the joint session were congruent with the other parts of the course. As a result, the joint session was seamlessly infused into the ongoing curriculum and experienced as a matter of course, which has been highlighted as one of the strengths of the infusion model of international social work education (Asamoah et al., 1997), and an important aspect of curriculum design (Martin, 2003). By the time the students participated in the session they already had been introduced to basic interviewing and engagement skills and were familiar with the learning strategies of role play and feedback. This meant that the groundwork for the joint session had been laid, and the students were able to focus on the novel aspects of the session.

Another strength of this initiative was the fact that the two faculty involved were familiar with each other, with each other's curricula and practice contexts, and had had the experience of working collaboratively within their own schools in curriculum design and delivery. This allowed the two facilitators to model a relaxed, friendly, and open communication style to the participants, which appeared to contribute to the creation of a rapport between the two cohorts. This connection was also an important motivator. Both faculty were committed to working out any initial difficulties and were able to use their connections with university services to access the necessary technical support.

Utilizing the case material from each country in a student role-play demonstration and follow-up discussion also put the students directly into a collaborative learning experience where the practice similarities and differences came alive through what they saw, heard, and then reflected upon together. Video conferencing technology allowed for a unique learning experience that would not be possible with other web-based methods that rely more on written forms of expression. The wide-angle lens and audio capacity of the cameras facilitated the joint discussion by allowing the 25 U.S. students and 16 Irish students to see one another as a group and to zoom in on individuals when they spoke.

While there are many positive aspects associated with video conferencing in international social work education, there were challenges experienced during this video conference that could also pose difficulties for others who might embark on this type of initiative. As noted, the signal connection was briefly lost during the session, and although it was reconnected quickly, the event did disrupt the flow of the session, and perhaps was responsible for a few of the students' "lower comfort" ratings. In follow-up discussions with IT about strategies to reduce the likelihood of a disruption, it was suggested that a network technician could be assigned at both sites solely to monitor the connection. Given the critical role of technology for this teaching methodology, schools of social work interested in using video conferencing to further the internationalization of their curriculum must be prepared to advocate for university investment in the technology and IT support necessary to ensure a smooth implementation. The calculation of the actual cost of the IT resources is difficult, as they were provided as part of each university's support services. Irrespective of this integrated IT support structure, having an IT technician available solely to monitor the connection may have implications for the number of video conferencing sessions that could be held per course. The operation of the camera, however, is a task that could be easily learned by a student, which would be one way to reduce the amount of IT resources necessary.

Another challenge when using international video conferencing technology involves the time differences. Since video conferencing occurs synchronously, a time that works for both sets of students must be found. The key to dealing with this particular challenge lies again in the preparation, since addressing institutional barriers to adjusting class schedules takes time. Nonetheless, it was our experience that, once the initiative was understood by all parties affected, creative problem solving around scheduling occurred. It is important to note, of course, that we were adjusting the schedule for only one class session. If multiple video conferencing sessions were planned, the institutional challenges might have proved more difficult.

Whenever a new initiative is introduced that will draw on limited resources or require ongoing administrative adjustments, as this type of initiative does, a clear and upfront understanding of the educational benefits is important. We have found that the students themselves (and the participating IT staff) were effective ambassadors for this initiative. After the first video conference, word spread quickly about this novel international experience. An article also was written in a school newsletter about the initiative and included a student interview about the experience. A stated commitment to ongoing evaluation of the learning outcomes for participating students also is critical to the process of maintaining support for the additional resources that may be needed.

Language is a further challenge that may be encountered in the development of an international education initiative. While it was not an obstacle in this example, as both sets of students spoke English, there was the need for adjustment to degrees and types of accents. There also was confusion at times due to the use of unfamiliar colloquial vocabulary. Preparing students beforehand to speak as slowly and clearly as possible and having faculty members and students prepared to repeat what was said if not clear are strategies that can finesse this obstacle.

Finally, a challenge that must be recognized in future replication of this experience between other universities involves the "digital divide." As defined by Abels (2005), the term refers to the handicaps universally faced by economically struggling universities as well as by developing nations that may not have the requisite technology to participate on an equal footing with first-world countries. The universities that participated in this project had equivalent and advanced IT capacities. If video conferencing, as well as other forms of distance education, was to be adopted on a larger scale by social work programs to further internationalization, the digital divide must be addressed to ensure that the opportunity to engage in virtual international collaborative learning does not just occur between universities in wealthy nations but that also includes social work students and educators at universities in poorer and developing countries.

The strengths and challenges of our experience provide some preliminary guidelines. While we believe that most social work courses have the potential to benefit from distance education collaboration, we believe it is critical that the faculty involved develop a relationship beforehand and become familiar with one another's courses and syllabi. This will allow them the opportunity to strategically select a class session that will likely provide optimal sharing of similarities and differences, whether that be in practice, policy, or research. Equally important, students need to be well prepared beforehand for the joint exercises and discussion and committed to similar readings and lecture material. The size of the classes might also rule out certain courses, since a class size of more than 25 students might not be able to be fully captured on camera.

Study Limitations

This pilot study involved a very small sample, mostly qualitative feedback, and did not have any type of comparison group. The response rate of 50% from the Irish students (versus 72% for the American students) also was disappointing in particular since the discussion and verbal feedback were positive. The Irish group was small and very manageable, so they may have found the submission of a written questionnaire to be an unnecessary additional task since they had multiple opportunities to discuss the experience with their fellow students and the facilitator in subsequent sessions. In retrospect, the response rate might have been increased if more time had been allotted for them to complete their evaluation immediately after the session. In light of these design limitations, the feedback results cannot be generalized beyond the experience of the students who participated in the study. In addition, in order to assess the impact on the students with respect to whether this experience increased their appreciation of global social work issues, additional measurement tools would need to be developed to track this anticipated outcome.

Future Directions

Despite these limitations, this project demonstrated the learning that is possible between social work students from different countries by giving them the opportunity through video conferencing to have a joint, virtual, synchronous classroom experience. Given the generally positive feedback received, we plan to continue the use of the videoconference as an inaugural cross-national encounter and to learn from the challenges encountered.

To further enhance the international aspect of this course and deepen the students' cross-national learning experience, we plan to provide more opportunities for them to interact individually and in small groups prior to and after the joint session by using other forms of asynchronous distance learning technology, such as discussion boards, file sharing, and video streaming. While in this pilot project both professors individually delivered similar lecture material to their students prior to the video conference as part of the preparation, in the future these preparation activities could be shared by having each professor and/or other international expert prepare a PowerPoint lecture with audio that would be shown to both classes. This addition would result in an even richer international experience, allowing the students to have multiple opportunities to learn cross-nationally from one another (and their respective professors) but in an asynchronous fashion not constrained by time differences and the technical support resources inherent in video conferencing.

In addition to expanding the types of technology to further the international conversation among the students, we also plan to conduct more sophisticated research on learning outcomes. In particular, we would like to better understand whether and how the learning from the virtual, face-to-face, cross-national sessions is similar to or different from the learning outcomes when solely using asynchronous technologies in cross-national education. Our very preliminary findings here suggest that there is value in this educational experience, but without a comparison group and more quantifiable outcome measures, we cannot say for certain how this method compares to other online methods available for enhancing international social work education.

REFERENCES

Abels, P. (2005). The way to distance education. In P. Abels (Ed.), *Distance education in social work: Planning, teaching and learning* (pp. 3–22). New York, NY: Springer Publishing Company.

Asamoah, Y., Healy, L. M., & Mayadas, N. (1997). Ending the international-domestic dichotomy: New approaches to a global curriculum for the millennium. *Journal of Social Work Education, 33*, 389–340.

Bontempi, J., Runyan, C., & Heath, J. (1999). Training by satellite: Planning and evaluating a video conference for injury prevention practitioners. *Journal of Community Health, 24*(6), 451–466.

Boyle, D. P., Nackerud, L., & Kilpartrick, A. (1999). The road less travelled: Cross-cultural, international experiential learning. *International Social Work, 42*(2), 201–214.

Bye, L., Prom, K., & Tsybikdorzhieva, B. I. (2006). Utilizing technology to infuse international content into social work curriculum: A Siberian correspondent model. *Journal of Teaching in Social Work, 26*(3/4), 41–55.

Carrilio, T. & Mathiesen, S. (2006). Developing a cross border, multidisciplinary educational collaboration. *Social Work Education, 25*(6), 633–641.

Carter-Anand, J., & Clark, K. (2009). Crossing borders through cyberspace: A discussion of a social work education electronic exchange pilot project across the Atlantic. *Social Work Education, 28*(6), 583–597.

Cincatta, N. F., Tokatlian, N., & Miller, J. (2006). The international exchange program in the first person. *Social Work in Health Care, 43*(2/3), 193–197.

Coe, J. R., & Elliot, D. (1999). An evaluation of teaching direct practice courses in a distance education program for rural settings. *Journal of Social Work Education, 35*(3), 353–365.

Coe-Regan, J. A., & Freddolino, P. (2008). *Integrating technology into the social work curriculum*. Alexandria, VA: Council on Social Work Education

Cogburn, D., & Levinson, L. (2003). U.S.–Africa virtual collaboration in globalization studies: Success factors for complex, cross national leaning teams. *International Studies Perspectives, 4*, 34–51.

DeJong, P., & Berg, I. K. (2001). Co-constructing cooperation with mandated clients. *Social Work, 46*(4), 361–365.

DiClemente, C. C., & Velasquez, M. M. (2002). Motivational interviewing and the stages of change. In W. R. Miller & S. Rollnick (Eds.), *Motivational interviewing—Preparing people for change* (pp. 201–216). New York, NY: Guilford Press.

Ekblad, S., Manicavasagar, V., Silove, D., Baanhielm, S., Reczycki, M., Mollica, R., & Coello, M. (2004). The use of international videoconferencing as a strategy for teaching medical students about transcultural psychiatry. *Transcultural Psychiatry, 41*(1), 120–129.

Ford, K. A., & Rotgans-Visser, R. J. (2005). Internationalizing social work education using Blackboard 6: INHOLLAND University, NL and James Madison University. *Journal of Technology in Human Services, 23*(1/2), 147–165.

Gilin, B., & Young, T. (2009). Educational benefits of international experiential learning in an MSW program. *International Social Work, 52*, 36–47.

Hendriks, P., Kloppenburg, R., Gevorgianiene, V., & Jukutiene, V. (2008). Cross-national social work case analysis: Learning from international experience within an electronic environment. *European Journal of Social Work, 11*(4), 383–396.

Hollister, D., & McGee, G. (2000). Delivering substance abuse and child welfare content through interactive television. *Research on Social Work Practice, 10*, 417–427.

Holmes, R. H., & Mathews, G. (1993). Innovations in international cross-cultural social work education. *Arete, 18*(1), 43–47.

Johnson, A. K. (1999). Globalization from below: Using the Internet to internationalize social work education. *Journal of Social Work Education, 35*(3), 377–393.

Larsen, A., Sanders, R., Astray, A., & Hole, G. (2008). E-teacher challenges and competences in international comparative social work courses. *Social Work Education, 27*(6), 623–633.

Martin, P. (2003). Key aspects of teaching and learning in arts, humanities and social Sciences. In H. Fry, S. Ketteridge, & S. Marshell (Eds.), *A handbook for teaching and learning in higher education: Enhancing academic practice* (pp. 301–323). London, UK: Kogan Page.

Midgley, J. (2001). Issues in international social work: Resolving critical debates in the profession. *Journal of Social Work, 1*(1), 21–33.

Miller, W. R., & Rollnick, S. (2002). *Motivational interviewing—Preparing people for change.* New York, NY: Guilford Press.

Mounsey, A. L, Bovbjerg, V., White, L., & Gazewook, J. (2006). Do students develop better motivational interviewing skills through role-play with standardized patients with student colleagues? *Medical Education, 40*, 775–780.

Nagy, G., & Falk, D. (2000). Dilemmas in international and cross-cultural social work education. *International Social Work, 43*(1), 49–60.

Panos, P. (2005). A model for using videoconferencing technology to support international social work field practicum students. *International Social Work, 48*, 834–841.

Petracchi, H., & Patchner, M. (2000). Social work students and their learning environment: A comparison of interactive television, face-to-face instruction, and the traditional classroom. *Journal of Social Work Education, 36*(2), 335–347.

Powell, J., & Robison, J. (2007). The 'international dimension' in social work education: Current developments in England. *European Journal of Social Work, 10*(3), 383–399.

Raymond, F. B. (2005). The history of distance education in social work and the evolution of distance education models. In P. Abels (Ed.), *Distance education in social work: Planning, teaching and learning* (pp. 23–42). New York, NY: Springer Publishing Company.

Rooney, R. H. (1992). *Strategies for work with involuntary clients.* New York, NY: Columbia University Press.

Rotabi K., Gammonley, D, Gamble, D., & Weil, M. (2007). Integrating globalization into the social work curriculum. *Journal of Sociology and Social Welfare, 34*(2), 165–185.

Saleebey, D. (2008). *The strengths perspective in social work* (5th ed.). New York, NY: Pearson/Allyn & Bacon.

Vernon, R., Vakalahi, H., Pierce, D., Pittman-Munke, P., & Adkins, L. (2009). Distance education in social work: Current and emerging trends. *Journal of Social Work Education, 45*(2), 263–276.

Wilke, D., & Vinton, L. (2006). Evaluation of the first web-based advanced standing MSW program. *Journal of Social Work Education, 42*, 607–620.

York, R. (2008). Comparing three modes of instruction in a graduate social work program. *Journal of Social Work Education, 44*(2), 157–172.

Yuen, A. (2009). Rising to the challenge: Global social work education. *International Social Work, 52*(1), 119–121.

Part 3: Teaching and Conducting Research

A Comparison of Student Knowledge and Attitude toward Research: Are Main Campus Students Different from Those in a Hybrid Environment?

RACHEL L. BUCHANAN and DEBORAH A. MATHEWS
Department of Social Work, Salisbury University, Salisbury, Maryland, USA

The trend toward the use of distance education in teaching social work students has been rapidly growing over the past two decades. A constant issue of concern is related to student outcomes. This paper reports on a longitudinal quasi-experimental study assessing the differential knowledge and attitude toward research between social work students taking a research methods course in one of two modalities: traditional classroom versus distance setting. Both bachelor's and master's degree students participated in this 2-year study. Descriptive statistics and results of inferential tests as well as implications for future study are presented in this paper.

INTRODUCTION

Just a decade ago, the use of distance technology to provide students with a degree in social work at both the undergraduate and graduate levels was a phenomenon embraced by a relatively small number of large public institutions with combined BSW-MSW programs (Siegel, Jennings, Conklin, & Napoletano Flynn, 1998). However, as technology has improved, distance education is becoming more common in social work programs (Coe & Elliott, 1999; Wilke & Vinton, 2006; York, 2008).

A recent survey of the current status of distance education in social work education shows this changing picture. Vernon, Vakalahi, Pierce, Pittman-Munke, & Adkins (2009) found that 61% of BSW programs and 83% of MSW programs are currently either "delivering, developing, or contemplating" (p. 267) distance education course delivery. This is a significant increase over the findings from a 1995 survey sponsored by the Council on Social Work Education in which less than half (42.9%) showed interest in distance education (Lockhart & Wilson, 1997). The impetus behind this rapidly growing trend seems directly related to growing institutional pressure for programs to expand their pedagogical options in response to the increasing number of students who are forced to balance the demands of full-time employment and family responsibilities with their need and desire for higher education (Crowell & McCarragher, 2007; Freddolino & Sutherland, 2000; Vernon et al., 2009). The academic horizon seems to be shifting from the more traditional model of students coming to the university to the university going to its students. This trend is only expected to increase in the foreseeable future.

The literature from the years 1998 through 2009 illustrates that the nature of distance education delivery has also evolved. Wilson (1999) notes that the use of distance education in social work has developed over a series of three phases: off-campus instruction (where traditional face-to-face delivery is provided by faculty traveling to off-campus sites); distributed education (through the use of technology such as interactive television); and computer-mediated education (online web-based learning). This is not inconsistent with Siegel and colleagues (1998), who initially found the primary technology used was either interactive or one-way television delivery. This trend seems to have changed a decade later when Vernon et al (2009) noted that over half (63%) of surveyed BSW programs and three-fourths (76%) of MSW programs were offering a hybrid form of delivery (a combination of face-to-face instruction and technology). The emerging popularity of the hybrid, or *blended*, form of delivery seems fueled by the belief that this approach offers social work students the best of both worlds: traditional teaching and use of technology (Ayala, 2009; Garrision & Kanuka, 2004).

As the use of technology in social work education has evolved, so have concerns about the quality of experience a student will have in a virtual academic environment (York, 2008). Although the range of these misgivings has varied, there has been a primary focus on comparing traditional students with their peers in a distance setting with respect to variables such as the classroom experience (Freddolino & Sutherland, 2000; Petracchi & Patchner, 2000) and educational outcomes (Hisle-Gorman & Zuravin, 2006; Schoech & Helton, 2001; Thyer, Artelt, Markward & Dozier, 1998; Wilke & Vinton, 2006). The research on distance education courses historically has compared outcomes from these delivery systems with those of traditional face-to-face social work courses. Although not the focus of this paper, it is interesting to note that there are some social work educators who would argue that there may be an inherent problem in assuming that traditional social work courses have been assessed rigorously enough to assume their own worthiness as a basis for effective comparison (Quinn & Fitch, 2011).

ATTITUDE

Within the world of social work education, it would seem to be an accepted fact that the research curriculum elicits more student disdain, greater performance anxiety, and less content interest than any other area of the social work curriculum (Adam, Zosky, & Unrau, 2004). It also is widely agreed that this negativity is historic and more pervasive in social work than with same age peers in other academic disciplines (Adam et al., 2004; Epstein, 1987, 1996; Green, Bretzin, & Leininger, 2001). This generally negative attitude toward research is exacerbated by students' pervasive belief that the content is not relevant to their future as practitioners (Green et al., 2001) and fueled by a lack of confidence in their ability to master the concepts and skills (Adam et al., 2004).

This observation complicates the life of a social work research educator, who often is met by a group of students with significant anxiety, an inability to connect research to practice, and a high fear of failure. One might couple this inherent challenge with the findings of Moore (2005), who surveyed 81 social work faculty members and found the generalized belief that live instruction is superior to that found in an online environment. These several factors have created a climate in which research faculty often are conflicted about the potential impact of teaching in a web-assisted environment.

LEARNING OUTCOMES

The social work literature strongly suggests that there is little to no difference in learning outcomes (operationally defined as course-level grade performance) between distance learners and their on-campus counterparts (Coe & Elliott, 1999; Petracchi & Patchner, 2001; Wilke & Vinton, 2006; York, 2008). In fact, York "could not find any scientific studies that revealed superior outcomes for traditional instruction compared with the ITV format" (p. 159) and goes on to note that some research has suggested that instruction via the Internet actually produces *superior* outcomes when compared to traditional models.

At least two studies have been conducted comparing MSW students taking a research methods course in a traditional versus a distance setting. Neither found any significant difference in course outcomes (Dalton, 2001; Petracchi & Patchner, 2000). This finding compares with a study (Faul, Frey,

& Barber, 2004) of MSW students taking a foundation research course where, although the students in the traditional course demonstrated slightly greater content outcome knowledge, there was no statistically significant difference between the cohorts. Both groups showed a statistically significant gain in research knowledge.

CURRENT STUDY

This paper will report on a quasi-experimental study conducted over two academic years to assess the differential knowledge about and opinion toward research between social work students taking a research methods course in an on-campus setting when compared to students taking the same course at a distance site. Students at the distance setting were at one of three off-campus sites, which ranged from 67 to 183 miles from the main campus. Although the specific configuration of the class connections varied, the satellite students were always "in class" with either their peers on the main campus or with students at a second satellite site.

The course delivery for both groups was "blended." This meant that half of the weekly content was delivered through the use of a course management system, with the additional half coming from "live" instruction. The difference between the two groups was that the students in the satellite setting had only in-person contact with an instructor twice a semester; all other classroom instruction time was delivered through interactive television. Students at distance sites, however, were able to fully interact with faculty through microphone-equipped classrooms, which also contained PowerPoint and video capabilities and a document camera for displaying overheads. Regardless of setting, all students were taught by experienced tenure-track faculty.

At this university, undergraduate and foundation MSW students are required to pursue a two-course research sequence. The first course is an introduction to the scientific method, with a focus on learning basic concepts, mastering research vocabulary, differentiating among experimental designs, and understanding various sampling approaches. The second expects students to learn the intricacies of single-subject design to help them better evaluate their own practice. For this study, students were surveyed midterm of the second course about their knowledge and opinions related to the first course.

METHODS

Over the course of 2 years (Wave 1, $N = 62$ and Wave 2, $N = 61$), students at a mid-size combined social work program in the mid-Atlantic region of the

United States, who were enrolled in spring semester sections of Social Work Research II at either the undergraduate or graduate level and across all four campuses, were invited to participate in this study. After obtaining university IRB approval, the investigators went to each section of the Research II classes (Wave 1, $N = 4$; Wave 2, $N = 5$) to introduce the study. During these sessions, the investigators discussed the informed consent process, confidentiality, what would be required, and the extra credit incentive. (All students who participated would receive at minimum one extra credit point for the Research II class; the maximum number of extra points to be awarded was five. The number of points awarded was based on the number of items students got correct in the knowledge section of the survey.) In order to ensure that student responses could not be connected to their names, a third party (not one of the researchers or instructors) scored the knowledge section of the survey, reported the extra credit totals for each student in the classes, and de-identified the dataset prior to passing it along to the researchers. To access the survey, students were e-mailed a link to the informed consent and online survey; another link to the informed consent and online survey was placed in the course management program used by all of the Research II instructors.

Measure

A modified version of the Kirk-Rosenblatt Research Inventory (1981) was used for this study. (The Kirk-Rosenblatt Research Inventory is a measure designed to assess social work students' opinion, knowledge, and beliefs about research.) The only modifications were the removal of any knowledge questions that were not covered in the Social Work Research I course. Two main sections of the Inventory were the focus of this study: Opinion of Social Work Research and Knowledge of Social Work Research.

Opinion of social work research

The opinion scale contains 15 items all measured on a five-point Likert scale: *strongly agree, moderately agree, agree, moderately disagree, and strongly disagree*. Examples of items include "The only reason I would enroll in social work research is because it is required"; "I feel that social workers should be able to evaluate their own practice"; and "Social work research is not particularly useful to the practitioner providing direct services." After the recoding of negatively worded items, student responses for all 15 items were summed together to form a total opinion toward social work research scale with a theoretical range of 15 to 75; a higher score would indicate a more positive opinion toward social work research. Cronbach's alpha for Wave 1 was 0.83; for Wave 2, it was 0.81.

Knowledge of social work research

The knowledge scale consists of 30 true/false items pertaining to basic research methods topics. Examples of items include "an operational definition of a concept indicates the way that the variable will be measured"; "stratified samples are non-probability samples"; and "in evaluative research, the intervention is referred to as the dependent variable." Student responses to the 30 items were reviewed; incorrect responses were coded "0" and correct responses as "1." After this coding process, the responses for each student were summed together to form a total knowledge score, with a theoretical range of 0 to 30; a higher score would indicate greater knowledge of social work research. Cronbach's alpha for Wave 1 was 0.69; for Wave 2, it was 0.76.

RESULTS

Information was gathered from students in two distinct settings: main campus and the three satellite sites. For Wave 1, the three satellite groups were all of comparable size (see Table 1 for information on Wave 1 and Wave 2 demographics). The majority of the students were under the age of 30, both at the main campus and satellite sites; however, there was a greater distribution of ages at the satellite sites compared to the main campus. The majority of the students were female, with the distributions being similar

TABLE 1 Demographics of Wave 1 ($N = 62$) and Wave 2 ($N = 61$)

	Main Campus		Satellite Site	
	Wave 1 ($N = 40$)	Wave 2 ($N = 38$)	Wave 1 ($N = 22$)	Wave 2 ($N = 23$)
Age				
20–23	19 (47.5%)	16 (42.1%)	3 (13.6%)	5 (21.7%)
24–30	12 (30.0%)	11 (28.9%)	10 (45.5%)	10 (43.5%)
31–35	6 (15.0%)	4 (10.5%)	2 (9.1%)	3 (13.0%)
36+	3 (7.5%)	7 (18.4%)	7 (31.8%)	5 (21.7%)
Gender				
Male	3 (7.5%)	7 (18.4%)	1 (4.5%)	2 (8.7%)
Female	37 (92.5%)	31 (81.6%)	21 (95.5)	21 (91.3%)
Race/Ethnicity				
Asian American	1 (2.5%)	1 (2.6%)	0 (0.0%)	1 (4.3%)
Black/African American	4 (10.0%)	7 (18.4%)	4 (18.2%)	3 (13.0%)
White/Caucasian	34 (85.0%)	27 (71.1%)	18 (81.8%)	18 (78.3%)
Hispanic	0 (0.0%)	1 (2.6%)	0 (0.0%)	0 (0.0%)
Other	1 (2.5%)	2 (5.3%)	0 (0.0%)	1 (4.3%)
Program				
BSW	26 (65.0%)	23 (60.5%)	13 (59.1%)	13 (56.5%)
MSW	14 (35.0%)	15 (39.5%)	9 (40.9%)	10 (43.5%)

across both settings. Students were predominantly White, with there being no noticeable differences in race among the sites. The majority of the students were senior undergraduates. There were no categorical differences in the demographic breakdown for Wave 2 from Wave 1.

Opinion toward Research

An independent *t*-test was run to determine whether there were any significant differences in student opinion of social work research based on the site at which the student took their Research I class (i.e., main campus or satellite). For Wave 1 data, there was a statistically significant difference in opinion between the two sites—$t\ (60) = 2.21, p < 0.05$—with the main campus students showing a more positive opinion with a mean score of 57.43 ($SD = 8.11$) versus 52.86 ($SD = 7.14$) for the satellite students. This picture changes when we look at students by program, with there being no significant difference for the undergraduate students; however, a significant difference for the graduate students based on the sites was found: $t\ (21) = 3.45, p < .05$. Students on the main campus had a mean score of 62.64 ($SD = 4.43$), and the satellite students had a mean of 55.22 ($SD = 5.89$). For Wave 2, there were no significant differences in opinion either by site location or program status. See Table 2 for more information.

With the finding of significant differences between BSW and MSW students at each site, we ran an additional analysis to determine whether there was a general program level difference between the groups, not solely by

TABLE 2 Independent *t*-Test Comparing Overall and Site-Level Opinion of Social Work Research for Wave 1 and Wave 2 across the BSW and MSW Programs

	n	*M*	*SD*	Difference	*t*	*p*
All – Wave 1	62					
Main Campus	40	57.43	8.11	4.56	2.21	0.03
Satellite	22	52.86	7.14			
BSW – Wave 1	39					
Main Campus	26	54.62	8.30	3.39	1.23	0.23
Satellite	13	51.23	7.68			
MSW – Wave 1	23					
Main Campus	14	62.64	4.43	7.42	3.45	0.002
Satellite	9	55.22	5.89			
All – Wave 2	61					
Main Campus	38	55.42	8.25	−0.14	−0.07	0.95
Satellite	23	55.57	7.11			
BSW – Wave 2	36					
Main Campus	23	53.57	7.89	−0.36	−0.13	0.90
Satellite	13	53.92	8.28			
MSW – Wave 2	25					
Main Campus	15	58.27	8.22	0.57	0.20	0.85
Satellite	10	57.70	4.81			

TABLE 3 Independent *t*-Test Comparing Program-Level Opinion of Social Work Research for Wave 1 and Wave 2

	n	*M*	*SD*	Difference	*t*	*p*
All – Wave 1	62					
BSW	39	53.49	8.16	−6.25	−3.18	0.002
MSW	23	59.74	6.16			
All – Wave 2	61					
BSW	36	53.69	7.90	−4.35	−2.22	0.031
MSW	25	58.04	6.90			

site. As indicated in Table 3, MSW students consistently had a statistically significant higher opinion toward social work research than BSW students, across both waves of data.

Knowledge of Social Work Research

In order to test for differences in knowledge across site locations, an independent *t*-test was conducted. For Wave 1, there was a statistically significant difference in knowledge across both sites: $t(60) = 2.00$, $p = .05$. Main campus students showed a greater level of knowledge ($M = 21.75$, $SD = 4.01$) as compared to the satellite campus students ($M = 19.68$, $SD = 3.70$). When these data were looked at by program, while not statistically significant ($p = 0.058$), there was a difference seen across sites for the BSW program; the mean score for students on the main campus was 20.42 ($SD = 3.43$) and for satellite students was 18.23 ($SD = 3.00$). For MSW students, there was no statistically significant difference in knowledge scores. However, it should be noted that main campus students had higher knowledge scores ($M = 24.21$, $SD = 3.95$) than satellite students ($M = 21.78$, $SD = 3.73$). In Wave 2, however, there were no significant differences in knowledge of social work research across site location or program. See Table 4 for more information.

Given the findings regarding opinion based on program status, analysis was conducted to see whether there were any statistically significant differences in knowledge across the two programs and waves of data. For Wave 1, a statistically significant difference was found between BSW and MSW students; with MSW students scoring significantly higher than their peers at the undergraduate level. However, the same difference was not seen in Wave 2. See Table 5 for details.

DISCUSSION

Web-enhanced instruction within the world of higher education is growing and changing the face of how social work education is being delivered (Coe

TABLE 4 Independent *t*-Test Comparing Overall and Site-Level Knowledge of Social Work Research for Wave 1 and Wave 2

	n	*M*	*SD*	Difference	*t*	*p*
All – Wave 1	62					
Main Campus	40	21.75	4.01	2.07	2.00	0.050
Satellite	22	19.68	3.70			
BSW – Wave 1	39					
Main Campus	26	20.42	3.43	2.19	1.96	0.058
Satellite	13	18.23	3.00			
MSW – Wave 1	23					
Main Campus	14	24.21	3.95	2.44	1.48	0.16
Satellite	9	21.78	3.73			
All – Wave 2	61					
Main Campus	38	20.79	5.24	0.44	0.36	0.72
Satellite	23	20.35	3.27			
BSW – Wave 2	36					
Main Campus	23	21.48	5.02	0.79	0.48	0.64
Satellite	13	20.69	4.17			
MSW – Wave 2	25					
Main Campus	15	19.73	5.57	−0.17	−0.09	0.93
Satellite	10	19.90	1.60			

TABLE 5 Independent *t*-Test Comparing Program-Level Opinion of Social Work Research for Wave 1 and Wave 2

	n	*M*	*SD*	Difference	*t*	*p*
All – Wave 1	62					
BSW	39	19.69	3.42	−3.57	−3.74	0.000
MSW	23	23.26	3.97			
All – Wave 2	61					
BSW	36	21.19	4.68	1.39	1.18	0.245
MSW	25	19.80	4.37			

& Elliott, 1999; Crowell & McCarragher, 2007; Faul et al., 2004; Freddolino & Sutherland, 2000; Wilke & Vinton, 2006; York, 2008). Over the past two decades, a relevant question has evolved from being "should social work education be taught using technology" to "what are the outcomes associated with the use of distance education?" In the latter part of the 1990s, there was a call for social work educators using distance education to empirically assess student-related impacts associated with this growing trend.

Prior to 1998, many researchers found distance education to be less effective than education in traditional settings. Research after 1998, however, generally indicates that educational outcomes across these two modalities have become more balanced (Zhao, Lei, Yan, Lai, & Tan, 2005). Data from our current study are generally consistent with the other post-1998 findings. The one difference that did appear between our two settings was in the

Wave 1 data: There was a difference across settings, but it was present only for undergraduate students.

In considering why this difference occurred in the Wave 1 data, the literature presents two plausible explanations. The first (and simpler) explanation is that the difference was found due to the nature of the undergraduate students in Wave 1. As noted by Diaz and Cartnal (1999), students who perform best in an online setting possess a distinct set of learning traits, which includes the ability to be academically independent and an intrinsic motivation toward learning. While the research course (as noted) is not completely online, it is blended with an hour's worth of online work per week. It could be that the students in the distance settings did not possess these characteristics to the same degree and, therefore, performed more poorly. This cohort specificity in our findings could explain why a different outcome was found in Wave 2.

A competing explanation is that the nature of the instruction and overall course delivery was better in the second year. Zhao and colleagues (2005) proffer that distance education programs become better over time as the instructors master the learning process, receive more training on the dynamics of teaching in virtual environments, and gain a command of the technology.

The Wave 2 findings indicate that there was no difference in *knowledge* across sites, which is consistent with preexisting studies (Faul et al., 2004; Patchner, Petracchi & Wise, 1998; Petracchi & Patchner, 2000; Royse, 2000; Stocks & Freddolino, 1998; Westhuis, Ouellette, & Pfahler, 2006; Wilke & Vinton, 2006). There have not been as many studies completed to date that look at students' *opinions* toward research; nonetheless, the findings from our research are consistent with two previous studies comparing live instruction with instruction via interactive television (Petracchi & Patchner, 2001; Petracchi et al., 1998).

When considering the data related to students' opinion of research, the findings are similar to that of knowledge; there was a difference based on site in Wave 1, but no difference was found in Wave 2 data. When comparing Wave 1 data strictly across sites, there was a statistically significant difference between the two settings, with main campus students' opinion being higher than that of their peers at the satellite settings. When looking at program status (undergraduate versus graduate), there was no difference between main campus and satellite students in the undergraduate program; however, there was a statistically significant difference among graduate students, with those on the main campus having a higher opinion of research than those at the satellite sites.

Although our research question initially was solely focused on campus versus off-campus student performance, the differences that appeared interestingly were program-level, not site-specific. In reviewing some of the literature regarding program-level performance differences, there is evidence that graduate students demonstrate more self-regulated learning characteristics than do their undergraduate peers (Guri-Rosenbilt, 1999; Moore & Kearsley, 2004; Nesler, 1999). This fact could suggest that online and hybrid learning may be more suited to graduate than undergraduate students. Specific to social work research, there is general agreement that students typically regard research courses from a negative perspective and enter the courses with a high level of anxiety and low sense of confidence (Adam et al., 2004; Epstein, 1987; Hardcastle & Bisman, 2003). This may suggest that graduate students are more able to regulate this anxiety than undergraduates. If this should be the case, then the tendency of social work programs to treat senior undergraduates and foundation-level graduate students similarly could disadvantage the former. Ultimately, it may be that online or hybrid research courses currently are more suited for graduate students.

LIMITATIONS

There are several limitations to this study, which need to be discussed. First, the reliability for the knowledge scale for Wave 1 was just below 0.70 (0.69). This raises some question about the dependability of this measure; however, the reliability for Wave 2 was 0.76, which is more acceptable but still not very high. A second limitation is that we cannot account for differences between instructors' techniques in our analysis. It may be that some instructors were more or less comfortable with the distance education setting (or the research content), and this affected the students' results both on knowledge and opinion. A third limitation is the change in the structure of the course from Wave 1 to Wave 2. While there were positive changes in outcomes between the waves, we do not have information on students' opinions of the course material presentation, so we cannot control for these possible differences. The fourth limitation is the small size of our sample and the use of nonprobability sampling techniques.

A major strength of the study was that all of the instructors (both in Wave 1 and Wave 2) used the same syllabus, online materials, textbook, and assignments. While we cannot control for differences in teaching style, we do know that students were participating in an internally uniform curriculum. Another strength is that we do have data across multiple points in time. This factor allows us to have more information about the different cohorts and to see whether there were changes over time.

CONCLUSION

Since 1998, there has been a growing body of literature comparing student outcomes between social work courses offered in traditional face-to-face settings and those offered in a distance format. The vast bulk of this research shows that there is no statistically significant difference in outcomes, meaning that distance education is an effective alternative format for social work education. This study supports this growing body of literature.

As noted by Ayala (2009), perhaps it, therefore, is time to move on from researching the usefulness of the modality to looking more closely at the effectiveness of the different types of technology available for teaching social work research content across different settings. In short, it may be time to move beyond "should we do this" to "which technology should be embraced?"

Another area that may prove worthy of additional research is whether online and hybrid learning is equally suitable for both undergraduate and graduate students. As the trend grows toward fully online master's programs, one wonders whether the approach will be adopted by undergraduate programs as well. Determining whether undergraduate students have suitable characteristics and learning styles for this type of pedagogical environment is paramount before the trend is embraced by baccalaureate programs.

REFERENCES

Adam, N., Zosky, D., & Unrau, Y. (2004). Improving the research climate in social work curricula: Clarifying learning expectations across BSW and MSW research courses. *Journal of Teaching in Social Work, 24*(3/4), 1–18.

Ayala, J. (2009). Blended learning as a new approach to social work education. *Journal of Social Work Education, 45*(2), 277–288.

Coe, J. A., & Elliott, D. (1999). An evaluation of teaching direct practice courses in a distance education program for rural settings. *Journal of Social Work Education, 35*(3), 353–365.

Crowell, L., & McCarragher, T. (2007). Delivering a social work MSW program through distance education: An innovative collaboration between two universities. *Social Work Education*, 26(4), 376–388.

Dalton, B. (2001). Distance education: A multidimensional evaluation. *Journal of Technology in Human Services, 18*, 101–115.

Diaz, D. P., & Cartnal, R. B. (1999). Students' learning styles in two classes: Online distance learning and equivalent on campus. *College Teaching, 47*(4), 130–135.

Epstein, I. (1987). Pedagogy of the perturbed: Teaching research to the reluctant. *Journal of Social Work Education, 4*(1), 5–18.

Epstein, I. (1996). In quest of a research-based model for clinical practice: Or, why can't a social worker be more like a researcher? *Social Work Research, 20*(2), 97–100.

Faul, A., Frey, A. J., & Barber, R. (2004). The effects of web-assisted instruction in a social work research methods course. *Social Work Education, 23*(1), 105–118.

Freddolino, P. P., & Sutherland, C. A. (2000). Assessing the comparability of classroom environments in graduate social work education delivered via interactive instructional television. *Journal of Social Work Education, 36*(1), 115–129.

Garrison, D. R., & Kanuka, H. (2004). Blended learning: uncovering its transformative potential in higher education. *Internet and Higher Education, 7*, 94–105.

Green, R.G., Bretzin, A., & Leininger, C. (2001). Research learning attributes of graduate students in social work, psychology, business. *Journal of Social Work Education, 37*(2), 333–341.

Guri-Rosenbilt, S. (1999). *Distance and campus universities: Tensions and interactions*. Oxford, UK: IAU Press.

Hardcastle, D. A., & Bisman, C. D. (2003). Innovations in teaching social work research. *Social Work Education, 22*(1), 31–43.

Hisle-Gorman, E., & Zuravin, S. (2006). Teaching social work research: A comparison of web-based and in-class lecture methods. *Journal of Technology in Human Services, 24*(4), 77–93.

Lockhart, L., & Wilson, S. (1997). Distance education: A summary of survey results. *Social Work Education Reporter, 45*(2), 5.

Moore, B. (2005). Faculty perceptions of the effectiveness of web-based instruction in social work education: A national study. *Journal of Computers in Human Services, 2*(3/4), 53–66.

Moore, M. G., & Kearsley, G. (2004). *Distance education: A systems view* (2nd ed.). Belmont, CA: Wadsworth Publishing Company.

Nesler, M. S. (1999). Factors associated with retention in a distance based liberal arts program. (ERIC No. ED442440).

Patchner, M. A., Petracchi, H. E., & Wise, S. (1998). Outcomes of ITV and face to face instruction in a social work research methods course. *Computers in Human Services, 15*(2/3), 23–38.

Petracchi, H. E., & Patchner, M. A. (2000). Social work students and their learning environment: A comparison of interactive television, face-to-face instruction, and the traditional classroom. *Journal of Social Work Education, 36*(2), 335–346.

Petracchi, H. E., & Patchner, M. A. (2001). A comparison of live instruction and interactive televised teaching: A 2 year assessment of teaching an MSW research methods course. *Research on Social Work Practice, 11*, 109–117.

Rosenblatt, A., & Kirk, S. A. (1981). Cumulative effect of research courses on knowledge and attitudes of social work students. *Journal of Social Work Education, 17*(2), 26–34.

Royse, D. (2000). Teaching research online: A process evaluation. *Journal of Teaching in Social Work, 20*(1/2), 145–158.

Quinn, A., & Fitch, D. (2011). Considering construct validity in distance educational research in social work education: Suggestions for a multivariate approach to researching efficacy. *Journal of Social Work Education, 47*(2), 321–336.

Schoech, D., & Helton, D. (2001). Qualitative and quantitative analysis of a course taught via classroom and internet chatroom. *Qualitative Social Work, 1*(1), 111–124.

Siegel, E., Jennings, J. G., Conklin, J., & Napoletano Flynn, S. (1998). Distance learning in social work education: Results and implications of a national survey. *Journal of Social Work Education, 34*(1), 71–80.

Stocks, J. T., & Freddolino, P. P. (1998). Evaluation of a world wide web-based graduate social work research methods course. *Computers in Human Services, 15*(2/3), 51–69.

Thyer, B. A., Artelt, T., Markward, M. K., & Dozier, C. D. (1998). Evaluating distance learning in social work education: A replication study. *Journal of Social Work Education, 34*(2), 291–295.

Vernon, R., Vakalahi, H., Pierce, D., Pittman-Munke, P., & Adkins, L. F. (2009). Distance education programs in social work: Current and emerging trends. *Journal of Social Work Education, 45*(2), 263–276.

Westhuis, D., Ouellette, P. M., & Pfahler, C. L. (2006). A comparative analysis of online and classroom based instructional formats for teaching social work research. *Advances in Social Work, 7*(2), 74–88.

Wilke, D., & Vinton, L. (2006). Evaluation of the first Web-based advanced standing MSW program. *Journal of Social Work Education, 42*, 607–620.

Wilson, S. (1999). Invited commentary: Distance education and accreditation. *Journal of Social Work Education, 35*, 326–330.

York, R. (2008). Comparing three modes of instruction in a graduate social work program. *Journal of Social Work Education, 44*(2), 157–172.

Zhao, Y., Lei, J., Yan, B., Lai, C., & Tan, H. S. (2005). What makes the difference? A practical analysis of research on the effectiveness of distance education. *Teachers College Record, 107*, 1836–1884.

A National Research Survey of Technology Use in the BSW Teaching and Learning Process

BRITTANY BUQUOI, CARLI McCLURE, JOSEPH W. KOTRLIK, KRISANNA MACHTMES, and J. C. BUNCH

School of Human Resource Education and Workforce Development, Louisiana State University, Baton Rouge, Louisiana, USA

The purpose of this descriptive-correlational research study was to assess the overall use of technology in the teaching and learning process (TLP) by BSW educators. The accessible and target population included all full-time, professorial-rank, BSW faculty in Council on Social Work Education–accredited BSW programs at land grant universities. BSW educators did not appear to be using technology in the TLP at an advanced or even moderate level. However, they were found to be more likely to incorporate technology in the TLP as the amount of technology available increased and as their constructivist teaching philosophy strengthened.

INTRODUCTION

Societies worldwide have become increasingly dependent on technology. In the past, communication among people had largely been dependent on written, verbal, and nonverbal cues. However, the introduction of new technologies has transformed the way in which people communicate, especially in education (Prensky, 2001), where much of the recent focus has been on the growing use of technology in the teaching and learning process (TLP). Specifically, in social work education, researchers have found that social work educators are increasing their use of technology in the TLP (Ballantyne, 2008; Dennison, Gruber, & Vrbsky, 2010; Shdaimah, 2009). Technologies used by social work educators increasingly included (1) imagery, (2) audio, and (3) digital video (Ballantyne, 2008; Shdaimah, 2009).

Newer technologies offer important opportunities for student interaction, collaboration, and engagement (Williams, Karousou, & Mackness, 2011). To measure university students' perceptions of emerging technologies, Murphrey, Rutherford, Doefert, Edgar, and Edgar (2012) measured levels of acceptance of Second Life, Twitter, content management systems (CMS), and social networking. They found a high level of acceptance for CMS use among university students but lower levels of acceptance for Second Life, social networking, and Twitter (Murphrey et al., 2012).

Boer, Campbell, and Hovey (2011) evaluated the use of Internet resources in three types of social work–blended learning courses. Their examination of courses in social work theory, interviewing and assessment, and integrative seminars detailed use of online videos, publication resources, and discussion forums. They found Internet-based resources offered benefits of flexible scheduling, but some traditional face-to-face components were difficult to translate into online equivalents, such as community building, skills practice, and measurement of student involvement. The blended nature of the courses allowed face-to-face meetings to offset some of these concerns, especially the ability of instructors to evaluate student abilities (Boer et al., 2011). However, the growing use of online resources to enhance face-to-face instruction has raised questions about the value that technology adds to the learning experience (Jones, 2010). Nevertheless, research has confirmed that technology supports student learning when integrated into the TLP (Vannatta, Beyerbach & Walsh, 2001; Saunders & Klemming, 2003).

While the use of technology offers great benefits, negative perceptions among educators can prevent or delay its adoption into the TLP (Jones, 2010; Perron, Taylor, Glass, & Margerum-Leys, 2010; Sarnoff, 2005; Waldman & Rafferty, 2008; Zeman & Swanke, 2008). Trends in the use of technology specifically in social work instruction indicated the following barriers to its adoption in the TLP: (1) time restraints, (2) workload, (3) insufficient infrastructure, (4) adequacy of timely information, (5) training, (6) isolation, (7) lack of interaction, (8) physical and technological inaccessibility, (9) difficulty in the transmission of practice values, and (10) lack of high-speed Internet access (Jones, 2010; Perron et al., 2010; Sarnoff, 2005; Waldman & Rafferty, 2008; Zeman & Swanke, 2008). Moreover, Beaulaurier and Radisch (2005) cautioned that while the use of web-based content is increasing, many online sources suffer from incompleteness, inaccuracy, and lack of peer review.

When considering technology adoption, therefore, it is important to consider that educators may experience a degree of anxiety toward integrating technology into the TLP (Kotrlik & Redmann, 2005; Redmann & Kotrlik, 2004). Previous research indicated that technology use in the TLP decreased when anxiety toward technology use increased (Kotrlik & Redmann, 2005;

Lokken, Cheek, & Hastings, 2003). Further, older educators often experienced more anxiety toward technology use and hence used technology less frequently than their younger counterparts (Lokken et al., 2003).

Beaulaurier and Radisch (2005) concluded that there has been little research in the field of social work education regarding integration of new technologies in the classroom despite the Council on Social Work Education (CSWE) accreditation standards for technology integration. If social work educators want to be successful in the TLP, they must realize that technology has become a necessity to younger generations, and the importance of integrating technology into their teaching competency (Lokken et al., 2003; Prensky, 2001). Finally, a helpful study conducted by Peckham and Iverson (2000) found that technology use produced more motivated, productive, and empowered students, which are essential qualities for future social workers to employ in their practice.

THEORETICAL FRAMEWORK

The framework undergirding this study was Rogers's (2003) diffusion of innovation theory. Rogers defined *an innovation* as ". . .an idea, practice, or object that is perceived as new by an individual or other unit of adoption" (p. 12). Practice was operationalized as the integration of technology in the TLP by BSW educators. To that end, determining how BSW educators are integrating technology into the TLP might provide insight toward developing strategies to encourage the adoption of technology by them.

Rogers (2003) found that five key attributes contribute to an innovation's rate of adoption, relative advantage, compatibility, complexity, trialability, and observability. Relative advantage can be described as BSW educators' perceptions of the degree to which the practice of integrating technology into the TLP supersedes the practice of traditional methods of instruction. If an individual perceives the relative advantage of one innovation to be greater than another, the individual is more likely to adopt. Compatibility conveys how individuals perceive the innovation will match their current values, previous experiences, and probable felt needs. Specifically, if BSW educators perceive the use of technology as compatible with their values, previous experiences with technology, and their felt need to be an effective instructor, they are more likely to adopt the practice of integrating technologies in the TLP (Rogers, 2003).

Rogers (2003) defined complexity as an individual's perception of the difficulty level associated with understanding and using an innovation. Unlike relative advantage and compatibility, complexity is negatively associated with rate of adoption. For example, if BSW educators perceive technology to be "user-unfriendly" or a contributor to anxiety, they may choose not to move forward. Conversely, if BSW educators perceive the level of difficulty and anxiety to be minimal, they are more likely to adopt. Trialability is the process in which an innovation can be used on a trial basis by a potential adopter. The more opportunities afforded to "try" different technologies on a pilot basis, the more likely individuals are to adopt its use. Finally, observability represents the opportunity for a potential adopter to first see the results of a specific innovation implemented by others. Having the opportunity to observe colleagues and sister professionals who have adopted such technologies likely will increase the rate of adoption.

In addition to the five attributes proposed, it is important to understand the process an individual experiences when adopting an innovation. Rogers (2003) identified five stages in the decision-innovation process. During the first stage, knowledge, individuals are exposed to the innovation at which time they seek and process information regarding the innovation. Then, in the persuasion stage, the individual forms a favorable or unfavorable attitude toward the innovation based on prior knowledge gained. In the third—decision—stage, the individual posits the positive and negative outcomes of adopting or rejecting the innovation. After a decision has been made, the individual enters the implementation stage, or rejects the innovation. Finally, during the confirmation stage, individuals confirm their decision and continue implementing the innovation. We hypothesize that an understanding of where BSW educators are within the innovation-decision process can help to facilitate and support the adoption process of a technology innovation.

PURPOSE AND OBJECTIVES

The purpose of this descriptive-correlational research study was to assess the overall use of technology in the TLP by full-time BSW educators at land grant universities. The research objectives were to determine BSW educators' (1) personal and professional characteristics (age, gender, years of professional experience, faculty rank, tenure status, sources of technology training, and teaching philosophy); (2) use of technology in the TLP; (3) perception of barriers toward the use of technology; and (4) perceived anxiety toward the use of technology, and to determine whether a relationship existed between their use of technology and selected personal and professional characteristics, and whether some of these variables explain BSW educators' acceptance and use of technology in the TLP.

METHOD

Population

The population included all full-time, professorial-rank BSW faculty in CSWE-accredited BSW programs at all 1862 and 1890 land grant universities. Land grant colleges and universities were designated by their state legislatures or Congress to receive the benefits of the Morrill Acts of 1862 and 1890 (APLU, 2012). The original mission of these institutions was to provide a practical education for the working class. Over the years, however, these universities have evolved into robust institutions of higher education that are mandated to serve the entire state where they are located with a broad range of academic and professional curricula. Public and private land grant universities were used in previous research with the same instrument and contributed to the authors' decision to use this universe as the population for this research study, as well (Kotrlik & Redmann, 2005). They also were selected as the population for study due to their diversity and the opportunity to uniformly secure representation from all 50 states (APLU, 2012).

Due to the relatively small size of this population (N = 152), a census was utilized. Twenty-four BSW educators were identified as frame errors (e.g. educators who were no longer working at the university or who were not tenured [or faculty members] and hence removed from the accessible population. As a result, a revised accessible population of 128 was used in this study. Usable responses were collected from 61 of the 128 BSW educators for a 47.7% response rate.

Instrumentation

Permission was received from the authors to modify the instrument designed by Kotrlik and Redmann (2005), which had measured availability and adoption of technology; technology training; perceived barriers to the implementation of technology; and, perceived technology anxiety. Specific items and scales were selected from this instrument and grounded in the theoretical base of the study. (Additional items were added after a review of the literature.) An expert panel of faculty and doctoral-level social work graduate students evaluated the instrument for face and content validity. The instrument then was pilot-tested with 38 land grant university adjunct social work faculty. Minor changes to the instrument were made based on the expert panel recommendations and the results of the pilot test.

The instrument included three scales measuring three constructs: (1) use of technology, (2) perceived barriers to the use of technology, and (3) perceived anxiety toward the use of technology in the TLP. The first construct included 22 items that were rated on a five-point summated scale that ranged from 1 = *Not like me* to 5 = *Just like me*. The second construct included 5 items on a four-point summated scale that ranged from 1 = *Not a barrier* to 4 = *Major barrier*. The third construct included six items on a five-point summated scale that ranged from 1 = *No anxiety* to 5 = *Very high anxiety*. Finally, 11 items were used to identify demographic and professional characteristics, which included four items to measure teaching philosophy, using a five-point summated scale that ranged from 1 = *Not like me* to 5 = *Just like me*, and one item each to measure age, gender, years of professional experience, faculty rank, tenure status, and sources of technology training. An additional item was added for participants to select all technology they were currently using in teaching from a list of 23 researcher-identified technologies. All scales (except the teaching philosophy scales) possessed exemplary reliability according to the standards for scale reliability published by Robinson, Shaver, and Wrightsman (1991). The two teaching philosophy scales possessed only minimal reliability; however, this is not unusual for scales that contain only two statements (Kaplan & Saccuzzo, 2001).

Data Collection

Data collection began after receiving university Institutional Review Board approval. A SurveyMonkey Internet questionnaire was sent to the target population in accordance with the tailored design method developed by Dillman, Smyth, and Christian (2009). Data collection included a pre-notice e-mail message and three Internet surveys. At the end of the third week, a random sample of the remaining non-respondents were contacted via telephone and e-mail to solicit participation.

To control for non-response error, an independent-samples *t*-test was used to compare the BSW educators' summated means for the dependent variable technology use in the TLP by response wave. The participants who responded to one of the three e-mail collection efforts were considered to be early respondents and participants who responded after the telephone follow-up were considered to be non-respondents since they did not respond to the three e-mailed surveys. No statistically significant difference existed between the respondents and non-respondents for technology use in the TLP ($t = 1.32$, $p = .19$). Therefore, it was concluded that the sample was representative of the survey of the universe, and the non-respondents were combined with the respondents for further analyses.

Data Analysis

The data for Objectives 1 through 4 were analyzed using descriptive statistics and the data for Objective 5 using Pearson correlation coefficients. The strength of relationship for the Pearson coefficients was interpreted using Davis's (1971) conventions. The data for Objective 6 was analyzed using forward multiple regression with the dependent variable used in this analysis being the summated mean for the technology use in the TLP scale. As listed in the objectives, 11 potential explanatory variables were initially identified. However, due to the limitations for forward multiple regression inherent in the limited number of cases, only variables that were significantly correlated to BSW educator's technology use in the correlational analyses for Objective 5 were used in the exploratory forward regression analysis. This decision was made because the number of observations was not adequate to include all variables in the analysis according to the recommendations of Hair, Black, Babin, Anderson, and Tatham (2006). An *alpha* level of .05 was established *a priori* for all statistical analyses in the study.

FINDINGS AND RESULTS

Objective 1 sought to describe the BSW educators' personal and professional characteristics ($N = 61$). There were only 54 (88.5%) valid cases as a result of seven participants' not responding to the request for demographic information. Over half of the respondents (61.1%) were female; mean age was 52.0 years ($SD = 11.3$); and their years of teaching experience averaged 16.8 ($SD = 10.6$). Approximately one-third (21, 38.9%) were assistant professors, 19 (35.2%) were associate professors, and 14 (25.9%) were professors. Over one-third (22, 40.7%) reported they were on a tenure track, and 32 (59.3%) had received tenure. As for technology training, over three-fourths (49, 80.3%) were self-taught, over two-thirds (42, 68.9%) attended technology workshops/conferences, and over two-thirds (44, 72.1%) used colleagues as a source of training. Almost one-third (19, 31.1%) of the participants used webinars for technology training, and less than one-fourth (13, 21.3%) had enrolled in a specific college course.

The mean number of technologies used by faculty while teaching was 8.70 ($SD = 2.72$) of 23 technologies listed (Table 1). The top five technologies reportedly used were the instructor's school e-mail (59, 97%), Internet at school (57, 93%), student's school e-mail (55, 90%), Internet at home (55, 90%), and web-based course management systems (53, 87%). All of the other technologies were used by fewer than half of the faculty, with the bottom 12 technologies being used by fewer than one-third.

The faculty members were asked to respond to four statements about their teaching philosophy (Table 2). Two of the statements were based on behaviorist teaching philosophy, and two were based on constructivist teaching philosophy.

Objective 2 aimed to describe the BSW educators' use of technology in the TLP measured by 22 items that were rated on a five-point summated scale. The data were interpreted using the interpretation ranges presented in Table 3. Analysis of the scale composite mean ($M = 3.39$, $SD = .76$) revealed they consider the use of technology in the TLP to be "Some" like them. The two top-rated statements ("Very much like me") were "I allow my students to submit assignments in electronic form (instead of paper)" ($M = 4.00$, $SD = 1.25$) and "I expect my students to use technology to enable them to be self-directed learners" ($M = 3.97$, $SD = .87$). The lowest-rated statement was "I encourage students to use various personal digital devices, smart phones, or tablet computers in class" ($M = 2.44$, $SD = 1.34$), which indicates

TABLE 1 Technology Used by BSW Faculty in the Teaching/Learning Process

Instructional Technologies	*N*	%
Instructor's school e-mail	59	96.7
Internet at school	57	93.4
Students' school e-mail	55	90.2
Internet at home	55	90.2
Course management system (Moodle, Blackboard, Angel, Web CT, etc.)	53	86.9
DVD or CD players	45	73.8
Smart phone (iPhone, Android, Blackberry, etc.)	25	41.0
Teleconference (Adobe Connect, Skype, ooVoo, etc.)	24	39.3
Computer lab with Internet access	24	39.3
CD or DVD recorder	22	36.1
Tablet computer (iPad, Galaxy Tab, Xoom, etc.)	22	36.1
Online forum	19	31.1
Digital video camera	14	23.0
Digital photo camera	14	23.0
Texting	13	21.3
Online chat (Live)	10	16.4
Facebook	8	13.1
Interactive white board (Smart Board, Numonics, Promothean, TouchIT, Mimi, etc.)	6	9.8
QR (Quick Response) codes	2	3.3
Twitter	2	3.3
Console gaming (Wii, Xbox, Nintendo DS, etc.)	1	1.6
Virtual worlds/simulations (Second Life, OpenSim, etc.)	1	1.6
Desktop computer gaming	0	0.0

Note. $N = 61$. Number of technologies used: $M = 8.70$, $SD = 2.72$.

TABLE 2 Teaching Philosophy of BSW Faculty

Teaching Philosophy Statements	*N*	*M*	*SD*
Behaviorist Construct	54	3.95	.72
My teaching philosophy reflects my belief that students learn most effectively through INSTRUCTOR-STUDENT interaction.	54	3.83	.91
My teaching philosophy reflects my belief that students learn most effectively when given opportunities to INTERACT WITH CONTENT AND THE INSTRUCTOR.	54	4.07	.75
Constructivist Construct	54	3.69	.74
My teaching philosophy reflects my belief that students learn most effectively when provided opportunities to INTERACT WITH CONTENT AND CONSTRUCT THEIR OWN LEARNING.	54	3.70	.84
My teaching philosophy reflects my belief that students learn most effectively through STUDENT-STUDENT interaction.	54	3.69	.95

Note. 1 = *Not like me*; 2 = *Very little like me*; 3 = *Some like me*; 4 = *Very much like me*; 5 = *Just like me*.

the faculty felt this statement was "Not like me," although the somewhat high standard deviation indicates that considerable variation existed in the responses to this item.

Objective 3 sought to determine BSW educators' perceived barriers regarding their use of technology in the TLP (Table 4). Analysis of the

TABLE 3 Technology Use in the Teaching/Learning Process by BSW Faculty

Statements	*M*	*SD*
I allow my students to submit assignments in electronic form (instead of paper).	4.00	1.25
I expect my students to use technology to enable them to be self-directed learners.	3.91	.87
I assign students to use the computer to do content related activities.	3.84	1.05
I model the use of record keeping software for my students.	2.51	1.49
I encourage students to use various personal digital devices, smart phones, or tablet computers in class.	2.44	1.32
Construct Mean	3.39	.76

Note. Five examples of instruments in the scale have been provided in this table to protect the original authors' instrument content. Scale interpretation: 1.00 to 1.49 = *Not like me*; 1.50 to 2.49 = *Very little like me*; 2.50 to 3.49 = *Some like me*; 3.50 to 4.49 = *Very much like me*; and 4.50 to 5.00 = *Exactly like me*.

TABLE 4 Perceived Barriers to Using Technology in the TLP Perceived by BSW Faculty

Statements	*M*	*SD*
Enough time to develop lessons that use technology.	2.73	.89
Availability of effective instructional software for the courses I teach	2.40	.96
Availability of technology for the number of students in my classes.	2.38	1.04
Availability of technical support to effectively use educational technology in the teaching/learning process	2.38	1.06
Administrative support for integration of technology in the teaching/ learning process.	2.25	1.04
Construct Mean	2.43	.79

Note: Scale interpretation: 1.00 to 1.49 = *Not a barrier*; 1.50 to 2.49 = *Minor barrier*; 2.50 to 3.49 = *Moderate barrier*; and 3.50 to 4.00 = *Major barrier*.

summated mean ($M = 2.43$, $SD = .79$) revealed that they encountered only minor barriers to the use of technology in the TLP. Faculty reported that "Enough time to develop lessons that use technology" was their most serious barrier and rated it moderate ($M = 2.73$, $SD = .89$). The other four items listed were rated as minor barriers. The data were interpreted using the interpretation ranges reported in Table 4.

Objective 4 sought to describe BSW educators' perceived anxiety toward the use of technology (Table 5). Analysis of the construct mean ($M = 1.84$, $SD = .63$) revealed they experienced only some anxiety when using technology in the TLP. Faculty reported they experienced "Some anxiety" with all statements in the scale, with the highest anxiety rating reported for "How anxious do you feel when you attempt to use new options on various technologies?" ($M = 2.17$, $SD = .84$).

Objective 5 sought to determine if a relationship existed between the BSW educators' use of technology in the TLP and selected variables as listed in Table 6 Statistically significant relationships existed between technology use in the TLP and four variables. A very strong positive association existed between technology use and two variables: "number of technologies used in

TABLE 5 Perceived Anxiety Experienced by BSW Professors When Attempting to Use Technology in the TLP

Statements	*M*	*SD*
How anxious do you feel when you attempt to use new options on various technologies?	2.17	.84
How anxious do you feel when you try to use new technologies?	2.00	.87
How anxious do you feel when you cannot keep up with new technologies?	1.98	.69
How anxious do you feel when you try to learn technology related skills?	1.78	.84
How anxious do you feel when you think about your technology skills compared to the skills of other instructors?	1.61	.79
How anxious do you feel when someone uses a technology term that you do not understand?	1.52	.69
Construct Mean	1.84	.63

Note: Scale interpretation: 1.00 to 1.49 = *No anxiety*; 1.50 to 2.49 = *Some anxiety*; 2.50 to 3.49 = *Moderate anxiety*; 3.50 to 4.49 = *High anxiety*; and 4.50 to 5.00 = *Very high anxiety*.

TABLE 6 Relationships between the Use of Technology in the TLP, Perceived Barriers to the Use of Instructional Technology, and Perceived Anxiety toward the Use of Instructional Technology

Personal and Professional Characteristics	Relationship with Technology Use		
	r	*p*	Effect Size Interpretation
Number of technologies used	.61	<.001	Very strong association
Teaching philosophy: Constructivist[a]	.50	.000	Very strong association
Teaching philosophy: Behaviorist[a]	.42	.001	Moderate association
Technology anxiety[a]	−.32	.019	Low association
Age[a]	−.22	.118	—
Years professional experience[a]	−.17	.230	—
Tenure status[b]	−.07	.636	—
Barriers to technology use[a]	−.05	.701	—
Faculty rank[b]	−.05	.732	—
Gender[b]	.04	.770	—
Sources of technology training[a]	.04	.777	—

Note: The correlation coefficient also serves as the effect size coefficient. Effect sizes for statistically significant correlations interpreted according to the set of descriptors by Davis (1971): .70 or higher = *Very strong association*; .50 to .69 = *Substantial association*; .30 to .49 = *Moderate association*; .10 to .29 = *Low association*. Alpha set *a priori* at .05.

[a]Pearson correlation.

[b]Point biserial correlation.

the TLP" and the "strength of the faculty's constructivist teaching philosophy." A moderate positive association existed between technology use and the "strength of the faculty members' behaviorist teaching philosophy." Finally, a low negative association existed between technology use and the faculty members' "technology anxiety." No statistically significant relationships existed for the other variables.

Objective 6 was analyzed using forward multiple regression to determine whether a relationship existed between the BSW educators' use of

TABLE 7 Forward Multiple Regression Model Summary for Technology Use in the TLP

				Change Statistics				
Variables	R^2	Adjusted R^2	*SE*	R^2 Change	*F* Change	df1	df2	*P* of *F* Change
Types of technology used in instruction	.38	.375	.61	.38	31.40	1	52	.000
Constructivist teaching philosophy	.50	.48	.55	.12	12.80	1	51	.001
Variables in the Regression Model				*B*	β	SE	t	*P*
Types of technology used in instruction				.15	.52	.03	5.03	.001
Constructivist teaching philosophy				.38	.37	.11	3.58	.001

technology in the TLP and the four variables found to be significantly related to technology use in Objective 5. It was decided *a priori* to use only those variables in the regression analysis that were significantly correlated to technology use because there was minimal chance that the other variables had the potential to have any substantial effect size on the dependent variable. (Hair et al. (2006) state that the minimum ratio of cases to potential explanatory variables is 5:1.) There was no evidence of multicollinearity in the regression analysis. Two of the variables explained 50% of the variance in the composite mean for the Technology Use in the TLP scale: constructivist teaching philosophy and number of technologies used in teaching (R^2 = .50, R^2_{adj} = .48; Table 7). According to Cohen (1988), the variance explained by the types of technology used in instruction (R^2 = .50) represents a large effect size, and the additional variance explained by the faculty's use of the constructivist teaching philosophy (additional R^2 = .12) represents a small effect size.

CONCLUSIONS, IMPLICATIONS, AND RECOMMENDATIONS

The most important conclusion that can be drawn from this study is that this population of BSW educators does not appear to be using technology in the TLP at an advanced or even moderate level. In fact, 61 BSW educators (at the 152 land grant universities used in this study) were not using the technologies listed at even a moderate level. This finding appears to contradict previous research that showed there has been a recent increase of technologies used in the TLP by BSW educators (Ballantyne 2008; Dennison et al., 2010; Shdaimah, 2009). Moreover, BSW educators in this study were minimally encouraging students to use various personal devices, smart phones, or tablet computers in class or administering student assessments through online quizzes or online document submission. Although the majority of the educators in this study used e-mail, the Internet, and course management systems, additional technologies (such as teleconference systems, computer labs, and online forums) were used by less than 50%. More surprisingly, interactive white boards and online forums, both entirely asynchronous, were used by fewer than one-fourth of the educators surveyed in this study. Perhaps the lack of integration of technology could be due to BSW educators' not perceiving a positive relative advantage to using technology in the TLP. According to Rogers (2003), if an individual does not perceive the new innovation to be better than the previous system, the individual is less likely to adopt it. Additionally, the nature of some courses could be another reason why these educators were not integrating technologies in the TLP. Specifically, courses such as social work practice may be better taught without use of certain technologies (Boer et al., 2011). Consistent with Rogers (2003), if individuals do not perceive an innovation to be compatible with their current values, previous experience, and probable felt needs, they also are less likely to adopt. The possible relationship between course content and the extent of technology integration in the TLP is an area in which further research is needed.

It seems that a majority of BSW educators in this study are only at the first stage of Rogers' (2003) decision-innovation process (i.e., knowledge). Without proper knowledge of technologies, and proper technology training, they are unable to move forward in the process of adopting new technologies. Additional opportunities for training may be beneficial in an effort to further the integration of technology in the TLP. According to Rogers, the opportunity to observe other professionals using an innovation could increase adoption. Yet, without proper training, educators are more likely to be unable to properly integrate technology in the TLP and increase student learning (Lawless & Pellegrino, 2007).

It is important to recognize that the most serious barrier identified was their having enough time to develop lessons that use technology, which is consistent with current research (Jones, 2010; Perron et al., 2010; Zeman & Swanke, 2008). Would an increase in training that could result in more efficient use of and greater confidence in the use of technology soften this barrier?

BSW educators in this study identify with both constructivist and behaviorist teaching philosophies. This may be due to the nature of BSW courses. For example, BSW educators may take a more hands-on constructivist approach in social work practice courses where they could be more of a facilitator of learning, providing students with opportunities to construct their own meaning and learning (Schunk, 2012). It is interesting that BSW educators in this study are not using technology more since they tend to follow a constructivist teaching philosophy, which is associated with students' finding and applying information and concepts from many sources, typically involving technology (Judson, 2006; Palak & Walls, 2009). On the other hand, an educator may identify more with a behaviorist approach when teaching a course that requires an emphasis on lecture, such as social policy (Schunk, 2012). Identifying the teaching philosophies of social work educators is a new endeavor and might fruitfully be further developed in future research.

Clearly, BSW educators in this study are not maximizing the technologies available for use in the TLP. Although only one-third of the CSWE accredited programs were used in this research study (and only 61 faculty participated), all CSWE-accredited programs follow the same standards, and thus it makes sense that elements of this study may apply to accredited CSWE baccalaureate programs in general. Further research is needed, however, to explore this hypothesis. It is possible that since BSW educators are mainly teaching themselves how to use the technologies they are currently using and this has not resulted in a substantial use of technology in the TLP, there may be a need for release time and additional training. Exploring these issues is worthy of additional research in order to maximize the potential learning experience for the students that can be facilitated by greater use of the emerging technologies in academia.

REFERENCES

Association of Public and Land-Grant Universities. (2012). *150 years of learning, discovery and engagement: The Morrill Act: 1862–2012*. Washington, DC: Author. Retrieved from http://www.aplu.org/document.doc?id=780

Ballantyne, N. (2008). Multimedia learning and social work education. *Journal of Social Work Education*, *27*(6), 613–622.

Beaulaurier, R., & Radisch, A. (2005). Responding to the CSWE technology guidelines: A literature review and four approaches to computerization. *Journal of Teaching in Social Work*, *25*(1), 129–150.

Boer, C., Campbell, S., & Hovey, A. (2011). When you come to a fork in the road, take it: Teaching Social Work practice using blended learning. *Canadian Journal of Learning and Technology*, *37*(3), 1–17.

Cohen, J. (1988). *Statistical power analysis for the behavioral sciences* (2nd ed.). Hillsdale, NJ: Lawrence Erlbaum Associates.

Davis, J. A. (1971). *Elementary survey analysis*. Englewood Cliffs, NJ: Prentice-Hall.

Dennison, S., Gruber, K., & Vrbsky, L. (2010). Research literature review on social work education instructional methods: 1998–2008. *Journal of Teaching in Social Work*, *30*(1), 399–419.

Dillman, D. A., Smyth, J. D., & Christian, L. M. (2009). *Internet, mail, and mixed-mode surveys: The tailored design method* (3rd ed.). Hoboken, NJ: John Wiley & Sons, Inc.

Hair, J. F., Black, W. C., Babin, B. J., Anderson, R. E., & Tatham, R. L. (2006). *Multivariate data analysis* (6th ed.). Upper Saddle River, NJ: Pearson/Prentice Hall.

Jones, P. (2010). Collaboration at a distance: Using a wiki to created a collaborative learning environment for distance education and on-campus students in a social work course. *Journal of Teaching in Social Work*, *30*(225–236). doi:10.1080/08841231003705396

Judson, E. (2006). How teachers integrate technology and their beliefs about learning: Is there a connection? *Journal of Technology and Teacher Education*, *14*(3), 581–598.

Kaplan, R. M., & Saccuzzo, D. P. (2001). *Psychological testing: Principles, applications, and issues* (5th ed.). Belmont, CA: Wadsworth/Thomson Learning.

Kotrlik, J. W., & Redmann, D. H. (2005). Extent of technology integration in instruction by adult basic education teachers. *Adult Education Quarterly*, *55*(3), 200–219. doi:10.1177/0741713605274630

Lawless, K. A., & Pellegrino, J. W. (2007). Professional development in integrating technology into teaching and learning: Knowns, unknowns, and ways to pursue better questions and answers. *Review of Educational Research*, *77*(4), 575–614. doi:10.3102/0034654307309921

Lokken, S. L., Cheek, W. K., & Hastings, S. W. (2003). The impact of technology training on family and consumer sciences teacher attitudes toward computers as an instructional medium. *Journal of Family and Consumer Sciences Education*, *21*(1), 18–32.

Murphrey, T. P., Rutherford, T. A., Doefert, D. L., Edgar, L. D., & Edgar, D. W. (2012). Technology acceptance related to second life, social networking, twitter, and content management systems: Are agricultural students ready, willing, and able. *Journal of Agricultural Education*, *53*(3). doi:10.5032/jae.2012.03056

Palak, D., & Walls, R. T. (2009). Teachers' beliefs and technology practices: A mixed methods approach. *Journal of Research on Technology in Education*, *41*(4), 417–441.

Peckham, J. D., & Iverson, M. J. (2000). Use of the Internet in Georgia's agricultural education programs. *Journal of Southern Agricultural Education Research*, *50*(1), 82–90.

Perron, B., Taylor, H., Glass, J., & Margerum-Leys, J. (2010). Information and communication technologies in social work. *Advances in Social Work*, *11*(1), 67–81.

Prensky, M. (2001). Digital natives, digital immigrants. *NCB University Press*, *9*(5), 1–6.

Redmann, D. H., & Kotrlik, J. W. (2004). Analysis of technology integration in the teaching-learning process in selected career and technical education programs. *Journal of Vocational Education Research*, *29*(1), 3–25.

Robinson, J. P., Shaver, P. R., & Wrightsman, L. S. (1991). Criteria for scale selection and evaluation. In J. P. Robinson, P. R. Shaver, & L. S. Wrightsman (Eds.), *Measures of personality and social psychological attitudes* (pp. 1–16). New York, NY: Academic Press.

Rogers, E. M. (2003). *Diffusion of innovations*. New York, NY: Free Press.

Sarnoff, S. (2005). Linking social work students to the wider world via an asynchronous learning network. *Journal of Teaching in Social Work*, *25*(1), 117–127.

Saunders, G., & Klemming, F. (2003). Integrating technology into a traditional learning environment. *Active Learning in Higher Education*, *4*(1), 74–86.

Schunk, D. H. (2012). *Learning theories: An educational perspective* (6th ed.). Upper Saddle River, NJ: Pearson/Merrill Hall.

Shdaimah, C. (2009). The power of perspective: Teaching social policy with documentary film. *Journal of Teaching in Social Work, 29*(1), 85–100.

Vannatta, R., Beyerbach, B., & Walsh, C. (2001). From teaching technology to using technology to enhance student learning: Preservice teachers' changing perceptions of technology infusion. *Journal of Technology and Teacher Education, 9*(1), 105–127.

Waldman, J., & Rafferty, J. (2008). Technology-supported learning and teaching in social work in the UK—A critical overview of the past, present, and possible futures. *Journal of Social Work Education, 27*(6), 581–591.

Williams, R., Karousou, R., & Mackness, J. (2011). Emergent learning and learning ecologies in web 2.0. *The International Review of Research in Open and Distance Learning, 12*(3). Retrieved from http://www.irrodl.org/index.php/irrodl/article/view/883/1686

Zeman, L., & Swanke, J. (2008). Integrating social work practice and technology competencies: A case example. *Journal of Social Work Education, 27*(6), 601–612. doi:10.1080/02615470802201630

Research on Webbed Connectivity in a Web-Based Learning Environment: Online Social Work Education

DORINDA NOBLE and AMY CATHERINE RUSSELL
School of Social Work, Texas State University, San Marcos, Texas, USA

This paper describes the preliminary data and analysis of how students in an online MSW program perceive their experiences, interactions, and responses to learning structure, material, and technology in the Web environment. The student perceptions, which have been used to refine the online program, highlight how important it is to students to feel a personal or webbed connection to faculty and other students in the Web environment. Rather than being a cold, sterile learning environment, the online learning world appears to be one that encourages professional webbed connectivity and relationship building.

Hortencia, age 35, works in a community health center in a small city. She wants to pursue her MSW but cannot move to an area where such a degree is offered because she has many obligations to her large extended family. When she learns that a university in the state offers the MSW online, she applies and is accepted. Though it takes her 4 years to complete the program, Hortencia continues to be grateful for the educational opportunity, since she saw no other way she could work toward an advanced degree. At times, she struggled with the technology, but one benefit for her was that she made relationships with her fellow students, even though she has never met most of them. The relationships continue to be important to her, and they were paramount while she was in the program. She also feels connected to her teachers, though she visited the campus only once and hasn't met most of the faculty who handled her classes. Now that she has graduated, Hortencia has taken a position as a unit supervisor and has improved her standard of living. She recently wrote and secured a sizeable grant for her agency. Hortencia describes the online MSW program as "life-changing."

THE GENESIS OF THIS ONLINE MSW PROGRAM

In 2004, the School of Social Work at Texas State University was awarded a grant from the Administration for Children and Youth to build an online MSW program for rural child welfare staff. It was a somewhat breathtaking adventure for the School's twelve full-time faculty, none of whom had ever developed or delivered an online course. Some faculty, in fact, openly resisted the enterprise, saying that online technology "could not possibly equate face-to-face teaching in quality."

A decade later, this School has doubled in number of faculty and students, and the online MSW program, which serves part-time students, is largely responsible for transforming this faculty and program. This change process was not always smooth, but its effects have been profound.

The original faculty who participated in the program learned how to negotiate the online learning environment by a hit-and-miss approach, with the help of various consultants whom the School hired to assist. The University's leadership, after two years, seemed to notice the program and hired course designers through the University's instructional technology services (ITS) to create a more sophisticated, organized approach to the School's online offerings. The School provided a faculty person with a course release over two semesters to develop the online courses, ranging from graduate level social policy to human behavior in the social environment. Prior to offering these courses, the faculty person worked closely with curriculum designers to ensure that each course contained a variety of learning methods, including:

- activities, such as focused learning games,
- YouTube segments,
- mini-lectures of 15 to 20 minutes,
- chat rooms, focused discussion forums, and student cyber lounges,
- videos of role-plays, staff meetings, and other scenarios as well as of experts performing professional tasks,
- video journaling for reflection and growth,
- tests of cognitive knowledge,
- synchronous discussion in which all participants are visible by camera on the screen and can hear all participants through microphone,
- virtual learning experiences through virtual reality environments, including Second Life, and

- working as a community to develop products through such instruments as Google Docs and Wiki.

Every session had one learning goal or more, and each goal had to be measured by an activity or assignment.

The result was online courses that were rich with interactive, fast-moving, diverse learning experiences. Faculty increasingly translated these kinds of activities to their on-campus classes as well, and the general quality of instruction at the School improved, becoming more lively and engaging.

The online program, which is offered in both synchronous and asynchronous modes (based upon learning activities and the variety of times zones in which students live), is based in a learning management system known as Sakai. All students and faculty have cameras and microphones on their computers to allow for direct, real-time communication with faculty and other students. Faculty have online office hours, and students also can phone faculty for personal consultations.

The integrity of the School's fieldwork program has remained solid. Students, who are placed across the nation in communities in which they live, receive faculty help in the initial placement process. Though field seminar classes and visits with agency supervisors are conducted online, field faculty visit almost all placements at least once during the student's field practicum. Though this personalized approach is costly, the School is committed to providing at least some face-to-face time with agency supervisors and field students. The School provides agency supervisors with computer cameras and microphones if they wish so that they can communicate with field faculty face to face via computer.

The School has graduated 115 online students, many of whom have achieved very solid careers. Several have secured large grants for their agencies or communities; many have assumed positions of leadership in social agencies; virtually all are licensed and active in the profession.

WHAT THE SCHOOL HAS LEARNED ABOUT ONLINE EDUCATION

Faculty Talents

Online instruction is a burgeoning element in higher education. In the decade that the School has been engaged in online education, the technology available has far outstripped the capability of many educators to keep abreast of the teaching possibilities. For several years, the School has hired only faculty who are either adept at online teaching or eager to learn it but has found that even enthusiastic online educators must constantly adapt to new innovations. Faculty members also find they must regularly return to the arduous task of course development, as they not only incorporate new technology but also update course material. Updating courses, of course, is a task in classroom delivery as well, because the ubiquity, immediacy, and transparency of information has made teaching and learning an ever more complex endeavor (Isenberg & Fletcher, 2012).

Even though most studies have shown that online courses can be as effective as classroom courses (Tallent-Runnels et al., 2006), it is clear to the School that teaching online is substantially different from teaching in a traditional classroom. While the classroom environment allows for some spontaneity, online delivery requires far more scripting and planning. Online teaching is less likely to highlight a faculty member's engaging personality than would be the case in a classroom environment, where faculty may be able to sparkle with their acting ability and their engagement skills. Thus, some faculty members who have less charisma in the traditional classroom actually may be able to function better in an online environment, particularly if their organizational skills and attention to detail help them attend to the demands of the modality.

Faculty Time

Faculty consistently report that developing and delivering an online course is more time-consuming than functioning in a traditional classroom environment. A special demand emerges when the online course involves multi-generational learners (as is true for the School), in which the MSW student population includes roughly the same number of students younger than 30, students between 30 and 40, and students older than 40. Older learners tend to tolerate technology, while learners who are in their thirties will likely embrace it. Younger learners, who have grown up using technology for banking, paying bills, getting the news, connecting with friends, and playing games, assume that technology will be part of their education (Isenberg & Fletcher, 2012). The School has found that more mature learners (and even some learners in their thirties) are generally less sophisticated and comfortable in the online environment. How easily students are able to navigate the technology naturally will have a great impact on how smoothly class logistics proceed.

Faculty Commitment

Faculty not only must be adept at using the technology, they must be tolerant of the drudgery that working online sometimes generates. Learning to competently use technology nevertheless is an increasingly important part of professional growth (Collins, Cook-Cotone, Robinsoon, & Sullivan, 2004). Faculty must view the computer as a helpful servant in the process of transmitting and manipulating information, not as the primary player in the online educational process. Faculty also must accept online media as a tool to connect people, understanding that informal learning also will take place among students through social networking media, outside of the framework of the formal course. In fact, the School's online student cohorts have developed close relations. For instance, when one online student lost her son to an accident, the rest of the online cohort rallied around her and provided both emotional and concrete support, albeit from a distance.

Faculty Philosophy

Faculty who excel at online education tend to be constructivist in orientation, a philosophy that underscores the centrality of the learner's intentions, experiences, and cognitive strategies. They believe that adult learners construct different cognitive structures based on their previous knowledge and experience and that it is wise to create a rich and diverse learning environment to accommodate learners' different experiences (Reeves & Reeves, 2008).

The constructivist orientation also leads faculty to evaluate their role in the learning enterprise. Online teaching allows faculty to move out of the traditional role in which the instructor is "center stage," the party who holds and dispenses knowledge. Rather, the faculty place responsibility for learning here on the learner; the instructor increasingly becomes the facilitator of learning. With the help of the faculty person, the adult learner becomes responsible for recognizing, assessing, and organizing information into knowledge. The computer is responsible for what it does best: performing calculations, storing information, and retrieving it as the learner requires (Reeves & Reeves, 2008).

Student Experiences of Online Learning

Because the currency of online learning is language, the School has found that online students become adept at communication. Whereas classroom students sometimes may exhibit some difficulties in writing and speaking, online students quickly develop more specific and extensive vocabularies. Their writing skills are enhanced because they are practicing writing, and their verbal skills improve because of frequently being in front of the camera.

Because students are remote from one another, they often seem to feel emboldened to express true feelings. Such an atmosphere allows them to venture into examining their perceptions and values. Faculty, while encouraging free communication, must also ensure that students are safe from collegial disrespect (Regan & Youn, 2008). Sometimes, faculty have to protect themselves and their time from prolonged discussions. One faculty member was overwrought when a single reading generated 140 postings from 15 students. He explained to the students that they could continue to chat about the matter, but he was exiting the discussion. It has become clear from our experience that all online students tend to participate much more in discussions than do their on-campus counterparts, where it is easier for a few vocal students to dominate discussions.

Students are expected to work in groups on learning activities and products. They exchange information and learn about one another: the remote communities in which they live, the jobs they hold, and the challenges they face. This exchange invariably leads to multicultural understanding. This group process, and indeed the entire online learning environment, should be conceptualized as a process, not a one-time event (King & Stewart, 2012). Online students give many indications that they need and want webbed, interactive relationships with their fellow students and faculty since online learning is inherently a solitary endeavor, and students need to feel that they are in a connected community of learning.

METHODOLOGY FOR THE STUDY OF STUDENT PERCEPTIONS

The School, through the University's ITS, did a lengthy study of how students perceived the online curriculum, both in content and delivery. The results of this study have helped the faculty shape and refine the curriculum and pedagogical process. The data and analysis, in which students responded to a range of quantitative and qualitative queries about their learning experience, interactions, curriculum structure and materials, technology, and ultimate learning, point the way to future investigation and improvement.

Study Design

This research study design is mixed-methods and pre-experimental, focusing on one group: online graduate-level social work students (Engel & Schutt, 2013). The study presents student perception surveys, findings, and the analysis of both quantitative and qualitative data collected over the three years (from fall 2008 to fall 2011) in which the bulk of the School's more sophisticated online course development occurred. Although the data is longitudinal in nature, the research is presented in a cross-sectional format.

This study was deemed exempt by the University's Institutional Review Board from full or expedited review under federal exemption category 1(ii): research conducted in established educational settings on instructional strategies.

Measurement

The study's primary measurement is a student perception survey that covers responses from students in 11 courses containing 11 sections. The School developed these courses with intense support from the University's ITS department. As part of this support, the ITS created a perception measurement tool that students completed after the newly developed course was first delivered. Faculty built the instrument into the course, and some instructors gave students an extra credit incentive to complete the instrument. Student responses for the first group of courses were very high, as presented in the Results section.

The student perception measurement tool consists of six spectrums that are included in the quantitative and qualitative data analyses: overall experience (9 questions), quality of online learning interactions (8 questions), course structure and organization (5 questions), teaching and learning (10 questions), course materials (7 questions), and technology (2 questions). There are two categories of response items: 4-point ratings (*Agree*, *Tend to Agree*, *Tend to Disagree*, *Disagree*) and qualitative comments. Likert-scale response categories were coded 1 through 4, with 4 representing *Agree*.

Due to the range and to the large number of survey questions, this paper presents only specific and most relevant data, all of which the School has used to enhance online course delivery and curriculum.

Sample

The sample consists of graduate social work students enrolled in the first iterations of online MSW courses developed in partnership between the School and ITS. This sampling is purposive/criterion, non-probability sampling.

Data Analysis

Faculty researchers analyzed quantitative data through SPSS version 18 to assess the student responses collected from 11 online courses. Researchers analyzed and present herein descriptive statistics, with correlations, to explore possible associations between response categories. Additionally, they conducted regressions to explore possible models of student satisfaction and learning from online course delivery. Some survey questions were particularly interesting, such as overall satisfaction, instructor interaction, technology perceptions, and other areas relevant to possible course improvements. This statistical analysis translates into useful information for social work educators and parallels the study's examination of how the School's online curriculum developed.

Researchers conducted qualitative data analysis in a traditional manner through first- and second-level coding (Grinnell & Unrau, 2006). Coding, as defined by Rubin and Babbie (2008), is "classifying or categorizing individual pieces of data" (p. 460). Researchers coded apparent first-level themes and present them in this paper, with more theoretical and second-level themes presented afterward.

STUDY RESULTS

As noted, this study examined 11 sections of 11 online graduate social work courses, delivered over 3 years. Six foundation courses were included

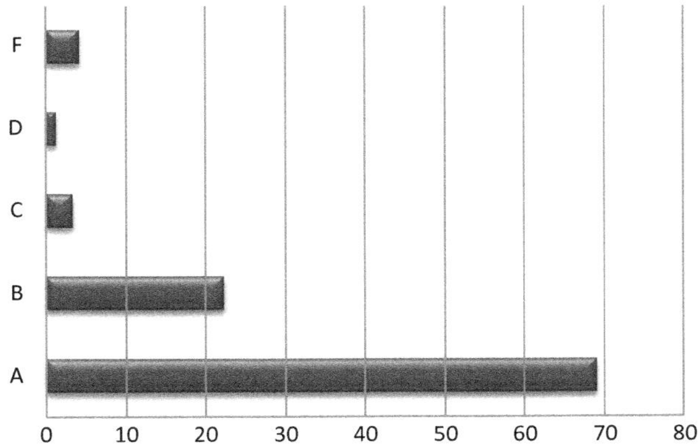

	A	B	C	D	F
Grade Distribution Percentages	69	22.3	3.3	1.2	4.1

FIGURE 1 Grade distribution percentages ($N = 242$).

and covered these topics: (1) policy, (2) human behavior and social environment, from conception to young adulthood, (3) foundation practice in working with individuals and families, (4) foundation practice in interviewing and communication skills, (5) research, and (6) human behavior and social environment from adulthood through death. The five advanced courses involved (1) diagnostic assessment, (2) advanced policy, (3) supervision and management, (4) organizational assessment, and (5) grant writing and resource development. Of the 242 students in these 11 classes (not including Incomplete grades), 92% responded ($n = 222$), an excellent response rate. Students were encouraged but not required to complete the survey.

The School collected this data for three purposes: (1) to enhance and improve online course delivery and content, based on student perception and feedback, (2) to assess and measure student learning outcomes for the School's reaccreditation process, and (3) to guide ITS in its partnership with the School toward developing and delivering high-quality online education. This feedback loop from students has allowed the School to streamline its outcome measurement, which benefits both the program's ability to refine its online offerings and the School's ease of access to student outcome measures. Because the School was preparing for its reaccreditation process with the Council on Social Work Education (CSWE) while also conducting this study, the researchers matched competencies and practice behaviors with the online course delivery. The survey questions relate directly to the explicit curriculum and the knowledge, skill, and values inherent in student learning, as mandated by CSWE Educational Policy and Academic Standard (CSWE, 2008).

Quantitative Results

This paper presents the means and percentages of primary interest from the 11 courses, which include course grades and mean responses to overall satisfaction with the course, instructor interaction, and manageability of the online course. Descriptive statistics reveal that the majority of students performed at an "A" level in course grade distribution, which includes all grades recorded for the 11 courses ($n = 242$). Incomplete grades are not included, but all grades are included even if the student did not complete the perception survey (see Figure 1). Only 10% were not satisfied with the technical assistance they received when experiencing problems ($n = 1$). Ninety percent ($n = 9$) of the means reported in the student perception surveys reveal that students agreed or tended to agree that they were satisfied with the technical assistance they received when experiencing problems with technology.

Student perception survey results from four courses (two foundation and two advanced courses) are presented in Table 1. The percentages reported are the highest across all four response categories (agree, tend to agree, tend to disagree, and disagree). These percentages show a majority of positive responses to the list of questions presented. Both policy courses and the one organizational assessment course revealed more dispersion among responses. However, there is only one percentage that reveals a majority of negative feedback to the questions asked in the survey. Additionally, this outcome reflects what social work instructors know about how students traditionally may dread and resist policy and research courses. This is apparent in contrast to percentages for Foundation Practice II, of which nearly all percentages fall in the highest positive response category (*Agree*).

The one item that revealed disagreement was in one course (Advanced Social Policy) regarding helpful instructor feedback. Students disagreed with the response category "The instructor's answers to my questions and feedback on assignments helped me better understand course content" and the ability of the instructor to clarify assignment content in one advanced course ($M = 2.48$, *Tend to Disagree*). This finding may imply that students expect instructors to be available and more effective when there is confusion over course assignments. This outcome contrasts with more positive answers when students were asked to respond to "I am satisfied with the quality of interaction with the instructor" ($M = 2.85$, *Tend to Agree*). All other means in these response categories across the four courses showed that students agreed or tended to agree when asked about overall satisfaction in the course, including the pace, difficulty, and manageability of the workload. Moreover, they had a positive attitude toward course content.

Instructor Interaction Correlations

Correlation coefficients were computed among 12 variables that signified overall satisfaction with the course, manageable workload, classmate

TABLE 1 Comparisons of Four Online Courses

	Online Course Means and Percentages*			
Item Responses for Online Field Tests	Social Welfare Policy $N = 30$	Foundation Practice II $N = 14$	Advanced Social Policy $N = 20$	Organizational Assessment $N = 15$
Overall, I am satisfied with this course.	3.17 50% Tend to Agree	3.93 93% Agree	3.50 50% Agree	3.53 53% Agree
I would recommend this course to others.	3.23 43% Agree	3.93 93% Agree	3.55 55% Agree	3.47 53% Agree
Overall, the pace of this course is about right.	2.80 33% Tend to Agree	3.93 93% Agree	3.25 65% Tend to Agree	3.40 47% Agree/Tend to Agree
Overall, the difficulty level of this course was about right.	3.30 50% Tend to Agree	3.86 86% Agree	3.65 65% Agree	3.47 53% Tend to Agree
The workload for this course was manageable.	2.70 30% Agree	3.71 71% Agree	3.30 45% Agree	3.40 47% Agree/Tend to Agree
I have a positive attitude toward the course subject matter at the end of the course.	3.37 53% Agree	3.71 79% Agree	3.50 55% Agree	3.47 53% Agree
I am satisfied with the quality of interaction with the instructor.	2.93 37% Tend to Agree	3.93 93% Agree	2.85 35% Tend to Agree	3.40 47% Agree/Tend to Agree

(Continued)

TABLE 1 (Continued)

Item Responses for Online Field Tests	Online Course Means and Percentages* Social Welfare Policy *N* = *30*	Foundation Practice II *N* = *14*	Advanced Social Policy *N* = *20*	Organizational Assessment *N* = *15*
I am satisfied with the quality of interaction with my classmates.	3.27 43% Agree	3.64 71% Agree	3.95 95% Agree	3.53 53% Agree
I felt supported and helped in this online learning environment.	3.13 40% Agree	3.64 64% Agree	3.35 50% Agree	3.53 53% Agree
The content of this course is well structured and organized.	2.87 47% Tend to Agree	3.86 86% Agree	3.35 45% Agree	3.47 53% Tend to Agree
I was able to master the material in the assignments.	3.13 63% Tend to Agree	3.64 64% Agree	3.35 55% Tend to Agree	3.47 53% Tend to Agree
The instructor's answers to my questions and feedback on assignments helped me better understand course content.	3.10 47% Agree	3.86 86% Agree	2.42 30% Tend to Disagree	3.47 53% Agree
The online discussion forums helped me to learn and understand the course content.	3.10 47% Tend to Agree	3.43 57% Tend to Agree	3.60 60% Agree	3.33 67% Tend to Agree

*Highest percentages are reported and means reported for ordinal scales ranging from 1 (*Disagree*) to 4 (*Agree*).

TABLE 2 Correlations among Overall Satisfaction and Instructor Interaction ($N = 11$)

	Overall Satisfaction with Online Course
Quality of interaction with instructor	.864**
Frequency of interaction with instructor	.872**
Felt supported and helped in online environment	.936**
Discussion forums kept student connected to instructor and classmates	.860**
Instructor effectively facilitated discussion forums	.797**
Instructor's answers to questions on assignments helped understanding of content	.908**
Instructor's answers to questions were timely	.643*

*$p < .05$. **$p < .01$.

interaction (2 variables), online learning attitudes and support, technical assistance, and instructor interaction (5 variables). A p value of less than .05 was required for significance. The significant correlations are presented in Table 2 for the relationships between overall satisfaction with the course and instructor interaction variables. These coefficients are very close to one and show strong relationships between the instructor's interactions with students across seven variables and students' overall satisfaction with the online course. Although not significant, it is interesting to note that five correlations computed for associations between technical assistance satisfaction and instructor interaction variables were negative coefficients. This may mean that when online students experience technical problems, they may rely more on instructor interaction.

Predictors of Student Satisfaction

Researchers conducted two multiple regression analyses to predict overall satisfaction with the course and technical assistance satisfaction. The overall course satisfaction analysis included instructor interaction variables as predictors (instructor's answers were timely, instructor's answers helped understanding, instructor effectively facilitated forums, satisfaction with frequency of instructor interaction, satisfaction with quality of interaction with instructor). The regression equation was significant: $R^2 = .948$, adjusted $R^2 = .896$, $F(5,5) = 18.235$, $p > .01$. Based on these results, instructor interaction variables, in combination, appear to be strong predictors of student satisfaction. In Table 3 indices are presented to show strength of the individual predictors. Only one variable was statistically significant: Instructor's answers to questions were timely ($p < .05$). The correlations among instructor interaction variables ranged from .643 to .908. It is tempting to say that only instructor's timely answers is the most useful predictor; however, because all variables are significantly correlated, the complete model reveals strong predictors together as an indicator of student satisfaction.

TABLE 3 Bivariate and Partial Correlations of Student Satisfaction Predictors

Predictors	Correlation between Each Predictor and Student Satisfaction
Quality of interaction with instructor	.864
Frequency of interaction with instructor	.872
Instructor effectively facilitated discussion forums	.797
Instructor's answers to questions on assignments helped understanding of content	.908
Instructor's answers to questions were timely	.643*

*$p < .05$.

The second regression was conducted on technical assistance satisfaction as the dependent variable, selecting only cases when students agreed they were satisfied with this assistance, and included the same set of instructor interaction variables as the first regression. This equation was not significant: $R^2 = .634$, adjusted $R^2 = .342$, $F(4,5) = 2.170$, $p = .209$. The regression findings may suggest that instructor variables are better predictors of overall satisfaction with an online learning course, as opposed to predicting whether students were satisfied with the technical assistance they received when experiencing problems.

In sum, the quantitative results reveal that student perceptions of instructor interaction have an impact on their satisfaction with the online course, learning, and delivery of content in the online environment. Instructor interaction (whether it is timely, frequent, or effective in helping students understand content) has a very significant impact on student satisfaction in the online learning environment. Additionally, instructor interaction presents predictors to the students' overall satisfaction with the online course.

Qualitative Results

The perception survey offered students qualitative response options after each quantitative question. Students could choose to elaborate on their quantitative response. The survey offered approximately 30 qualitative responses per course, and students did not hesitate to identify what they liked least or most, including suggesting improvements. In the analysis, there were no themes linked to specific courses, other than that students highly commended some instructors for their interactions with students and highly praised the course content. However, this feedback was not linked to specific topics or to whether the course was foundation or advanced. What was evident in the qualitative data analysis is that patterns and themes fell along two spectrums: *content* and *process*. In content, responses related to what was contained within the course, such as materials, video mini-lectures, and the topic of the course itself. Process revealed responses related to how the online course was delivered and the tasks and knowledge required to navigate an online course.

Themes: What Students Liked Most

Students responded on two spectrums to the open-end question of what they liked most in the course. The first area related to content, while the second related to process. Students responded that they most liked course content, multicultural components, the textbook, the interesting assignments, course materials and their variety (such as transcripts, mini-lectures, role-plays, lesson notes, and assignments that had students working directly with agencies). For example, one student noted he was able to conduct "grant work with an agency." A student in another course referred to most liking the "course assignments and interviewing." Another student identified that she most appreciated "the range of ideas and exposure to different ideas."

When addressing the delivery of the course and process-related issues, students overwhelmingly stated that what they liked best was the interaction with and the prompt response time from the instructor. Students also reported that they liked doing individual work, working at their own pace, having flexibility, working from a syllabus that was clear, engaging in group interaction, participating in discussion forums, relating directly to the instructor, and using multiple media tools. The most frequent qualitative comment that students identified as the thing they liked most was feedback from the instructor, response time, and attention from the instructor when returning grades and comments as well as when clearing up questions. For example, one student said what she liked most how "well laid out" the course was and that the student therefore "knew what to expect." Other students identified liking the process such as "the supportive nature of instructor," "the professor's detailed feedback and quick response," and "communication with the professor was timely and excellent."

Themes: What Students Liked Least

Students responded primarily on one spectrum to the open-end question of what they liked least in the course, which was with regard to course process and delivery. The only exception related to the amount of materials, not the materials themselves. In other words, it was not the course content they liked least, but it was how much material the course contained that they disliked—which may be viewed as process. Some students reported that there was too much content to process through the semester, a response that is reported as typical by Siebert and Spaulding-Givens (2006). If responses were favorable to the instructor, there were fewer "liked least" responses for these courses.

Students gave patterned responses in the process and delivery of the online courses, making such comments as we need more feedback, we had problems meeting with and coordinating with group members, there is a lot of group work, I had technology problems, the instructor was not available, there was too much reading, test questions need to be improved, there are too many assignments, and the workload is too heavy.

Similar to the fact that students most liked instructor interaction, they inversely least liked the lack of instructor interaction, which was the primary theme in the least-liked elements. Some students desired more feedback from the instructor, more live time, and wanted the instructor to be more available.

Students' Suggestions for Improvement

Students responded primarily along one spectrum to the open-end question requesting their suggestions for improving the course. If responses were favorable to the instructor, there were fewer suggestions for improving the course.

Students commented that the online course could be improved by assigning less group work, improving the continuity of lectures, giving more feedback, providing examples of and more explanations about assignments, offering more thorough and detailed instructions, giving technology training in preparation to taking an online course, providing more video mini-lectures from the professor, giving more time to complete exams, and improving technology and its user-friendliness.

The primary themed response for improving the course reflected what students liked least in the course—lack of interaction with instructor—and the most frequent kind of suggestion was more time and interaction with the instructor. Students primarily felt the instructor's role and interaction would improve the online course, which included quick grading and feedback turnaround as well as more personalized interaction with students. Surprisingly, but reflective of this theme, students requested more lectures from their instructor.

Second-Level: Theoretical Codes

Second-level (or theoretical) codes emerged from the qualitative data analysis across all three open-end questions and related to (1) flexibility, (2) immediacy, (3) clarification, and (4) interaction. Flexibility reflects students' comments that they need to work on their own, at their own pace, when they can. Immediacy was overtly represented in students' comments that they need quick and thorough responses to questions and that when they reach out for assistance from the instructor, they need the instructor to respond to them urgently. The third code of clarification reflects that students need their online courses to be very clear and assignments to be delineated in such a way that they feel confident that they understand what is expected. A primary repetitious code dealt with instructor interaction, or connectivity to the

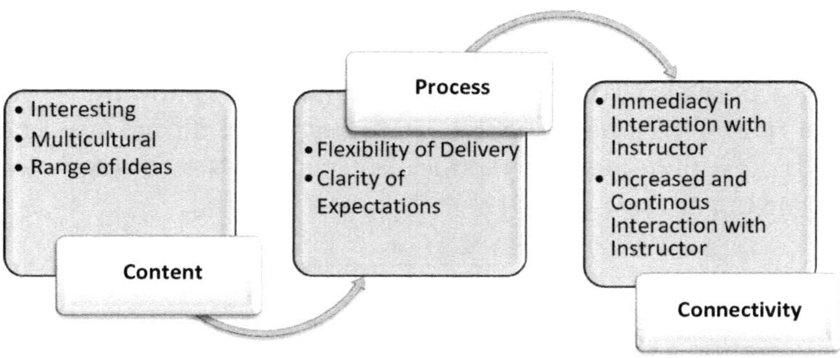

FIGURE 2 Online content and process typology.

instructor. Online learners need and want substantial interaction with their instructor; that much is clear. It highlights the fact that learners need connectivity to the instructor and face time. Interestingly, all theoretical codes deal with process, not content. A typology reflecting the first- and second-level coding is shown in Figure 2 for coded qualitative themes and patterns.

Taken together, the quantitative results demonstrate that student perceptions of the quality and quantity of interaction with their instructor are of utmost importance, and the qualitative results support this interaction in greater depth and detail. Although the quantitative results imply that few areas need improvement, the qualitative findings provide more exploration of student need. Primary findings from both quantitative and qualitative data analysis reveal that time invested by the instructor is a major determinant of effective online learning and student satisfaction within the online learning environment.

WHAT THIS STUDY MEANS TO THE SCHOOL AND TO ONLINE EDUCATION

The predominant finding of this study, both in qualitative and quantitative data, is that instructor connectivity can make or break a class. This interaction or connectivity seems to revolve around the amount of time such faculty spend with students, the timeliness with which they respond to students, and the clarity of their responses. This paramount conclusion strengthens the notion that online students long for webbed connections. Though they are communicating through technology, they want personal, individualized relationships with members of their community in general and with faculty members in particular.

The School has harvested student responses and used them to improve its online option. Faculty also have developed more specialized in-house assessment strategies to further strengthen and refine the program. In this way, the School has helped to create a learning community in which students and faculty collaborate on defining the learning process and outcomes. The School is increasingly moving away from teacher-driven learning and toward a partnership between students and faculty. It is expanding its arsenal of multi-media instructional approaches, a strategy that allows the brain hemispheres to better integrate knowledge and produces a stronger foundation for learning (King & Stewart, 2012).

Future Research

Since the inception of the School's online program, faculty have gathered data continually, every semester. The School now needs to compile and analyze this data in more structured ways.

Faculty recognizes that the student perception survey needs to be strengthened so that it more clearly highlights the difference between content and process, particularly in terms of understanding how instructor interaction increases student learning. The quantitative findings of the student survey revealed that students, in fact, were very positive about course content. In fact, what interaction they expect from faculty may not have a great deal to do with actual learning, since the course content and delivery are already developed before students take the course. Future measurement should try to discriminate whether (and to what extent) faculty interaction really affects student learning. It could be that faculty interaction is more important to student satisfaction than to student learning. And, it is unclear from the current data whether students want more personal interaction from faculty just for themselves or whether they want more interaction with the whole student cohort.

The School also is developing plans to expand the feedback loop by formally conducting interviews (and collecting qualitative data) from faculty and from course designers about how well they perceive the online program is functioning. Harvesting more information from these gatekeepers will give the School a better-rounded assessment of the process.

Another element that the School needs to develop are more reliable measures to delineate between content and process. This would include factors to measure what is actually needed for students to master the course content and what students expect from the instructor. These factors would help faculty and administration to better assess whether specific faculty should be investing their talent in on-campus or online instruction.

Faculty Preference for On-Campus or Online Courses

Because of the differences between these delivery modalities and because they each draw on different talent pools, some faculty may be better suited for either on-campus or online courses. Of the seven faculty who developed the courses included in this study, students exhibited little consistency in selecting favorite faculty.

Faculty who teach online consistently report that it is a time-consuming endeavor. The School is currently giving course releases to faculty to update existing online courses with new technology, new content, and new textbooks.

Hortencia's story, told at the beginning, illustrates the need for online education as an equalizing force in social work education and for building a more robust work force in the human services. The School continues to contend with the challenges and enjoy the transformative rewards of building a high-quality online graduate education program. Hortencia is one example of an adult learner who developed strong relationships in a Web-based learning environment. Though the modality is modern, the end result of learning and building relationships is timeless.

REFERENCES

Collins, J. L., Cook-Cottone, C. P., Robinson, J. S., & Sullivan, R. R. (2004). Technology and new directions in professional development: Applications of digital video, peer review, and self-reflection. *Journal of Educational Technology Systems, 33*(2), 131–146.

Council on Social Work Education. (2008). *Educational policy and accreditation standards*. Alexandria: VA: Author.

Engel, R. J., & Schutt, R. K. (2013). *The practice of research in social work* (3rd ed.). Los Angeles, CA: Sage.

Grinnell, R. M. Jr., & Unrau, Y. A. (2006). *Social work research and evaluation: Quantitative and qualitative approaches* (7th ed.). New York, NY: Oxford Press.

Isenberg, S., & Fletcher, G. (2012). The new classroom of multigenerational learners: Using androgogical principles in 21st century online learning. In C. J. Boden-McGill and K. P. King (Eds.), *Conversations about adult learning in our complex world* (pp. 79–90). Charlotte, NC: Information Age Publishing.

King, K., & Stewart, S. (2012). Facilitating transformative learning opportunities in higher education contexts for adult learners in online and virtual spaces. In C. J. Boden-McGill and K. P. King (Eds.), *Conversations about adult learning in our complex world* (pp. 291–308). Charlotte, NC: Information Age Publishing.

Reeves, P. M., & Reeves, T. C. (2008). Design considerations for online learning in health and social work education. *Learning in Health and Social Care, 7*(1), 46–58.

Regan, J. A. R., & Youn, E. J. (2008). Past, present, and future trends in teaching clinical skills through Web-based learning environments. *Journal of Social Work Education, 44*(2), 95–115.

Rubin, A., & Babbie, E. R. (2008). *Research methods for social work* (6th ed.). Belmont, CA: Brooks/Cole.

Siebert, D. C., & Spaulding-Givens, J. (2006). Teaching clinical social work skills entirely online: A case example. *Social Work Education, 25*(1), 78–91.

Tallent-Runnels, M. K., Thomas, J. A., Lan, W. Y., Cooper, S., Ahern, T. C., Shaw, S. M., & Ziaoming, L. (2006). Teaching courses online: A review of the research. *Review of Educational Research, 76*, 93–135.

A Process Evaluation of an Online BSW Program: Getting the Student Perspective

CAROLYN McALLISTER
School of Social Work, California State University, San Bernadino, California, USA

This paper reviews the student perspectives of an online BSW program. The structure of this program is presented, along with findings from a mixed-method evaluation of four matched BSW courses where each instructor taught both the online and face-to-face sections. Although there are no identified differences in performance, grades, or retention, students report differences in developing instructor and classmate relationships and in overall course satisfaction. Qualitative findings highlight the advantages of the flexibility of online education, tempered by challenges in making connections and fewer spontaneous interactions. Implications for online course development are discussed.

INTRODUCTION

Distance education has been available since the creation of correspondence courses, which began to proliferate in the United States during the latter part of the nineteenth century. Subsequently, multiple shifts and additions to distance education have occurred, most recently involving the emergence of an online format (Moore & Kearsley, 2011). The past decade has seen a move toward online education in the United States becoming a major part of the academic landscape. In their report on the status of online education in America, Allen and Seaman (2013) note that, in 2012, 32% of college students (6.7 million) reported taking at least one course online, compared to 9.6% of college students in 2002 (1.9 million).

The number of online courses and programs in social work continue to grow at a dramatic pace across the United States, although there are no firm statistics to determine how many social work students are exposed to online education. In 1998, Siegel, Jennings, Conklin, and Napoletano Flynn conducted a national study on distance education social work programs. Sixteen percent of programs reported using some form of distance education, but online education was not reported except as a mechanism to send curricular materials. Approximately a decade later, Vernon, Vakalahi, Pierce, Pittman-Munke, and Adkins (2009) found that 41% of BSW and 52% of MSW programs offered at least one distance education course, and the majority of them were online. As of December, 2012, the Council on Social Work Education (CSWE) listed five BSW distance education offerings; as of July, 2013, 22 MSW program options. The majority of these programs report some online components, and seven MSW and three BSW programs list themselves as having fully online programs (CSWE, 2013). In addition, since BSW students take the majority of their undergraduate coursework outside of social work major courses, it is likely that these students experience online course rates quite similar to the overall rates in the United States (Allen & Seaman, 2013).

The region where California State University, San Bernardino is located includes large areas of isolated rural communities. Similar to other social work programs, many potential social work students are working part- or full-time, have children and other family obligations, and historically have not been able to complete a face-to-face program (Oliaro & Trotter, 2010; Wilke & Vinton, 2006). As the only public university in the area with an accredited BSW or MSW program, our commitment as a school has been to meet the unmet community need for social workers. In 2009, Morris and Poirier completed a needs assessment of San Bernardino, Riverside, and Inyo County social service agencies, consisting of focus groups, surveys of employees, and interviews with administrators. They determined that rural areas had serious unmet needs in their BSW and MSW workforce. Further, the majority of the over 2,000 employees surveyed wanted a BSW or MSW degree but were unable to access traditional, on-campus programs. Based on those results, we began a BSW online offering that now has completed the second of 3 years it will take for the first full set of online classes.

A major goal for the school of social work is to provide an equivalent, high-quality experience to students taking the online version of any social work class, and therefore it is important to receive feedback about the strengths and challenges of online courses during implementation. One unique feature of the BSW online implementation is that most online and face-to-face classes have been taught simultaneously by the same instructor. This offered a unique opportunity to measure differences in experiences and outcomes based on teaching format. The focus of this evaluation was on the individual student's experience of taking the course, although overall outcomes of courses in the different formats were examined. Although grades are one criterion of measure, there are many other important factors to consider. This paper reports the findings of an exploratory evaluation and is based on four courses that have been taught both online and face-to-face (eight class sections in total). Findings from this study will help inform the future direction of this program and examine factors important for online education more broadly that have been minimally examined in the social work literature to date.

LITERATURE REVIEW

Grade and Performance Outcomes in Online Coursework

Research on social work online education primarily has focused on performance and grade outcomes for students taking online classes in comparison to those enrolled in traditional, face-to-face formats. Results of these studies have been mixed. A number of them have shown no difference in outcomes based on grade or performance outcomes (Ouellette, Westhuis, Marshall, & Chang, 2006; Petracchi, Malllinger, Engel, Rishel, & Washburn, 2005; Siebert, Spaulding-Givens & Siebert , 2006; Schoech & Helton, 2002; York, 2008). These studies align well with research in other fields showing no differences in performance or outcomes between online and face-to-face sections of courses (e.g., Beard, Harper, & Riley, 2004; Brown, 2012; Dutton, Dutton, & Perry, 2001; Pucel & Stertz, 2005). Additionally, two online social work programs retrospectively compared outcomes of their online and face-to-face cohorts. Wilke and Vinton (2006) found students in the first online advanced standing program generally showed similar outcomes to the face-to-face students. Oliaro and Trotter (2010) found that students in a distance BSW program, although demographically different from the on-campus student cohort, had grades equal to other part-time on-campus students.

On the other hand, several studies have provided a more negative outlook for student success in an online environment, finding that these students have poorer outcomes (Faux & Black-Hughes, 2000; Hisle-Gorman & Zuravin, 2006; Marson, Weil, & Marson, 2010). In addition, in the Wilke and Vinton study (2006), the online advanced standing students had poorer outcomes in fieldwork, although it was argued that demographic differences between cohorts may have been the primary cause. These findings align with studies focusing on the perspectives of faculty. That is, in at least two studies, social work faculty report perceiving online education to be less effective than virtually all other teaching formats, and caution colleagues who are teaching online, particularly practice method courses (Moore, 2005b; Vernon et al., 2009).

Student retention is an important additional outcome to consider. Students taking an online course may be less likely to complete them (e.g. Allen & Seaman, 2013; Brown, 2012; Dutton et al., 2001; McPhee & Söderström, 2012). The reasons for reduced retention have not been well studied. One possibility advanced by university administrators is that the online environment may require better organizational skills (Allen & Seaman, 2013). Further research in this area is needed to understand how educators can support online course completion and increase student retention.

Student Perspectives Regarding Online Learning

The perspective of students taking online courses is important to assess; yet only a few studies have focused on student satisfaction. The largest advantage reported by students to date is the flexibility offered in an online environment (Beard et al., 2004; Bellefeuille, Martin, & Buck, 2005; Benbunan-Fich & Hiltz, 2003; Madoc-Jones & Parrott, 2005). Studies are mixed with regard to students reporting feeling as though they were able to connect well with their faculty and peers (Olario & Trotter, 2010; Wilke & Vinton, 2006) versus feeling less well connected (Benbunan-Fich & Hiltz, 2003; Madoc-Jones & Parrott, 2005). Finally, while students generally do not report feeling less satisfied with pursuing an online version of the course (Pucel & Stertz, 2005), some studies report students stating that, all things being equal, they preferred a face-to-face environment to an online environment (Brown, 2012; Siebert et al., 2006).

Factors Leading to Quality Online Education

Educators in social work are engaged in a discussion on how to create an online educational environment beneficial to student learning and ways to use online environments to teach important social work skills (Anderson-Meger, 2011; Ayala, 2009; Benbunan-Fich & Hiltz, 2003; Maidment, 2005; Moore, 2005a; Siebert & Spaulding-Givens, 2006). A key element is using the online platform to promote a constructivist, student-centered learning environment where classes are designed around a student driven learning process rather than a "sage on the stage" approach (Ayala, 2009; Bellefeuille et al., 2005; Maidment, 2005; Moore, 2005a; Siebert & Spaulding-Givens, 2006). Anderson-Meger (2011) argues that online learning can be an excellent format to develop critical thinking. A blended approach (using online and face-to-face elements) is believed to enhance both online and face-to-face environments (Ayala, 2009). Reeves & Reeves (2008), in their review of the structure of an online health and social work education course, for example, provide important dimensions to consider when designing an online course, including theories of teaching and learning, orientations to goals and tasks, source of motivation, teacher role, support for metacognition and collaborative learning, cultural sensitivity, and the class structure. In addition, Cohen (2003) offers a comprehensive framework to evaluate distance education. Her six factors for evaluation are the process of teaching and learning, developing a community of learners, the instructor, the student, implementation of the course, and technology use.

Research on the factors important to quality online education is quite limited and has focused primarily on particular aspects of the learning environment. One study found that increased participation in discussion boards and similar class exercises led to higher grades in hybrid courses (DeNeui & Dodge, 2006). Another study found that factors associated with the instructor, such as instructor availability, effort to develop a community of learning, and availability to students, led to better online student outcomes (Benbunan-Fich & Hiltz, 2003). However, most studies continue to focus on grades as a primary outcome measure and do not look at the experiences of students or faculty. Our study, an exploratory investigation focusing on the beginning stages of implementing an online BSW program, attempts to go beyond looking solely at outcomes to also examine how students experience the process of taking online courses when compared to the face-to-face experience. Factors specifically examined were the process of teaching and learning, developing a community of learners, and the technology used; all are based on Cohen's (2003) model.

METHOD

This paper presents findings of a mixed-method (multi-methodology) evaluation of four equivalent BSW courses where the same instructor taught online and face-to-face sections of the course in the same academic year. Upon completion of each course studied, data were gathered using an online, anonymous survey of students and review and comparison of student grades in each course. Because the courses evaluated were taught by seasoned instructors with prior experience teaching the course, the key focus was to evaluate the experience of students taking the online section when compared to students in the face-to-face section.

The goals of this evaluation were to

- enhance the educational experience of online and face-to-face students;
- ensure that online courses were not leading to poorer student outcomes;
- learn more about student experiences in online versus traditional in-person courses;
- see how students report their study habits and use of classroom materials in online and in person formats; and
- find ways to build strong personal connections in an online environment.

Participants

The participants were students enrolled in one of the two sections (online or face-to-face) of each social work course offered. The students in the Introduction to Social Work course were pursuing a wide variety of undergraduate majors, while students in all other courses were upper-division students enrolled in the BSW program. (There are two sections in the BSW program, and students are assigned to a cohort that then determines which of two sections they will take.) The majority of students in both online and face-to-face sections concurrently were taking another face-to-face social work course. Overall, students in the BSW program are in their twenties (75%) or thirties (18%) or were 40 or older (7%). Approximately 50% identify as Hispanic/Latino, 25% as Caucasian, 16% as African American, 1% as Asian American, and 8% either as multi-ethnic or declining to disclose ethnicity. Approximately 90% are female and 10% are male. Participants in the online and face-to-face sections studied had no significant differences in demographic characteristics in terms of age, race/ethnicity, and gender and were representative of the total BSW population of this program.

Data Collection and Analysis

University IRB approval was obtained before beginning this study. The surveys were delivered using Survey Monkey to ensure separation from course content and were overseen by a faculty member not teaching the course being evaluated. (The only exception to this process was the face-to-face version of Introduction to Social Work, where the survey was passed out along with the final exam.) In the final week of each course, a request to participate in the study was sent by e-mail to all students enrolled in the courses, and a link to the Survey Monkey survey was placed on each class Blackboard site. In addition, administrative data was used to collect student grades.

Questions on the survey included a series of Likert scale items asking for participants to state their level of agreement (*strongly disagree, disagree, agree, strongly agree*) on statements in five areas: communication with faculty and classmates; study patterns during the course; perspectives on class assignments; satisfaction with the course; and technology/format used. Open-end questions allowed students to discuss the strengths and challenges of the course based on format and to give qualitative feedback. (See Table 1 for the list of survey questions.)

Survey results then were downloaded into SPSS 19 (2010). Analysis was completed using Mann Whitney U tests, comparing results of each question between the online and face-to-face class sections. *T*-tests were completed on the final grades of each class to determine differences based on course setting. Open-end responses were coded to uncover categories of responses and facilitate content analysis.

TABLE 1 Survey Items

Area of Study	Questions Asked
Communication with Faculty and Classmates	I got to know the instructor while participating in this class. The feedback provided by the instructor enhanced my learning in this class. How often the student communicated by: e-mail, phone and in person with this instructor (separate question for each). I got to know other students while participating in this class. I learned about professional communication in this class. How often the student communicated with classmates by: e-mail, phone and in person (separate question for each).
Study Patterns during the Course	How often did you use your course textbook? How often did you complete assigned readings? How much time did you spend reading course materials each week? How much time did you spend on assignments each week? (online only) How long did you spend online each week?
Perspectives on Class Assignments	The textbook enhanced my learning in this class. The additional readings enhanced my learning in this class. The exam(s) were good assessments of my learning in this class. The discussion boards enhanced my learning in this class. The discussion boards enhanced my peer communication skills in this class.
Satisfaction with the Course	Overall, I am satisfied with this course. Overall, I feel prepared for additional social work courses.
Technology/Format Used	The technology used in this course was easy to master. The technology support given in this class was helpful. I felt (Moodle/Blackboard depending on the course) was a good program for this class. I prefer taking classes online. Would you have preferred to take this class in another format? What made you choose your answer? What do you think are the advantages of taking the class in the format you did? What are the disadvantages of taking the class in the format you did?

Note. Specific questions were tailored to the assignment and course materials assigned in each course.

FINDINGS

Courses Evaluated

Introduction to Social Work was taught during fall 2010 face-to-face and spring 2011 online by the same instructor. It is taken by majors and non-majors. Study participation by students in the online section of this class was low. Social Welfare Policy I was the first of the two sequence courses taken by BSW program juniors and was taught as an online and a face-to-face course in fall 2011 by the same instructor. Social Welfare Policy II is the second of the two sequence course taken by BSW juniors, and both sections were taught as an online and face-to-face course in winter 2012 by the same instructor (who also taught Social Welfare Policy I). Finally, Human Behavior in the Social Environment (HBSE) I is the first of the two sequence courses

TABLE 2 Overview of Courses Studied

Class Name	Term Taught	Number of Participants: Online	Percent Participation	Number of Participants: Face-to-Face	Percent Participation
Introduction to Social Work	Fall 2010 (face-to-face) Spring 2011 (online)	8	32%	40	80%
Social Policy I	Fall 2011	19	79%	14	58%
Social Policy II	Winter 2011	10	43%	17	77%
HBSE I	Fall 2012	15	63%	12	44%

taken by BSW juniors and was taught primarily online (there were three in-class sessions) as well as face-to-face in fall 2012 by the same instructor. All online classes were designed to be asynchronous. Table 2 provides an overview of courses evaluated and participation rates for each class section.

Grades in Each Course

Grades were compared between online and face-to-face sections for all four courses. No course grades showed a statistically significant difference between the online and face to face sections.

Quantitative Findings

Four of the five main areas under study provided significant findings. These included communication with faculty and classmates, study patterns during the course, perspectives on class assignments, and satisfaction with the course. Table 3 presents these findings by course evaluated and area of study and puts forward the median scores in each section of the course. Only findings with significant differences are shown in the table.

Communication with Faculty and Classmates

All four courses had at least one survey item showing significant differences between online and face-to-face sections in the area of communication with faculty and classmates. All items were in the direction of online students' being less satisfied. In the Introduction to Social Work course, students in the online section felt they got to know their classmates less well than the students in the face-to-face section ($U = 235.5, p = .02$). In the Social Policy I class, students in the online section reported that they did not feel they got to know the instructor as well as students in the face-to-face section ($U = 213.0, p = .003$) and were less likely to find feedback from the instructor useful ($U = 2140, p = .012$). Students in the online section of the Social

TABLE 3 Quantitative Findings by Area of Study and Course Evaluated

Area Studied	Question	Course	Median Online Course	Median Face-to-Face Course	Mann-Whitney *U* Statistic	*p* Value
Communication with Faculty and Classmates	I got to know the instructor while participating in this class.	Social Policy I	Disagree	Agree	213.0	.003
		Social Policy II	Disagree	Agree	108.0	.001
	The feedback provided by the instructor enhanced my learning in this class.	Social Policy I	Disagree	Agree	214.0	.012
	How often did you e-mail the instructor?	HBSE I	Once a week	One or two times	48.5	.041
	How often did you phone the instructor?	HBSE I	More than once a week	About every other week	43.5	.021
	I felt I got to know other students while participating in this course.	Intro to SW	Agree	Strongly agree	235.5	.02
Study Patterns during the Course	What proportion of outside readings assigned did you complete?	Intro to SW	Half to three quarters	Quarter	59.5	.017
		HBSE I	Three quarters	Always	122.5	.046
Perspectives on Class Assignments	The midterm examination was a good reflection of my learning in this course.	Social Policy II	Strongly disagree	Agree	128.0	.008
	The advocacy worksheets substantially guided me through the advocacy project.	Social Policy II	Agree	Strongly agree	129.0	.002
Satisfaction with the Course	Overall, I am satisfied with this course.	Social Policy I	Disagree	Agree	211.0	.017
		Social Policy II	Disagree	Agree	121.5	.013
	Overall, I feel prepared for additional social work courses.	HBSE I	Agree	Strongly agree	49.0	.047

Note. Only items with significant differences between formats are included in this table.

Policy II class also felt they did not come to know the instructor as well. Finally, online students in the HBSE I course reported communicating with the instructor by e-mail ($U = 48.5$, $p = .041$) and telephone ($U = 43.5$, $p = .021$) more frequently.

Study Patterns during the Course

Students in two of the four courses reported different study patterns based on class format. In the Introduction to Social Work course, students online reported reading assignments other than the textbook in a higher proportion ($U = 59.5$, $p = .017$). The opposite was found in the HBSE I course, with online students reporting completing readings beyond of the textbook at a lower proportion ($U = 122.5$, $p = .046$).

Perspectives on Class Assignments

Students in one course reported differences based on perspectives of class assignments. Students in the online section of the Policy II stated that project worksheets were less helpful with their major advocacy project ($U = 129.0$, $p = .004$) and were less likely to agree that the midterm was a good reflection of their learning in the course ($U = 128.0$, $p = .010$).

Satisfaction with the Course

Three classes had differences in the area of course satisfaction and preparation. Online students in the Social Policy I ($U = 211.0$, $p = .017$) and Social Policy II ($U = 121.5$, $p = .013$) courses felt less satisfied with the course overall. Students in the face-to-face section of the HBSE I course felt better prepared to take other social work classes ($U = 49.0$, $p = .047$).

Technology and Format Used

There were no differences between online and face-to-face sections on any question in this area. In the area of technology format used, students were generally satisfied with the learning management system used for the courses (instructors used the learning management systems in online and face-to-face sections). Both online and face-to-face sections in all four classes reported preferring face-to-face courses.

Qualitative Findings

All students were asked for feedback pertaining to the advantages and disadvantages of taking the class in the format they were assigned. Results fell into four main categories of advantages and disadvantages of online versus face-to-face education.

Advantages of online education

The primary advantage of online education cited was flexibility. Some ways students illustrated this flexibility were "the class fit in their schedule," "allowed them to balance working and going to school," "work at their own pace," "materials for the class easily retrieved," and "not having to meet on a regular basis." A second advantage noted in all online classes was the reduction in transportation time and cost. In all online classes, however, some students felt that there were no advantages to online education.

Disadvantages of online education

The most common disadvantage to online education mentioned was the challenge in communication and exchange with the classmates and instructor. A common response from students in online classes was the lack of personal interactions with the instructor. Other comments were on having to wait to receive feedback and feeling the feedback given often was not sufficiently clear. Students also reported having trouble communicating with classmates. Other disadvantages noted included feeling confused about what they were learning, concern about the potential for cheating, difficulty in using the technology, and struggling with environmental distractions (not specified) when taking the class online.

Advantages of face-to-face education

The primary advantage noted by students in all face-to-face classes centered on the theme of communication and interaction with classmates and the instructor. The most common advantage noted was the ability to connect with and to receive immediate feedback from the instructor. This cohort also said the face-to-face lectures felt "more personal." Some student comments focused on being less able to procrastinate and having built-in reminders of assignments (because they needed to bring the work to class).

Disadvantages of face-to-face education

The most common disadvantage noted for students taking the face-to-face course was that there are no disadvantages to face-to-face classes! A few students in both classes, however, reported that class length and frequency were potential disadvantages. Very few students noted challenges with transportation.

DISCUSSION

Key Findings

Continued support for the "no difference" Hypothesis

The first finding is that none of these four courses showed significant differences in grades between students in online and face-to-face sections. None of these instructors, when asked, subjectively felt that students from the online or face-to-face sections of their class "performed differently." Because the assessments for online and face-to-face sections were essentially equivalent, it appears that taking these courses online did not lead to different academic performance outcomes. These findings are important to this program as they provide some level of comfort to those instructors teaching online (or preparing to teach online) that BSW students can perform equally well in an online environment. The data also support prior studies suggesting this variable need no longer be the primary focus of research (Ayala, 2009).

Students place high value on the in-the-moment communication present in face-to-face classes

A central observation offered by students was that they perceived the online environment to be missing the spontaneity and contemporaneous feedback of the face-to-face classroom. Remarkably, this theme was not reported in the literature reviewed for this paper. Many students felt they learned more face to face because they could have their questions answered immediately and instructors added more to their class lectures. This finding, of course, can be perceived as a flip side to the major advantage of online education, which students stated to be the flexibility of an asynchronous modality. Moreover, because they can be working on the class at any time, online students could not expect the teacher to be available when they were actually studying. Some students expressed a consequent anxiety by stating they felt uncertain of their learning in the online environment due to lack of instant feedback. This feedback is similar to that from other studies, showing some students feel less secure about their learning in the online environment, even in cases where their grades are equivalent (O'Brien et al., 2012; Ouellette et al., 2006; Pucel & Stertz, 2005). This outcome is one that we will be further exploring in greater detail to determine whether there are ways students could feel they were getting more timely feedback and additional support in the online environment.

Ability to fit school into other responsibilities is the key advantage of online education

Students in this study overwhelmingly remarked on flexibility as the key advantage to online education. As the majority of all BSW students work in addition to going to school and up to one-third of our baccalaureate students have child or elder care obligations, having the flexibility to work at home, in the evenings, or on weekends was a variable they valued. However, one student made a statement that the ability to work at home posed a challenge, as that student did not have a quiet work environment there. This issue of study environment and the impact it has on the educational experience of all students is an intriguing area for potential future research.

Building a learning community: Still a work in progress

When the instructors worked to develop these online sections, significant time went into developing ways for students to connect with the instructor and with peers. Discussion boards (where students were evaluated for the quality of response and their interaction with others), rapid responses to e-mails, and group projects all were part of each course. In addition, in all but the Introduction to Social Work course, students met the instructors in person prior to the beginning of the course, and most of the students reported using the instructor's office hours at least one time per quarter. Yet, in three of the four online class sections, students reported not getting to know their instructor or peers well. As noted, one of the two most common responses regarding online delivery was a feeling of disconnection from their instructor and to a lesser extent, their classmates. This finding is also noted in other social work research of online courses (Olario & Trotter, 2010; Wilke & Vinton, 2006) and therefore is an area that this program will continue to explore, with continued student feedback.

Online students study to the same extent as face-to-face students

A number of questions in this study asked for the amount of time students spent studying and whether their study patterns would change if the course were taught in a different format. Students did *not* report study pattern differences by class format. Online students read approximately the same amount and spent about the same amount of time studying as face-to-face students. There were no complaints from the online students that they felt they needed to study more than their face-to-face peers.

Limitations

Given that this was a pilot and exploratory study looking at a first run of online classes, there naturally are limitations to using these findings to generalize to all online or face-to-face BSW learning experiences. Low participation rates, particularly in the online section of the Introduction to Social Work course, make it more likely that responses came from people holding more extreme positions with comparison to the rest of the class. Moreover, the very modest sample makes generalization problematical. Finally, it is possible that there are characteristics of the California State University, San Bernardino student population and setting that make these findings dissimilar to those of other universities. As an example, for many of our students, the online social work class was one of their first such experiences. Finally, two of the classes (Social Policy I and II) had the same student population and instructor, so overlap of opinions between the classes is likely.

CONCLUSIONS AND RECOMMENDATIONS

Recommendations for Online Teaching and Course Development

The clearest message coming from comparison of online and face-to-face students enrolled in these courses is the perception that online learning provides fewer opportunities for in-the-moment communication and spontaneous exchanges among students and faculty. This poses a challenge for asynchronous online teaching, particularly when students are working on the class at times that are convenient to them and may have questions at times the instructor is not available. All of the faculty involved had an electronic discussion board specifically for questions or comments about the course, and the students were instructed to ask and answer questions on these boards. This option provided a quick response time, but from a student perspective, could not fully compensate for being able to ask questions in person. In response, an option might be to add some synchronous elements to the course, such as videoconferencing sessions, providing some in-class sessions, offering chat room options, or finding creative ways to help students benefit more from asynchronous communication.

An additional finding was that communication by other forms (such as phone, e-mail, or setting up face-to-face meetings) generally did not increase in online sections. The only exception was in the blended classes, where students met with the instructor monthly. This appears to signify that students are not reaching out more often unless they have some face-to-face experience with the instructor on which to build the relationship. Faculty teaching online may want to proactively establish synchronous meeting times with their online students, by phone, videoconference, or face-to-face, to initiate a connection to each student. With group projects, faculty could require some synchronous communications as well. Such synchronous meetings may improve communications and relationships for both students and faculty. Instructors also might use discussion boards more assertively in order to stimulate additional communication between faculty and students and students with one another.

Recommendations for Future Research

As we continue to implement the online BSW option, and expand online offerings to the MSW program, we will continue to investigate its impact. One area of research will focus on learning more about the students, the impact of the study environment, and similar contextual issues, such as employment and family obligations, where greater understanding of need may contribute to an ever more successful educational experience in online and face-to-face environments. Finally, we will continue to examine similarities and differences between online and face-to-face modalities as we fold practice courses into our online curriculum.

CONCLUSION

Despite the fact that online education has become the main form of distance education and is experienced by ever-increasing numbers of students in higher education, research looking at the factors leading to a successful online experience for students is an area that deserves greater scrutiny. Although students in the online course sections studied received grades equivalent to those in face-to-face classes and did not need to spend additional study time to receive those grades, online sections in this study were not as satisfying to students for the reasons that came forward from our research. On the other hand, the ability for students to pursue a degree, despite time challenges and distance from campus, are strong reasons to support this alternative format, and it is our plan to do so, innovating on the basis of the feedback from our continuing evaluations.

REFERENCES

Allen, I. E., & Seaman, J. (2013). *Changing course: Ten years of tracking online education in the United States*. Babson Park, MA: Babson Survey Research Group. Retrieved at http://www.onlinelearningsurvey.com/

Anderson-Meger, J. (2011). Critical thinking and e-learning in social work education. *International Journal of Business, Humanities, and Technology*, *1*(2), 17–27.

Ayala, J. S. (2009). Blended learning as a new approach to social work education. *Journal of Social Work Education*, *45*(2), 277–288.

Beard, L. A., Harper, C., & Riley, G. (2004). Online versus on-campus instruction: Student attitudes and perceptions. *Tech Trends*, *48*(6), 29–31.

Bellefeuille, G., Martin, R. R., & Buck, M. P. (2005). From pedagogy to technology in social work education: A constructivist approach to instructional design in an online, competency-based child welfare practice course. *Child & Youth Care Forum*, *34*(5), 371–389.

Benbunan-Fich, R., & Hiltz, S. R. (2003). Mediators of the effectiveness of online courses. *IEEE Transactions on Professional Communication*, *46*(4), 298–312.

Brown, J. L. M. (2012). Online learning: A comparison of web-based and land-based courses. *The Quarterly Review of Distance Education, 13*(1), 39–42.

Cohen, V. L. (2003). A model for assessing distance learning instruction. *Journal of Computing in Higher Education, 14*(2), 98–120.

Council on Social Work Education. (2013). Distance programs. Retrieved from http://www.cswe.org/accreditation/information/distanceeducation.aspx.

DeNeui, D. L., & Dodge, T. L. (2006). Asynchronous learning networks and student outcomes: The utility of online learning components in hybrid courses. *Journal of Instructional Psychology, 33*(4), 256–259.

Dutton, J., Dutton, M., & Perry, J. (2001). Do online students perform as well as lecture students? *Journal of Engineering Education, 90*(1), 131–136.

Faux, T. L., & Black-Hughes, C. (2000). A comparison of using the internet versus lectures to teach social work history. *Research on Social Work Practice, 10*(4), 454–466.

Hisle-Gorman, E., & Zuravin, S. (2006). Teaching social work research: A comparison of web-based and in-class lecture methods. *Journal of Technology in Human Services, 24*(4), 77–93.

Madoc-Jones, I., & Parrott, L. (2005). Virtual social work education: Theory and experience. *Social Work Education, 24*(7), 755–768.

Maidment, J. (2005). Teaching social work online: Dilemmas and debates. *Social Work Education, 24*(2), 185–195.

Marson, S. M., Weil, G., & Marson, B. M. (2010). Teaching social work values and ethics online. *Journal of Social Work Values and Ethics, 7*(1). Retrieved from http://www.socialworker.com/jswve/spring2010/1forum.pdf

McPhee, I., & Söderström, T. (2012). Distance, online and campus higher education: Reflections on learning outcomes. *Campus Wide Information Systems, 29*(3), 144–155.

Moore, B. (2005a). Key issues in web-based education in the human services: A review of the literature. *Journal of Technology in Human Services, 23*(1/2), 11–28.

Moore, B. (2005b). Faculty perceptions of the effectiveness of web-based instruction in social work education: A national study. *Journal of Technology in Human Services, 23*(1/2) 53–66.

Moore, M. G., & Kearsley, G. (2011). *Distance education: A systems view of online learning* (3rd ed.). Belmont, CA: Wadsworth.

Morris, T., & Poirier, J. (2009). Needs assessment report: Title IVE child welfare distance education pilot project for eastern frontier regions of Southern California. Retrieved from http://calswec.berkeley.edu/sites/default/files/uploads/title_ive_ar_2008_2009.pdf

O'Brien, C., Hartshorne, R., Beattie, J., & Jordan, L. A. (2012). A comparison of large lecture, fully online, and hybrid sections of introduction to special education. *Rural Special Education Quarterly, 30*(4), 19–31.

Oliaro, L., & Trotter, C. (2010). A comparison of on-campus and off-campus (or distance) social work education. *Australian Social Work, 63*(3), 329–344.

Ouellette, P. M., Westhuis, D., Marshall, E., & Chang, V. (2006). The acquisition of social work interviewing skills in a web-based and classroom instructional environment: Results of a study. *Journal of Technology in Human Services, 24*(4), 53–75.

Petracchi, H., Mallinger, G., Engel, R., Rishel, C. W., & Washburn, C. (2005). Evaluating the efficacy of traditional and web-assisted instruction in an undergraduate social work practice class. *Journal of Technology in Human Services, 23*(3/4) 299–310.

Pucel, D. J., & Stertz, T. F., (2005). Effectiveness and student satisfaction with web-based compared to traditional in-service teacher education courses. *Journal of Industrial Teacher Education, 42*(1), 7–23.

Reeves, P. M., & Reeves, T. C. (2008). Design considerations for online learning in health and social work education. *Learning in Health & Social Care, 7*(1), 46–58.

Schoech, D., & Helton, D. (2002).,Qualitative and quantitative analysis of a course taught via classroom and internet chatroom. *Qualitative Social Work, 1*(1), 111–124.

Siebert, D. C., & Spaulding-Givens, J. (2006). Teaching clinical social work skills entirely online: A case example. *Social Work Education, 25*(1), 78–91.

Siebert, D. C., Spaulding-Givens, J., & Siebert, C. F. (2006). Teaching clinical social work skills primarily online: An evaluation. *Journal of Social Work Education, 42*(2), 325–336.

Siegel, E., Jennings, J. G., Conklin, J., Napoletano Flynn, S. A. (1998). Distance learning in social work education: Results and implications of a national survey. *Journal of Social Work Education, 34*(1), 71–80.

Vernon, R., Vakalahi, H., Pierce, D., Pittman-Munke, P., & Adkins, L. F. (2009). Distance education programs in social work: Current and emerging trends. *Journal of Social Work Education, 45*(2), 263–276.

Wilke, D., & Vinton, L. (2006). Evaluation of the first Web-based advanced standing MSW program. *Journal of Social Work Education, 42*(3), 607–620.

York, R. O. (2008). Comparing three modes of instruction in a graduate social work program. *Journal of Social Work Education, 44*(2), 157–172.

Part 4: Creating Intimacy and Interaction

Being an Elbow: A Phenomenological Autoethnography of Faculty-Student Collaboration for Accommodations

REGINA T. P. AGUIRRE and CHAD DUNCAN
School of Social Work, The University of Texas at Arlington, Arlington, Texas, USA

Hybrid and online courses and advances in assistive technologies make accommodating students with disabilities ever-changing, requiring innovation. This reality, coupled with students' reluctance to disclose disabilities, points toward a need for replacing accommodations directed at those with disabilities with universal design whereby they become accessible to all—virtually eliminating the need for accommodations. In this paper, a master's of social work student (Chad) and his instructor (Regina) document their collaborations to revise a social work research course to meet his request for accommodations to make options more universally accessible. These revisions are done through reflections from both Chad and Regina from a phenomenological autoethnographic perspective—depicting their lived experiences.

The purpose of this paper is twofold: (1) to document a faculty member and student's process of collaborating to develop accommodations through autoethnographic[1] student and faculty reflections from a phenomenological[2] perspective and (2) to document the strategies developed through these

---

1 "Autoethnography is an approach to research and writing that seeks to describe and systematically analyze (*graphy*) personal experience (*auto*) in order to understand cultural experience (*ethno*)" (Ellis, Adams, & Bochner, 2010, para. 1).

2 The phenomenological perspective focuses on depicting the lived experience of a phenomenon (Moustakas, 1994).

collaborations not only to accommodate the student but move toward universal design[3] in the hybrid classroom.

WHERE DO WE BEGIN?—WITH CHAD'S PERSPECTIVE

In writing this paper, Chad sent me a reflection e-mail titled "Reflections from a Mirror I Can't See." It introduces our story:

> Having a disability makes other people nervous. Professors tend to rely on the student to have all the answers. A breakdown happens when even the person with a disability does not know what to do. A natural assumption is the person with a disability knows how to use the assistive technology. Trouble-shooting, however, becomes a learned skill of survival with mixed results.
>
> In an ideal world, state agencies and disability services provide the resources needed for a student to be successful. Not so in reality. Self-advocacy is easy to preach but is another barrier in practice. Professors, who may have a bias or just indifference toward accommodations, can be a challenge for any person. I'm constantly aware that asking for an accommodation is asking professors to make an extra effort when preparing their lessons. If a professor doesn't do the accommodation, or the accommodation doesn't work, I'm timid to go back unless the lines of communication are open. I feel like Oliver Twist asking, "Please, Sir, may I have some more?" I don't want to get out of an assignment, or to have an added advantage. I've been afraid to go back to a professor because I worried my grade could be affected.
>
> I just want to be me. I don't want to be the blind guy. I hit two minority statuses in social work classes: male and disabled. Social Work professors make me laugh by stumbling to label my disability: "Visually impaired," "differently abled," "sight limited," or "disabled." My response: "I'm blind." I got Dr. Aguirre when she said, "We'll figure out how to work with your disability." I asked, "What disability?" Laughter opens a lot of lines of communication.

REGINA'S PERSPECTIVE—HOW REGINA LEARNED ABOUT STUDENT ACCOMMODATIONS

Early in my doctoral education, I was fortunate to take 6 hours of instruction on teaching methods. We spent much time on learning styles and integrating

[3] An approach to instruction where "accommodations" are actually integrated in a way that benefits all the students, increasing universal access (Center for Universal Design, 2011).

technology to create a classroom—whether face-to-face, hybrid, or online—that would engage students with different learning styles (i.e., visual, aural, and kinesthetic). This preparation certainly created a "comfort zone" for me in using technology to improve my students' experiences. However, it only laid the foundation for understanding how technology could assist in improving the experiences of students with disabilities.

Later in my doctoral program, one of my professors asked me to share my notes with another student in the program; we'll call him Chris. I agreed. Chris is legally blind so he could neither see PowerPoint handouts nor take his own notes. Though his condition was explained to me, I still don't feel I understand what it is like to be Chris. He appears sighted and does not use a cane. What I could understand was his need for clear notes and not being able to write them himself. I was very ill during much of my doctoral study and relied upon classmates for notes on more than one occasion—notes that were not as helpful as one would think! So, I determined I would take clear notes and sat next to Chris so he could tell me when he especially wanted me to note something of importance to him. I learned that if I took my notes on legal-size paper, Chris could use a device at home that magnified them sufficiently for him. I also learned that properly contrasting colors in PowerPoint presentations and websites (e.g., white background with very dark colored text) made an incredible difference. Over time, I learned how much more Chris had to do just to keep up with the sighted world, yet he didn't let it deter him—his motivation was to surpass us all. I developed a respect for him that carried over to my teaching when working to accommodate students with disabilities.

REGINA'S APPLICATION OF WHAT SHE LEARNED

I primarily teach courses on research methods. When I became an assistant professor, I taught several semesters before a student declared a disability, and subsequently most of these have been in the form of learning disabilities. The first such student only wanted me to know of it; she did not want accommodations. She had something to prove. I would learn ironically over time that she was more the "norm" than the "exception." Many students, I discovered, keep their disabilities to themselves and simply work harder to keep up. When things became difficult—usually around mid-semester—I'd suddenly learn of their disability. At the beginning of every semester, I would ask whether a student had a disability. I wanted to know so that we could collaborate to make the class a pleasant experience and promote success. I thought perhaps this would allay any fears students might have about disclosing. Aside from that, I believed ultimately that it was a student's right to self-determination to not disclose.

REGINA DOESN'T KNOW EVERYTHING—COLLABORATIONS TO DEVELOP ACCOMMODATIONS

With learning disabilities, I found that students who requested accommodations mainly needed extra time for tests and assignments. These accommodations were easy to make and required very little effort on my part. However, I would learn also that creating accommodations could be a challenging and exciting process, allowing for creative use of technology. This eureka moment started when I subbed for a colleague—we'll call her Professor Rosado. She'd be giving a quiz that night and there wasn't much I'd have to do. Professor Rosado explained that she gives the quiz via PowerPoint—one multiple-choice question per slide. The students write their answers on an index card, then exchange and grade—easy enough. Then she explained that one student, Chad, is blind and, for his sake, she reads each question aloud. I remember thinking that was interesting; I wondered how he wrote his answers—maybe a note taker. I didn't give it much more thought than that. I subbed the class and gave the quiz. I knew who Chad was—the cane was a giveaway. I noticed aside from that, like Chris, he appeared sighted—clear eyes, clear glasses, appropriately focusing on me when I spoke, turning his head toward others when they spoke. The cane was the only way I could know which student in the class was Chad. Chad would later share the following assessment of Professor Rosado's accommodation:

> This really worked for me. I didn't have to schedule to take my test someplace else. I didn't have to worry about technology. I got to be in class like all the other students. I loved not having to ask for an accommodation. The professor took the initiative to address the visual and auditory needs of the students.

The next semester, I held an optional orientation session for my online research class. It is the first of two required research courses in our MSW program, and there was a lot of material to cram into an 11-week summer session. I arrived early to set up, and Chad was there. My mind began racing. How would this work? How would he "see" Blackboard and all of the materials there? Though I use audio files of all my lectures to supplement the class, it is all accessed through a visual interface. I took a deep breath and told myself that Chad was the best person to answer my questions. I had a few minutes before starting so went to talk with him. With both confidence and humor, he explained that he was a Mac user and that the assistive technology built into his Mac and his iPad would read everything to him—awesome! I walked away to start the session awed at his jolly and confident attitude—and also felt affirmed in my die-hard fanaticism for the Mac.

As I presented the format for the class, and the ins and outs of its structure, I heard many deep and heavy sighs from Chad. I made a note to check with him after class for his thoughts. Chad shared an important piece of information—he'd be out of the country for part of the semester. Having traveled internationally, often struggling with spotty Internet access, I was concerned for Chad. I asked myself, *Is this because he's blind? Would you be concerned if he were sighted?* I resoundingly answered, *YES! I would be concerned if he were sighted!* I had taught the class often enough to know that technical difficulties are a plague and that the shortened summer session would only make it more likely. I asked Chad what he thought of taking it in the fall and explained why. He agreed. Of course, no solution is perfect. In the fall, I'd be teaching the class face to face in a 5-week session in November, which would meet 2 days a week for 4 hours, each at a different campus. He thought it might work better, so we pursued that plan.

BEGINNINGS—CHAD KNOWS EVERYTHING (WE THINK)

In September, I began thinking about how I would present 15 weeks of material in a 5-week class. I remembered, too, that I needed to think of Chad as I prepared. I embrace the universal design approach where "accommodations" are integrated in a way that benefits all the students (Center for Universal Design, 2011). My first concern was how Chad would navigate the hybrid format of instruction I use. With a 5-week class, the hybrid format was even more important since much would have to be done outside of the classroom. Blackboard is how I deliver supplementary readings, along with PowerPoint, other handouts, supplementary videos, and quizzes. Blackboard is also how students submit assignments. How would this work? My "start with the client" social worker voice said, *Ask Chad*. His e-mail follows.

> Dear Dr. Aguirre,
>
> Well, best laid plans of mice and men . . . Blackboard doesn't work with my screen reader (VoiceOver); CourseSmart's eBooks said their books are accessible but they are not; and I'm falling behind because I can't read the texts. Other than that, I'm peachy.
>
> You asked what would I need. Now is a perfect time for me to advocate for myself. When presenting (like one of my current professors), please don't do the following: (Points to PowerPoint) "Here's my email," and changes slides. "My office hours are . . . (again points to the PowerPoint)." This was after I gave the accommodation letter and she saw my 64-inch white cane.
>
> . . . I'm sure anything you will hand out can be sent to me in a digital format. Test/assessments: not sure how you want to do those. I'll have my iPad; you can send me it; I can open a webpage or doc; fill-in the blanks

> and send it back to you. You said you have mp3s of your presentations, which should work better than trying to use VoiceOver on PowerPoint. I can't hand write very well. I can write a word or phrase; yet, since I can't see my own handwriting, it can be harder to read. Rosado was able to read my answers on her weekly quizzes.
>
> All in all . . . if you are presenting something and there is a visual component, I can't see it. Verbalize it and I'm fine. Rosado didn't have to accommodate me because the way she runs her class, she verbalized for every type of learner . . .
>
> Thanks for being open to working with me.
>
> —Chad Duncan

The description in Chad's e-mail of my colleague's oversights regarding "seeing" the PowerPoint made my heart sink. I thought to myself: *We are social work educators; we should get it! I'm going to get it.* I began working on revisions per Chad's direction. Blackboard was not going to work for him because we have a version that is not compatible with his screen reader (though other Blackboard packages are). So I planned to put PowerPoints, supplementary readings, handouts, and mp3s of my lectures on a CD for him. I also decided to audio-record each face-to-face class session and share those files with Chad and the rest of the class—a universal design strategy: Provide accommodations to all. I figured it might be useful for all the students to be able to re-hear the classes since we were looking at a grueling semester of only 5 weeks, with two 4-hour sessions per week. For the textbook, I had been toying with a web-based e-book for some time. I reviewed the content and decided it was quite similar to the textbook I already was using. Knowing VoiceOver could read most websites, I revised my course readings to this text. This would fulfill another universal design goal since it would cater to those who need to hear the text, like students with learning disabilities such as dyslexia. Ah, but there were more questions!:

> Hi Chad,
>
> I'm working out what I'm planning to do for the class and I want to ask you a question:
>
> For in class testing (if I go that route), can you use the iPad to take a test in Blackboard? Are you able to use the iPad to take a test using a word document?
>
> —Regina T. P. Aguirre

As I read this now, I cringe to see that I continue to ask about Blackboard when he said it so clearly: "Blackboard doesn't work with my screen reader."

However, true to his demeanor, Chad did not speak of my oversight but offered a solution instead:

> A word document would be preferable. I have headphones that would allow the iPad to read to me and not disrupt the rest of the class. Thanks!
>
> —Chad

Since Blackboard testing was not an option, I decided to return to in-class testing for the first time in 5 years. It would be a small hassle for me but worth it for Chad to have a closer approximation to his classmates' experiences. So, I could breathe a sigh of relief since, in my mind anyway, we had resolved all foreseeable issues. Now it was time to wait and see how things would go. His response illustrated the impact of such a small alteration; it made me sigh.

> I really do appreciate your willingness to work with me. I have been self-advocating a lot lately and it has been rough. Lots of closed doors, land mines, & making little progress. I am looking forward to your class!
>
> —Chad

IMPLEMENTATION—ARE WE READY TO RUMBLE?

I set out for my first day of teaching a familiar class (research) in an unfamiliar setting (satellite campus I had never taught at before) with an unfamiliar time line (5 weeks compared to 15) while charting unfamiliar waters (collaborating with a student who is blind to make the class work). I arrived early, with Chad's materials in hand—PowerPoints, supplementary readings, handouts, and mp3s of my lectures all on a CD. I was confident that I had everything he needed. Students started trickling in; I wondered how it would be for Chad in a new building. Would someone walk him in? Would he be offended or take kindly to my showing him where the restrooms and snack machines were? Was there anything else I needed to discuss with him? So many questions! I decided to wait for Chad to tell me his needs . . .

. . . And breathed a sigh of relief when I saw him enter the room with a companion. I made my way to the back of the classroom where they were and alerted Chad that I was standing before him. He introduced his companion as his wife, Jennifer. I felt like hugging her. What if Chad didn't have her? Deep breath—you're here to teach! I handed Chad the CD and told him all that I promised was there. I reminded him that any issues that arose we would work out together, but that he would have to tell me of the issues first. (I find that students assume I know of the issues and are then disappointed when I don't resolve them in a timely and effective fashion. I may be a professor and I may have a doctorate, but I don't know everything!)

As I said this, Jennifer had a look on her face that I couldn't decipher. Chad looked stunned. I waited and they indicated to me that what I was doing was not what they were used to receiving—another blow to the heart. What I offered seemed the least I could do, and they perceived it as such a surprise. *It shouldn't have been! I didn't have many details but repeated comments like these from Chad, and now his wife, made me think that pursuing his MSW degree had been one challenge after another*. I suspected I would learn more over the 5-week semester but needed to start class. He took a seat in the back. I immediately thought: *No! Not the back—you need to hear me at least!* (He must have heard me since for the rest of the semester, he sat in the front row.) Jennifer excused herself and we began.

INTRODUCTIONS, DAY-TO-DAY BUSINESS

As I noted, this class was unique to me for several reasons, including length and setting, but these students were in a cohort. They had begun the master's program together and always had class in the same room on the same two nights each week with the same 44 people. So, I had to introduce Chad and myself to their culture. As usual, I was filled with questions. How do I introduce him? Do I explain why he's in the class? Do I go into detail about accommodations? I decided to tell it like it is but to choose my words carefully. I welcomed the students and asked them to welcome Chad. I noted that he was not part of their cohort and thanked them for allowing us both to join them. I mentioned matter-of-factly that Chad was blind and that he and I had come to the decision that this class and its format was the best option for him to complete his research requirement. Done.

I thought to myself, *remember, Chad has noted that professors often say things like "as you can see, here is my contact information" and move on without noting it*. I'd have to remember that for my lectures, too. I was relieved that I'm not one to use much clip art, but I made a mental note that I would have to describe any images in detail so he could conjure them in his mind's eye. Then the questions came: What would I have done if Chad were born blind? How would I explain visuals to him then? Breathe, Regina—today's problems are enough for today!

FIRST FAILURES, ON THE SECOND DAY OF CLASS

In a class with 45 students that lasts 4 hours, making sure I would mix lecture with other activities was essential. I planned class activities in which students had to read a particular article or handout and then complete an in-class assignment in small groups. The first activity was to read a paper on the ethical issue of informed consent in research and then have small group discussions about reactions and solutions for making informed consent effective. I decided to check with Chad via e-mail before the second class to make sure VoiceOver was working:

> The eBook is AWESOME! . . . PDF is a picture scan. My readers see it as a picture —not a document. Leo at the Disability Office might be able to run the PDFs thru a software that takes the PDF and translates it to text. I am honestly not sure if he can or how long the process takes to return. Thank you!
>
> —Chad

Regarding PDFs and the eBook respectively, Chad later explained:

> University accommodation offices typically have a program that can convert the picture PDFs to text-PDFs called Optical Character Recognition software.
>
> I'm having to train myself how to remember what I have heard. Where do I store that information? I don't have the luxury of skimming the material. It is all read to me in a monotone voice that doesn't stress one word or another. I feel like Charlie Brown listening to his teacher. I actually have to know the information.

My reactions: Ah, a success and a failure; no time in a 5-week class to wait on technologies unfamiliar to us:

> Ok. Don't worry then about that article. We'll work around that one and I'll make sure the new ones are the other type of PDF. There are some PDFs your text reader can read, right?
>
> —Regina T. P. Aguirre

And Chad's response:

> Here is an easy rule of thumb, if a single word or paragraph can be highlighted, then a screen reader can read it. I had my wife check that article. The page highlighted but she could not highlight a single word. Does that make sense? I sincerely appreciate the extra efforts you're making. Thank you!
>
> —Chad

So, I altered the class activity for the second day and read a portion of the article aloud. It is the portion I wanted the students to focus on, and the added attention to it drove home my intended lecture points. Issue resolved—though not as gracefully as I would have liked, but we weren't home free. I reminded myself we would handle new issues one at a time. Yet, there was that burning question—Why does Chad continue to emphasize gratefulness for "extra efforts?" Is this extra? It doesn't seem it should be. Laws are in place to protect Chad—to help him get what he needs so he can have as close to the same opportunities as the sighted. What have been his previous experiences that make him so surprised by what, in my mind, simply are "reasonable accommodations?"

GETTING TO KNOW CHAD—REVELATIONS

At the end of the next session, a student asked whether she could address the class with a question. I agreed. She indicated that her daughter was recently diagnosed with a learning disability and that she was preparing for her meeting with the school. She pleaded that if anyone had advice, ideas, or resources, to please share. She clearly was very concerned for her daughter and terrified she would "slip through the cracks." Chad piped up confidently and assertively. I expected him to offer advice from personal experiences with his own disability. So, I was floored when he noted that he had been a special education teacher for 14 years. He proceeded to offer her important information about the process, resources available in the state, and how to advocate for her daughter. This raised more questions for me about Chad and his experiences in our master's program. I wondered what I was missing. I would find out in the next class.

EPIC FAILURE—CHAD'S DESCRIPTION, NOT MINE!

The next class was our first in-class quiz. I had the Word document ready to e-mail to Chad at the beginning of class as I handed out the paper versions to his classmates. He was ready with his headphones and iPad. We were both confident. The quiz began, and I stood at my computer station, working on a different project. I noticed heavy sighs from Chad. He continued to rub his eyes as if he were trying to focus. I looked at my e-mail; he had sent me a message. It wasn't working. I had e-mailed it as a Word document attached to the e-mail, but it wasn't working. Why? He sent me instructions, so I complied and waited.

I could see it still wasn't working. I walked over to check on him, squelching my fears with a self-directed, in-my-head pep talk that we would figure it out. Something with his iPad had gone awry due to a software update he had recently downloaded. Deep breath—I don't understand what the settings should be and don't know the iPad platform to know what to do. I can't fix it. He asked for the paper version. I wanted to scream: *You are blind! I can't do that! I'm not helping you that way! I want to help you! I want you to succeed! You are a special education teacher and should know better.* I could see that he was very upset, and my gut told me that what I was missing was that he was not used to being blind. I don't know how I knew this, but I was fairly certain that blindness was new for Chad, but this wasn't the time to discuss that. I needed to use my crisis intervention skills: help him see that there were solutions. I realized I could provide an alternative. There was an e-library with a Mac in the building so I asked if that would work, and he said yes. I offered him my elbow to walk down the hall. He politely refused. My certainty mounted—newly blind, something to prove like my other students with disabilities. I screamed in my head: *Let me help you! Accept the help!* The rest of the experience is better explained by Chad from an e-mail to his friends he graciously shared with me for writing this paper; the subject line was Epic Failure. The italicized text are his inserted retrospective reflections:

> With clouded vision from the tears, I blew it last night. Taking regular long semester classes and now added this condensed [research] class . . . I knew it would be a challenge.
>
> We plotted out—she'd send me a Word doc of the test. I'd use my iPad, listen to it and write my answers. Once I finished, I'd send it back to her.
>
> I get the test. Pages (the Mac version of Word doesn't open)—I can't manipulate any of it. I shut down that program. I go back to Mail—save the file. I attempt to navigate to Pages (which is on my second of four screens). I only have one screen. No Pages. Nothing that I've had for the last year. It is all gone.
>
> Panic breathing sets in. Deep sighs. My ability to work my iPad is failing as stress builds. I grab my phone—her e-mail will be the first e-mail—hit reply. "Please highlight and copy the quiz and post in the mail message body so I can reply and answer the questions. Please."
>
> (rational thought, right?) . . . professor is a Mac user. She does it. I get the e-mail (stress had me screw that up and it took me five minutes) . . .
>
> The functions with VoiceOver are different. "Why? Why isn't this working!?!?!?!" More panic breathing and tears begin to fall.
>
> (Two tragic errors—I've ONLY been using my iMac and the iPad functions differently. I had not practiced with it. Problem Two—I've never updated an iPad—I didn't know what I was doing but it reformatted EVERYTHING—that's why I didn't have Pages) . . .
>
> In the e-mail, I have it working—kind of . . . it isn't reading me the sentence but each word . . . that's ok. I can get an answer in.

I touch the screen—I enter my first answer. SUCCESS! Next function to go to the next word . . . when I touched the screen—I turned a rotor. NOW my iPad is reading one letter at a time.

Tears & snot bubbles . . . uncontrollable breathing. Every time I try to type–my iPad is switching between British English and American English. I can't get it to stop. PANIC!

I give. I ask for the paper version . . . maybe I can see it. Blindness & tears . . . impossible.

I was so desperate to make it work that I asked for the paper version. I haven't been able to see words on a page in years. I felt like I had to have the answer. I didn't want accommodations to take it later. I wanted to be treated like all the other students but my own emotions couldn't accept the fact that I am blind.

. . . she finds a Mac in the building. She takes me to it. Someone has locked it down—no assistive functions.

Dr. Aguirre offered to lead me properly (offering an elbow) down the hallway to the one Mac computer but I wouldn't take her arm. I was still in the mind set like the classroom. I could do it on my own. I didn't need assistance as I bounced off the walls of the hallway. So strong was my will in order to not appear vulnerable; meanwhile, it was obvious I was drowning in denial.

She's going to walk me back to class. I have to boo-hoo cry. I asked for a few minutes and I'd make it back. I cry and text Jen. Deep breathing. Refocus . . . it ain't how ya fall off the horse, it is how you get back on the horse . . . Find the bathroom—just hope is the MEN'S room—at this point—It wasn't out of the question to screw that up. Blow my nose. Deep breathing. Focus.

Walk out to where my class should be. A helpful person tells me that the door I'm standing outside of is not my class. Losing my focus. Two girls come over and helpfully start telling me that it is the wrong class. "Aw. You're lost. Let's go down to the guard and find where you are suppose to be." FULLY BLOWN tears and panic breathing. LOST IT, again.

Door opens—"He's in this class." She grabs my jacket and pulls me in. Vapor locked—can't speak. Tears falling. I can only shake my head. "Do you want me to walk you to your seat?" I shake my head no and tap the wall. Mouth "Thank you." Someone brought me a chair. Listened to the lecture and slowly refocus . . . I got my breathing back. Asked an intelligent question about the lecture.

I purposefully ended class early. I wanted to talk with Chad. I asked him how he was doing. And he confirmed my suspicion—He was newly blind. In the class I had subbed earlier that spring, he lost his eyesight. It had been just a few short months. All I could think was WOW. He told me the details of the struggles he had in other classes and of losing his sight. In a later e-mail (for writing this paper), he gave me this description:

> During the spring of 2011, I lost the rest of my eyesight during class. There are good eye days and bad eye days. This was bad and I decided it was due to allergies. It progressed for two more days until the majority of my visual field was lost. Two days earlier, I could read a screen on a computer or my phone but now I couldn't.
>
> Eye specialists probed and scanned my eye for some cause and a way to treat it proved fruitless. I spent the week crying. In one of my other social work classes, the professor had the students practice some solution-based techniques. I knew not to think of my eyesight so I thought about baseball. I hate baseball. "I'm not going to think about my eyes," I repeated.
>
> The professor asked, "If you went to sleep. When you woke up and a miracle happened, what would you see?" The first thing in my head was, "I would be able to see." Before a tear fell in class, I got out the door next to me and got to the bathroom. I boo-hoo'd for a bit. With puffy eyes, I calmly walked back to my seat. I was sure I had gotten away with it until the person next to me whispered, "Have you grieved your eyesight yet?" BUSTED!

Chad knew blindness was coming. He had been losing his sight for a while. His moment of truth was, when he was still teaching, a student of his raised a chair at him, and he didn't see it. His administrator voiced concern for his safety. Chad chose to leave teaching and pursue his MSW degree before his sight was completely gone. I was amazed at him. And now understood better. His sight was leaving slowly. He could feign eye contact; his eyes were clear; he could still (barely) make out text messages (in very large font) on his phone. He appeared sighted, except for his cane. I realized that this coupled with his unfamiliarity (or unwillingness) in asking for help, was what spawned all the gratefulness. He was in a liminal space—not quite blind and not quite sighted. And how could he know what he needed in accommodations for in-class testing? He was a special education teacher for students who were emotionally disturbed—not blind. I tried to comfort him and let him know we would work it out. I asked him to go home and just breathe, relax, and take solace in knowing that I would work with him. I reminded him that he needed to advocate for himself with his instructors as he advocated for his students when he was a teacher. He sighed heavily.

There was more to that story, but we both went to our respective homes. I had solutions in mind but knew he needed time before I shared. Here is the e-mail he sent to me later:

> Jennifer & I came home. I had to cry some more.
>
> We did not get to plugging in my iPad. She promised we would put Pages back on and test it tonight.
>
> Safety nets for future in class tests . . . bringing PC laptop; will use iPad to read; and Jen is going to wait around to trouble-shoot or read to me. Not being John Wayne—I can get up to the university early on Tuesdays & Thursdays to take tests at the OSD Testing Center . . . if anything goes wrong, they can fix it.
>
> At some point, I have to accept that accommodations are there for a reason. I'm not John Wayne and John Wayne was a character . . . .I will work on my newly discovered human status and be more open to asking for assistance.
>
> Sincerely,
>
> Chad

When I read this, my reaction was that we could do better. I did not like the idea of a PC laptop that was unfamiliar to him or of his wife having to come in and help. I needed to find a solution where Chad could feel some independence and could see that though challenging, his disability is navigable, given enough ingenuity and collaboration. I wanted to empower him. In collaborating with Chad, I knew that his Mac was a better solution. In my asynchronous online class, students take their quizzes online, at home, on their own computers. I decided to go this route for the entire class. Everyone now would take their quizzes online via Blackboard. And Blackboard would not stop Chad. Chad would receive his in a Word document that VoiceOver could read to him and then he could type in his responses and send the document back to me. And thankfully, this worked. We had hit a home run—finally! And, this was another step toward universal design since it opened the door for others who might be assisted, for example, with test anxiety, by taking the exam at home.

EPIC SUCCESS—TOTAL ACCIDENT BUT STILL A SUCCESS

Two activities I do in class for the sessions on qualitative research method involve showing clips from the movies *Instinct* and *Awakenings*. Both provide illustrations of observation as a legitimate data collection technique. *Instinct* also demonstrates both ethnography and phenomenology in action so I showed this clip first. I didn't think anything of showing these in class—Chad could hear, so he would be fine. I have taught this class many times, and I practically know the clips by heart and rarely watch anymore. I usually catch up on e-mail or some other task. Thankfully, I did watch this time. I realized quickly that there was much imagery for the ethnography and observation illustrations that was not narrated in some form. I jumped in and described what was being shown on the screen. I hoped it would be enough and that I had problem-solved quickly enough for Chad to not feel slighted. I asked him after class, and he said that the strategy worked well. Sigh of relief! I certainly did not want to be like the colleague who forgot to describe her visuals; here's a description Chad shared of a similar situation that did not go so well for another colleague—there but for the grace of God and good preparation go I!:

> Here is part of a conversation I've been having with Jimmy today [Another blind student]. I had to share. Too funny. Yes, I thought the same thing but didn't speak up.
>
> Begin forwarded message:
>
> . . . yesterday, when Amy was demonstrating on the board, pointing at things and saying "this" and "that" . . . I know you were thinking the same thing I was. "What the hell is she talking about?"
>
> —Jimmy

TROUBLE-SHOOTING PDFs—NO EASY SOLUTIONS IN "SIGHT"

Not surprisingly, many of my assignments in the research class require students to read scholarly journal articles. I did not realize it but, though the PDFs were in formats that Chad's VoiceOver could read to him, the explanation of tables with data was not always logical—and to my dismay, the solution is in the hands of those who make the PDFs, not the persons using the assistive technology. Here is Chad's explanation:

> Publishers have the ability to format PDFs to read tables of information. The majority of tables are read from top to bottom of a column before it reads the next column to the right. The reader does not have the ability to read a row of information if the PDF is formatted to read by columns. However, some publishers format the PDFs to read by rows allowing the reader to read the information from the first cell on the left to the last cell on the right of a row.

> This difference is important because my books will list the diagnosis in the first column, symptoms in the next column, and treatments in the last column. So, I would hear all the diagnoses, start at the top of the symptoms, and then by the time I get to the treatments, I have no clue what diagnosis is related to the treatments. This can be avoided if the publisher formats the books properly which doesn't take a lot of effort.

PLANNING FOR THE FUTURE—THE SECOND RESEARCH CLASS

As we "wrapped up" the semester, Chad asked me about the second research class. My head began to spin. This class is more difficult; I don't teach it but know its content and delivery plan well. (At the time, I was chair of our research curriculum committee and oversaw implementation of all bachelor's and master's level research courses.) My first question to Chad was: Does VoiceOver work with SPSS?—the statistical program used in the course. Long story short, SPSS was going to be a problem. It currently interfaced only with JAWS, an assistive software that costs close to $1,000 and, at the time we inquired, it was said to not interface all that well with JAWS. I did not think it fair to ask Chad to purchase a "so-so" technology to use for one class session on one piece of statistical software he was unlikely to use in his career. I consulted with the committee and we agreed that the assignments in SPSS could easily be completed in Excel, which is compatible with VoiceOver. In our discussion, I asked whether we could make it a universal design decision—that is, make the assignments in the second research class be in Excel rather than SPSS for all the students. The argument I made was twofold: (1) universal design is sound pedagogy and (2) more of our students would use Excel in their practice than SPSS. The committee graciously agreed and changes were made.

POSTSCRIPT

Chad has continued to have struggles that he has shared with me. However, his triumph, that I hopefully had some part in, involves his assertiveness and persistence in asking for the help he needs. He does this continually, although he admits it is exhausting and emotionally taxing.

Here are a few examples that illustrate other important considerations for faculty in preparing their accommodations.

Classroom Management

I had to speak up in one class with an instructor who didn't have classroom management skills. As she talked, so did several students. When she would get louder, so would these students. I was frustrated, and interrupted the class. My attempt at self-advocacy felt more like a plea. If I have one sense and that sense is overloaded, something had to be done.

Technology—A Double-Edged Sword

Technology hinders. As laptops become a routine part of class materials, distractions have followed. A student was in the back, playing a game muted; however, the 12 mouse clicks per 10 seconds let everyone know that the student wasn't taking notes. As listening became more focused, the mouse clicks sounded like thunder, as the presentation quietly went on in the background.

Technology Prevents Epic Failures—At a Psychological and Financial Price

After our semester together, Chad sought services from a state agency to require more assistive technology. When we worked together, he had had only the technology built into his Mac and iPad. In seeking new technologies, Chad was required to undergo emotionally taxing psychological assessments of his mental stability and his intelligence. I was upset by this; Chad is blind and simply needs assistive technology. Why did he have to undergo psychological assessments and intelligence testing? It seems a simple eye test would have sufficed. The hassle paid off, though I'm still not sure why the testing was necessary:

> I actually took a test in class. The professor, who is not techno-confident, gave me an eight-page paper test. Using the technology provided [by a state agency], I used a camera to take pictures (scans) of the page; allowed a $1,000 program to translate it into words; had it read line by line of the paper; used a $,1000 program to navigate the computer to MS Word; and then typed my responses. At the end, I e-mailed the professor my answers.
>
> BELIEVE ME—our technofailure was RIGHT in my mind. Two things worked . . .
>
> a) Prayer—not to do the test—to have the mindset to work everything; and
>
> b) The technology did exactly what it was suppose to do.
>
> It was awesome. I customized the program that read the scans, to have a proper British male voice. Then the program that was reading and navigating the computer (JAWS) was in an average American accent. It was very cool to have it actually work.

> Thought I'd share my success . . . (I wouldn't have needed the camera or fancy British speaking program if the professor knew how to use email or a flash drive.) The cost for all of this tech—over five grand . . .

Chad's later assessment of the experience:

> I must say there is a whole extra level of test anxiety when relying on technology. "Is it going to work? What is my Plan B, C, & D?" I freeze up when I think about the skills it takes to cover auditory comprehension. I've used visual memory all my life. I would remember where on the page the information was located and visualize the words. I've had to rework my cognitive processing. It is almost like I hear it, visualize it, and store where in the chapter the information is located as a reference point. Almost making it a kinetic memory. "Depression? Oh, that was chapter eight, with diagnostic criteria, treatments, and then in about the middle are medications. THEN it talks about how it affects different populations." If I can do that, I usually can pull the information out of my memory.

WHO IS THE EXPERT—STUDENT OR PROFESSOR? BOTH!

I have tried to demonstrate that my main strategy with Chad was to ask him what he needed. I viewed him as the expert; of course, Chad's expertise is still growing since his blindness is so new. When Chad and I began working on this paper, our original title was "The Blind Leading the Blind"; here is Chad's perspective on this:

> When Dr. Aguirre proposed the title, "The Blind Leading The Blind," I saw myself as the latter. Even though I was throwing out how she could accommodate me, she had better answers. Just like when someone assists a blind person walking somewhere, one does not take the arm of the blind person, guiding from behind. The blind person takes the arm of the sighted person. If I were being led from behind, I would be vulnerable to anything. From behind, obstacles are avoided by the sighted person thus giving the person being led a warning of a desk, book, or step.

To me, this passage shows Chad's growth. When we began our journey, he would not even take my elbow. He did not want to be vulnerable. Now he is noting that the help of others actually protects him, rather than increases his vulnerability.

MAKING FACULTY UNDERSTAND—SELF-ADVOCACY ISN'T EASY

Working with Chad, my constant message has been *Advocate for yourself.* He has taught me the toils involved, making me more committed to universal design, where classes become accessible to all, minimizing the need for accommodations. Here are reflections from Chad that illustrate some of the issues:

> We Are Not Trained—and I (Dr. Aguirre) am Proof of That! As a former Special Education teacher, I was trained how to make accommodations but I don't know if professors have developed these skills.

When I invited Chad to write this paper with me, I shared with him an article that was similar in format, using phenomenology and autoethnography. However, I forgot to check that it was in a PDF format that his screen reader could use. I thought I had learned! Here's Chad's reaction to my continued struggle to get it right.

> I got the BIGGEST laugh!!!! I tried to read the article–it is the picture PDF but I burst into laughter and I tried & tried to make it work . . . then I realized the irony that you sent me a picture PDF–I am honestly still chuckling.
>
> Students with Disabilities Have More than the Disability to Overcome. Students with disabilities have to fill out more paperwork and be organized. Able-bodied students have to worry about recalling the information for the test. Students with disabilities have to coordinate with the professor and the disability accommodation office to get the test accessible, scheduled to be taken at the testing center, and/or use assistive technology to take the test. We have to reapply each semester for these services. Nice? It is a paper form that those of us who are blind cannot fill out ourselves.

DISCUSSION

As this paper demonstrates, the classroom environment is often an obstacle to learning for students with disabilities. Laws protecting such students are created and implemented with the goal of "leveling the playing ground." Such disabilities include learning disabilities, such as dyslexia, and physical disabilities, such as deafness and blindness. Higher education faculty are used to accommodating students in the traditional, face-to-face model of instruction with such allowances as extended time for tests and assignments and audio recordings of lectures. However, with the advent of hybrid and online courses, accommodating students with disabilities requires flexibility and innovation by faculty (Roberts, Crittenden, & Crittenden, 2011). The rapidly changing environment of higher education (and students' reluctance to disclose disabilities) point toward a need for greater use of the universal design approach to instruction where the classes are designed to be accessible to all, virtually eliminating the need for accommodations (Center for Universal Design, 2011). The purpose of this paper is twofold: (1) to document, through reflections, a faculty member's and student's process of collaborating to develop accommodations and (2) to specify the strategies developed through the collaborations not only to accommodate the student but move toward universal design as a standard for the hybrid classroom.

Recommendations

Though much of the accommodations have been described earlier in this paper, Chad had additional recommendations that will add to a faculty member's toolbox in moving toward making better accommodations. They also may assist faculty who find themselves in the position I did where the student did not always know what to suggest.

> Handouts in the Absence of Screen Reader Options. Since I can't see the presentation or the handout, pairing me with a competent student to describe the handout was helpful. Also, if a professor notices a table layout has a long list of categories, with examples in the following columns, asking another student to go over the table may be a simple accommodation that will help the blind student comprehend the information more effectively.
>
> E-Books. As I listen to my eBooks, I wish I could take notes. As a sighted person, notes were my visual reminder, but now I don't have that ability. Reading a simple chapter of thirty pages takes me a couple of hours. I have to go back over the chapter a second time to reinforce the material. Four hours of a monotone, computer generated voice can be annoying. I don't say that to get sympathy. It is a fact of life for a blind student. I am grateful to be able to learn independently rather than having to always ask a person to read to me.
>
> PDF v. Word Document for Providing Instructions. Having to write a paper with a framework [outline], like a specific case file format, a professor could send me documents that contained the format; however, it is difficult to listen to the PDF, remember the specifics of the format, and re-create the framework on a word processor. Ideally, if a professor would create a Word document with the framework or heading, I would not have to go back and forth, re-listening to the PDF.
>
> In-Class Group Activities. For group activities, a professor found a student willing to read the activity aloud and be a scribe. Rarely in my experience has this been put into practice and I'm therefore often forced to not participate, just listen.
>
> In-Class Presentations. When I have had to present in class, I prepare a PowerPoint or outline and ask someone to read the first word of each

section to cue me to the next section. Since it is a PowerPoint, I practice and memorize the slides.

Formatting Word Documents. Some instructors have sent me notes on drafts in different colors & font styles which screen reading programs will read differently. Bold, underlined, and italics are rarely picked up by screen reading software. VoiceOver's default setting announces the colors of the text. It can be used to draw attention. (This also is read aloud.) An asterisk (*) also draws attention.

Delivering E-Files. Professors have sent me accessible PDFs via e-mail; however, the files were in a zipped or condensed format. Had the professors provided separate emails for each file, burned a CD, or transferred the files to my flash drive, I could have navigated to the files more productively.

Conclusion

Providing accommodations can be daunting for faculty, especially when they involve advances in technology unfamiliar to the faculty member. Metaphorically, we can offer the students our elbows, but we may not always know where to lead. From a social work perspective, the logical approach is to "Start where the student is" by taking his or her elbow, but the student may be as ill-versed in available options as the faculty member. The key to successful accommodations evolves from collaboration between the faculty member and the student—just as the best treatment planning in a clinical setting is a collaborative one between clinician and client. Presented in this paper are various solutions employable by any faculty-student dyad. However, our experience here suggests a strategy for problems not addressed in our journey together—collaboration! In the end, Chad and I were each other's elbows.

REFERENCES

Center for Universal Design. (2011). Principles of universal design. Retrieved from http://www.ncsu.edu/project/design-projects/udi/center-for-universal-design/the-principles-of-universal-design/

Ellis, C., Adams, T., & Bochner, A. (2010). Autoethnography: An overview. *Forum Qualitative Sozialforschung/Forum: Qualitative Social Research, 12*(1), Art. 10. Retrieved from http://nbn-resolving.de/urn: nbn: de:0114-fqs1101108.

Moustakas, C. (1994). *Phenomenological research methods*. Thousand Oaks, CA: Sage.

Roberts, J., Crittenden, L., & Crittenden, J. (2011). Students with disabilities and online learning: A cross-institutional study of perceived satisfaction with accessibility compliance and services. *Internet and Higher Education, 14*, 242–250.

Introducing Case Management to Students in a Virtual World: An Exploratory Study

JOANNE LEVINE
Center for Distance Learning, Empire State College, State University of New York, Saratoga Springs, New York, USA

RUIFANG HOPE ADAMS
School for Graduate Studies, Empire State College, State University of New York, Saratoga Springs, New York, USA

This paper discusses a small, exploratory study introducing students to case management using role-plays conducted in a virtual world. Data from pre- and posttest questionnaires (to assess self-efficacy regarding a range of case management tasks) suggest students felt more confident in their abilities after virtual role-play participation. Also discussed is preparing students for learning in a virtual world, some best practices to consider when developing virtual world experience, and larger contextual issues of increased broadband access to avoid exacerbating educational disparities.

INTRODUCTION

Case managers in professional attire sit across from their clients, military family members, conducting intakes at the "Adirondack Human Services Agency." Manipulated by human service students, they are avatars in Second Life, and the agency exists only in a virtual world. Located in different geographical locations across the United States, students communicate in real time as they take turns role-playing a case manager and a client.

The above scenario provides a glimpse of a virtual role-play where case management students practice intakes using avatars. Introducing students to learning experiences in a virtual world is more important now than ever before as distance learning is now a normative part of the educational landscape; over 6.7 million students were taking at least one online course during the fall 2011 term, and 32% of higher education students now take at least one course online (U.S. Department of Education, 2011). Evidence shows it is possible to effectively teach helping skills at a distance using web-based learning environments (Adcock, Duggan, Nelson, & Nickel, 2006; Moreno, Mayer, Spires, & Lester, 2001; Nelson & Erlandson, 2008), and 77% of academic leaders rate the learning outcomes in online education as the same as or superior to those in traditional face-to-face settings (Allen & Seaman, 2013; U.S. Department of Education, 2011). Despite this fact, social work education is only beginning to explore the educational potential of virtual worlds (Adcock et al., 2006; Moreno et al., 2001; Nelson & Blenkin, 2007).

In this paper, we discuss an exploratory study introducing students to case management intakes using role-plays conducted in a Second Life virtual world. Also discussed is how to prepare students for this virtual learning exercise, some best practices to consider when developing an introductory virtual world experience, and contextual issues, such as increased broadband access to avoid exacerbating educational disparities in the expanding world of distance learning.

VIRTUAL WORLDS: CHARACTERISTICS AND USES

A virtual world is a highly graphical 2- or 3-D simulated interactive environment accessed online, on game consoles, or on mobile devices by multiple users via an online interface. Other terms for virtual worlds are digital worlds, simulated worlds, and Massively Multiplayer Online Role-Play Games (MMORPG). Avatars and their environments can be highly customized by the players, and the resulting real-life simulation allows opportunities for collaboration and interaction (Childress & Braswell, 2006; Yee, 2006).

Interaction and communication occur both asynchronously and synchronously (in real time) through text-based mediums (typically e-mail and discussion boards) among a network of people without constraints of time and place (Mayadas, 1997; Jones, 2007). Increasingly, communication through broadband connections (such as a cable modem) to the game manufacturer's server (e.g. Microsoft and Xbox Live) enables players to speak with one another in real time during role-playing sessions.

While numerous virtual worlds exist, all have the following characteristics (http://www.virtualworldsreview.com/info/whatis.shtml):

1. *Shared Space*: Many users are able to participate at once.

2. *Graphical User Interface*: Space is depicted visually, ranging in style from 2-D "cartoon" imagery to more immersive 3-D environments.
3. *Immediacy:* Interaction takes place synchronously in real time.
4. *Interactivity*: Users are able to alter, develop, build, or submit customized content.
5. *Persistence*: The world's existence continues regardless of whether individual users are logged in.
6. *Socialization/Community*: The formation of in-world social groups is permitted and encouraged (e.g., teams, guilds, clubs, and/or neighborhoods).

Virtual worlds enable thousands of people daily to engage in recreational role-plays; and increasingly, online role-plays are being used for educational purposes. Online role-play is an experiential and interactive format. Proficiency is attained by a collaborative inquiry-based interaction with other learners; teachers participate as co-learners and act as facilitators. Learning emerges through interactions with other students via the technology that mediates students' interactions, either asynchronously or synchronously (Nelson & Blenkin, 2007). Synchronous e-learning

> "supports work relations among learners and teachers as more social in real time" while asynchronous e-learning "makes it possible for learners to log on to an e-learning environment at any time and download documents or send messages to teachers or peers." (Hrastinski, 2008, p. 52)

MMORPGs also provide educators with opportunities for developing learning activities that closely replicate "real-world" experiences. Second Life, for example, is the most widely used MMORPG in educational settings. There is a wiki (a website that all users can contribute to and edit) devoted specifically to how this virtual world can be used for such endeavors (see http://wiki.secondlife.com/wiki/Second_Life_Education/Resources). This wiki includes links to sites providing training in Second Life, videos showcasing educators, and direct links to a sampling of the several hundred educational institutions with virtual campuses. Examples of educational institutions with virtual worlds in Second Life include the Virtual University of Edinburgh and The U.S. Centers for Disease Control and Prevention.

The Virtual World: An Exploratory Study

Participants were undergraduate students enrolled in an online course focused on case management, offered by a state college located in the northeastern United States. In this course, students learned the basics of client assessment, collaborative problem solving, treatment planning, referrals, treatment team participation, record keeping, and outcome evaluation.

One of the course requirements was participation in an 8-week synchronous role-play to help students understand the reciprocity that exists within the case manager/client/consumer relationship. Students who did not choose to do this in the virtual world (Second Life) used a synchronous chat function available in the course. The students decided what roles (case manager or client/consumer) each would assume for the first case. (The roles switched for the next case.) All students examined cases involving two military families, and overviews are presented below.

> Case 1: Martin is a 31-year-old ex-marine, honorably discharged following service in the war in Afghanistan. He is married to a woman he met while he was in basic training. They have two children, a boy and a girl. Martin planned to be a career military man until, while out on patrol with his team, there was an explosion from an improvised explosive device (IED). Two of his close friends were killed, and Martin was found unconscious with no memory. When medically stable, Martin was sent home to the United States for treatment where he was diagnosed with a traumatic brain injury. Three months after leaving Afghanistan, his memory was completely restored except for the IED incident. One month later, Martin was honorably discharged and happily returned home to his wife and children.
>
> Martin's wife has a much different perspective. She feels that Martin had increasingly become more irritable, withdrawn, and disconnected from her. When he did speak to her and their children, it was negative and hurtful. He started to drink, and his behavior was becoming more and more erratic.
>
> Case 2: Tonya is a 34-year-old mother of two young children. Her husband, Bobby, is a paramedic and also an Army Reservist. He was deployed to Iraq shortly after Thanksgiving for his second tour. Tonya has been finding it increasingly difficult to make ends meet, even though Bobby's job is paying the difference between his military pay and his employment's straight pay. Prior to leaving, Bobby borrowed money against his 401 K, thinking it would last long enough to compensate for the lack of funds. Tonya, a stay-at-home mom, is worried she won't be able to make ends meet as the money borrowed is going quickly. Not wanting Bobby to worry about anything, Tonya puts up a positive front telling him that everything is "fine." In reality, she feels hopeless and lonely. Their 9-year-old son also has been having anxiety attacks, thinking that his father is going to be killed.

The virtual role-play was about conducting a case management intake with Martin and Tonya. The focus was on understanding the importance of information gathering and how it can be helpful in assessing the needs of the client/consumer. Students were presented with additional scenarios to guide their role-plays about the case management intake.

Virtual World: Role-Play Preparation

Prior to the role-play in Second Life, students participated in an online orientation developed using instructional design principles derived from cognitive load theory. Cognitive load theory posits that our working memory is limited with respect to the amount of information it can hold as well as the number of operations it can perform on that information. A major implication, especially when one is learning a difficult task, is that limited working memory should be used efficiently (Gerven, 2003; Sweller, Merrienborer, & Paas, 1998). When designing instructional materials, such as the Second Life orientation, it is critical to remember the limitation of working memory and how instructional materials may impact it (Kalyuga, Ayres, Chandler, & Sweller, 2003). Several researchers have examined the effects of cognitive load theory and instructional design. Their findings suggest that when designing instructional platforms for complex constructs, it is essential to consider the diversity in the educational and life experiences of the learner and adapt technologies to minimize extraneous or ineffective cognitive load (Jong, 2010; Mayer & Moreno, 2003; Paas, Renkl, & Sweller, 2003; Renkl & Atkinson, 2003).

In the context of cognitive load theory, learning served as a scaffold from the more basic to the more complex. Students were trained to successfully master Second Life access, avatar creation, and avatar navigation. For example, students first were given information about how to open an account with Linden Lab (the creator of Second Life and its virtual world platform), register with Second Life, and download Second Life client site application software. A drop box also was set up in the course management system so that students could post their avatar names in a centralized place. This created a record of the students' names with their matching avatar names.

A group then was created in Second Life that included all of the participating students who were given access rights to the virtual case management agency: the Adirondack Department of Human Services. Access was only given to students and investigators participating in this study to prevent any uninvited public avatars in Second Life from entering and disrupting the students' role-play activities. Students then attended a one-to-one scheduled training with an instructional designer in Second Life to practice chat or voice discussion at least once before conducting their role-play activity.

To further help with mastering Second Life navigation, an instructional platform in Second Life was designed to include the same case scenarios for the intake role play as was found in the web-based case management course platform. A virtual role-play intake office, housed in the Adirondack Department of Human Services, was created to reflect a real-life environment. In this virtual space, students were able to engage in synchronous voice or chat discussions (Figure 1).

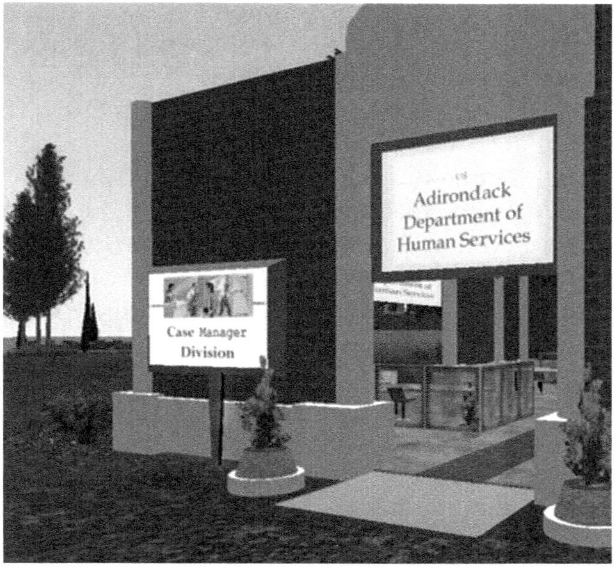

FIGURE 1 Adirondack Department of Human Services in Second Life.

Because virtual environments are very different than computer course management systems (Burgess, Slate, Rojas-LeBouef, & LaPrairie, 2010; Wang & Braman, 2010), it was important to make this introductory experience to a virtual world easily accessible to the students. Therefore, as soon as a student logged into Second Life during the scheduled time for the role-play, one of researchers immediately checked the student in, offered a teleport (direct and instant transportation), and guided her or his avatar directly to the virtual Case Management office location. By not proactively offering this assistance, these new users could have easily been overloaded and become lost and disorientated in Second Life (McKerlich & Anderson, 2007). Next, the avatars walked to the Adirondack Department of Human Services case management office and sat around an intake desk.

Inside the agency were two large posters that provided information needed to conduct the case management intakes. The role play session began with one student's avatar acting as a case manager and the other student avatar acting as the client. (For the second case, the pair reversed their roles.) Thus, everyone had an opportunity to assume the role of case manager and customer. Students communicated synchronously using either chat, voice or a combination of both.

Overview of Study

The study's objective was to explore whether participation in a virtual role-play could increase learners' feelings of self-efficacy (the belief that one can successfully perform the behavior in question) for tasks needed to conduct a case management intake. The theoretical framework was Bandura's theory of self-efficacy that enjoys a well-established body of empirical research support (Bandura, 1977; Bandura, Adams, Hardy, & Howells, 1980; Bandura, 1982; Sherer & Maddox, 1982).

Students were recruited from two online sections of case management and invited to participate via e-mails and course announcements. Students were informed that they would have to have adequate bandwidth (broadband) to participate. A total of 36 students were contacted, and 9 (25%) chose to participate. Institutional Review Board approval was granted, and informed consent forms were obtained from the study participants.

Study Design

Using a pre-and posttest design, students completed a 25-item self-efficacy scale during the first module of the course and again after participating in the role-play. A Likert-type scale was used for reporting whether *today* students felt very confident, confident, unconfident, or very unconfident in their ability to perform specific case management intake, assessment, and related tasks, such as developing a plan for providing case management; working collaboratively with a client; or responding empathetically to a consumer. All participants also completed a questionnaire about their demographics and their use of technology.

RESULTS

Demographics ($N = 9$) show all were female, with the majority (66%) ranging in age from 29 to 40, and some (22%) reporting they were a homemaker (Table 1) These demographics are typical for this college whose student body is largely composed of adult learners, 85% of the universe being 25 years old and over.

Participants' experience with technology (Table 2) shows that all used some type of social media, the majority had played online multi-user games, but only one reported any prior experience with virtual worlds. All students used broadband to access the Internet, which was consistent with the inclusion criteria for participation in this study.

Frequencies for the 25-item self-efficacy questionnaire were analyzed before and after the test for the 9 participants (Table 3). Items addressed perceptions of self-efficacy in three areas relevant to developing case management intake skills. The first area addressed basic case management tasks and skills, The second area focused on active listening skills and the third on foundational helping skill.

Pretest frequencies concerning mastery of case management tasks showed some students (22%) felt a lack of confidence regarding *providing*

TABLE 1 Demographic Overview

Item	Percent/Number ($N = 9$)
Gender	
Female	100% (9)
Age	
23–28 years	33% (2)
29–34 years	33% (3)
35–40 years	33% (3)
41–49 years	11% (1)
Employment Status	
Full-time	44% (4)
Part-time	22% (2)
Homemaker	33% (3)
Undergraduate Major	
Community/Human Services	89% (8)
Other Disciplines	11% (1)

TABLE 2 Technology Overview

Item	Percent/Number ($N = 9$)
Location of computer accessed for doing schoolwork	
Home	89% (8)
Work	11% (1)
Type of Internet access	
Broadband	100% (9)
Dial up	0
Age of computer	
Less than 1 year	44% (4)
More than 1 year	11% (1)
More than three years	33% (3)
Don't know	12% (1)
Online technologies used	
Social networking sites	100% (9)
Text messaging	89% (8)
Instant messaging	89% (8)
Cell phone for Internet access	78% (7)
Online multi-user games	67% (6)
Webinars	11% (1)
Virtual worlds	11% (1)

information for your client (33%) and *contributing to evaluation activities during the case management process* (22%). The majority (56%) reported not feeling confident about *assessing the social functioning of your client* and *developing hypothesis about the behavior of your client.* Posttest frequencies, however, showed all students felt greater confidence in their mastery of the above tasks.

Pretest frequencies about mastery of active listening skills showed that some students (11%) did feel confident about *giving feedback to your client,*

TABLE 3 Pre- and Posttest Frequencies for the Self-Efficacy Questionnaire

	Very Confident		Confident		Unconfident		Very Unconfident	
Item ($N = 9$)	*Pre*	*Post*	*Pre*	*Post*	*Pre*	*Post*	*Pre*	*Post*
1. Evidence ethical practices	11% (1)	22% (2)	56% (5)	78% (7)	33% (3)	—	—	—
2. Evidence best practices	—	33% (3)	78% (7)	78% (7)	22% (2)	—	—	—
3. Evidence diversity – competent practice	11% (1)	22% (2)	56% (5)	67% (6)	44% (3)	11% (1)	—	—
4. Develop a case management plan	11%(1)	56% (5)	44% (4)	44% (4)	44% (4)	—	—	—
5. Seek good fit between services and client's life	11% (1)	33% (3)	67% (6)	67% (6)	22%(2)	—	—	—
6. Give feedback to your client	—	67% (6)	89% (8)	33% (3)	11% (1)	—	—	—
7. Request feedback from your clients	—	56% (5)	78% (7)	44% (4)	22% (2)	—	—	—
8. Identify dynamics in your relationship with client	11% (1)	22% (2)	44% (4)	78% (7)	33% (3)	—	—	—
9. Work collaboratively with your client	22% (2)	56% (5)	78% (7)	44% (4)		—	—	—
10. Encourage participation of your client	33% (3)	56% (5)	44% (4)	44% (4)	22% (2)	—	—	—
11. Respond empathically to your client	33% (3)	67% (6)	56% (5)	33% (3)	11% (1)	—	—	—
12. Keep your client on task	33% (1)	22% (2)	78% (7)	78% (7)	11% (1)	—	—	—
13. Requesting information from your client	33% (3)	67% (6)	(56% 5)	33% (3)	11% (1)	—	—	—
14. Request disclosure of opinions and feelings from your client.	22% (2)	44% (4)	56% (5)	56% (5)	11% (1)	—	11% (1)	—
15. Provide information for your client	33% (3)	67% (6)	56% (5)	33% (3)	11% (1)	—	—	—
16. Disclose opinions and feelings with your client	11% (1)	44% (4)	56% (5)	56% (5)	33% (3)	—	—	—
17. Assess the social functioning of your client	11% (1)	33% (3)	33% (3)	67% (6)	56% (5)	—	—	—
18. Identify the personal characteristics of your client	11% (1)	22% (2)	56% (5)	78% (7)	33% (3)	—	—	—
19. Develop hypothesis about the behavior of your client	—	11% (1)	44% (4)	89% (8)	56% (5)	—	—	—
20. Develop overarching purpose and set goals, objectives, and outcome measures for your client	11% (1)	22% (2)	33% (3)	89% (8)	56% (5)	—	—	—
21. Employ contextual factors in interpreting individual behaviors	—	11% (1)	44% (4)	78% (7)	56% (5)	11% (1)	—	—
22. Conduct evaluation of one's leadership style	—	22% (2)	78% (7)	78% (7)	22% (2)	—	—	—
23. Engage in self-evaluation of personally selected performance goals	11% (1)	11% (1)	89% (8)	78% (7)	—	11% (1)	—	—
24. Contribute to evaluation activities during the case management process	22% (2)	22% (2)	67% (6)	78% (7)	11% (1)	—	—	—
25. Provide appropriate self-disclosure	22% (2)	56% (5)	33% (3)	44% (4)	44% (4)	—	—	—

responding empathically to clients, keeping your client on task, and *request disclosure of opinions and feelings from your clients*. Yet, a greater percentage of students (22%) did not feel confident about *requesting feedback from your client, encouraging participation of your client, disclosing opinions and feelings with your client* (33%; item 16), *identifying dynamics in your relationship with your client* (33%), *provide appropriate self-disclosure* (44%), and *assessing the social functioning of your client* (56%). In contrast, posttest frequencies showed no students reported feeling unconfident or very unconfident for *any* of the above items. Instead, students reported feeling very confident or confident for each item above.

Pretest frequencies for their mastery of foundational helping skills show a great majority of students (89%) felt very confident they could *engage in self-evaluation of personally selected performance goals*. In contrast, students reported a lack of confidence in their ability to *evidence best practices*, (33%) *evidence ethical practices, identify personal characteristics of your client, evidence diversity–competent practice* (44%), and *employ contextual factors in interpreting individual behaviors* (56%). Nevertheless, in the posttest responses, each student reported increased confidence in their mastery of each of the above helping skills.

DISCUSSION

This small exploratory study elicited valuable information about the benefits and challenges of teaching case management in a virtual world, which we hope will be helpful to consider for future efforts. The benefits of virtual-world role-play would appear to be both tangible and intangible. Intangible benefits arise from the accommodations for geographic constraint offered by virtual worlds. In this case, students from different parts of the state (and country) were able to role-play together. Exposure to diverse perspectives, born from different regions of this country and the world-at-large, is an intangible but extremely valuable learning experience. This would not have been possible in a face-to-face classroom.

Tangible benefits are suggested by posttest data and students' reflections. As discussed above, after the virtual role-play, students reported feeling more confident about a range of basic case management tasks, active listening expertise, and foundational helping skills. During the role-play, students were able to communicate in real time while observing the body language of their avatars and those of their classmates. As an experiential and interactive teaching method, this virtual role-play enabled learning by rehearsal, simulation, and feedback (Roschelle, 2010).

The beneficial nature of this learning experience is further supported by students' reflections. Through experiencing the dual perspectives of case manager *and* client, they developed greater empathy about the challenges experienced by both parties. One student commented, "I think this role play helps you to step into clients' shoes and see what they see. When the case manager asks a random question you understand how confusing it can be for the client who has no idea why it was asked." Another reflected, "By experiencing the intake process from the perspective of a disgruntled client, it taught me about what it might be like to be forced into a case management situation." Yet another observed,

> My case manager seemed a little passive and rushed to get the intake process over instead of asking questions about my past, present and future. I believe that case managers should not pacify their clients because the session will get lost; I believe this is what happened in my intake. I do empathize with the case manager because the intake process could be frustrating and tedious when you have a client that does not want to cooperate. In my next session as the client and the case manager I will listen more and do a lot less talking and try to provide more information.

Introducing case management in a virtual world also poses challenges. Students in this study were fortunate to participate in an online orientation through which they learned the skills needed for navigating in this virtual world. However, many human service programs may lack the institutional infrastructure for developing and implementing virtual world learning experiences (e.g., not having instructional designers, or a dearth of instructors knowledgeable about virtual worlds, and their potential for teaching and learning).

Another challenge lies in the need for broadband in order to access a virtual world without experiencing technical problems. While this study did not examine reasons for non-participation, interestingly, only 25% of case management students chose to participate in the virtual-world role-play. The inclusion criterion of broadband access may have been a barrier for some. While beyond the purview of this study, the lack of broadband access in the United States is a larger policy issue impacting distance learning. With an overall goal to help millions of Americans to have affordable access to broadband, a National Broadband Plan now is mandated by The American Recovery and Reinvestment Act of 2009. This Plan includes specific recommendations to support and promote online learning to address ". . . new demands of an information based economy" (National Broadband Plan, 2009). Educational achievement gaps are causing the United States, "when measured against international benchmarks, to lag significantly behind other advanced nations in preparing its students" (National Broadband Plan, Chapter 11: "Education," 2009). The growth of distance learning, including educational uses for virtual worlds, further highlights the need for access to affordable broadband technology for all of our citizens (Warburton, 2009).

Limitations of the Study

This was an exploratory study with several limitations. First, the sample size was small. Replication with a larger sample would enable meaningful statistical comparisons and provide additional qualitative data. Second, all participants were female. Third, the demographics of these undergraduate students were not representative since most were nontraditional adult learners. Finally, these students already were taking online courses, which necessitated some prior mastery of technology-mediated learning environments. All of these factors would hinder generalizing the findings to the larger population of undergraduate human service students.

Conclusion and Suggested Best Practices

The need to assess learning in virtual worlds will continue to evolve (Burgess et al., 2010). There also is a growing demand for virtual-world empirical studies both to guide the direction of instructional design in 3-D settings (Jarmon, Traphagan, Mayrath, & Trivedi, 2009), and the development of effective virtual world learning environments (Kluge & Riley, 2008; Nelson & Erlandson, 2008).

Finally, emerging from this exploratory study are some suggested best practices to consider when implementing an introductory educational experience in a virtual world.

1. *Select a virtual world that has already been used for educational purposes.* There are many virtual worlds from which to choose. Selecting one that has already been used for educational purposes (such as Second Life) makes it possible to network with other educators and receive assistance through a wiki, FAQ, or other forum specifically geared toward the needs of educators and educational institutions.
2. *Select a virtual world that is an open educational resource (OER).* OERs are free to use, thereby avoiding students or instructors incurring any additional fees for participating in a virtual world learning experience.
3. *Orient students to the virtual world prior to engaging in the learning experience.* It is important for students to be able to navigate their avatars and use communication tools prior to engaging in the formal learning experience. As discussed, consideration of the diversity of the learners' experiences and scaffolding learning new tasks (from the simplest to the complex) helps minimize ineffective cognitive load. If possible, collaborate with an instructional designer who can develop an online training component that will take these factors into account. If access to an instructional designer is not possible, point students to tutorials designed by the virtual world community to help new users.
4. *Provide clear inclusion criteria for technology requirements.* Virtual worlds require substantial bandwidth to work. Therefore, students and

instructors must know upfront what the technical requirements will be including whether the virtual world will work on either a PC or Mac. Unfortunately, some may not be able to participate in the learning experience if they do not have access to broadband or a compatible operating system. However, providing clear inclusion criteria for technology requirements will prevent frustration and possible abandonment of the virtual world learning experience.

REFERENCES

Adcock, A., Duggan, M., Nelson, E., & Nickel, N. (2006). Teaching effective helping skills at a distance: The development of Project CATHIE. *The Quarterly Review of Distance Education*, *7*(4), 349–360.

Allen, E. I., & Seaman, J. (2013). Changing course: Ten years of tracking online education in the United States. *Babson Survey Research Group*. Retrieved from http://www.onlinelearningsurvey.com/reports/changingcourse.pdf

Bandura, A. (1977). Self-efficacy: Toward a unifying theory of behavioral change. *Psychological Review*, *84*, 191–215.

Bandura, A. (1982). Self-efficacy mechanisms in human agency. *American Psychologist*, *37*, 122–147.

Bandura, A., Adams, N. E., Hardy, A. B., & Howells, G. N. (1980). Tests of the generality of self-efficacy theory. *Cognitive Therapy and Research*, *4*, 39–66.

Burgess, M. L., Slate, J. R., Rojas-LeBouef, A., & LaPrairie, K. (2010). Teaching and learning in Second Life: Using the community of inquiry (CoI) model to support online instruction with graduate students in instructional technology. *Internet and Higher Education*, *13*, 84–88.

Childress, M. D., & Braswell, R. (2006). Using massively multiplayer online role-playing games for online learning. *Distance Education*, *27*(2), 187–197.

Gerven, V. P. (2003). The efficiency of multimedia learning into old age. *British Journal of Educational Psychology*, *73*(4), 489–505.

Hrastinski, S. (2008). Asynchronous and synchronous e-learning. *Educause Quarterly*, *4*, 51–55.

Jarmon, L., Traphagan, T., Mayrath, M., & Trivedi, A. (2009). Virtual world teaching, experiential learning, and assessment: An interdisciplinary communication course in Second Life. *Computers & Education*, *53*, 169–182.

Jones, S. (2007). Adding value to online role-plays: Virtual situated learning environments. Paper presented at the Proceedings of the Australasian Society for Computers in Tertiary Education, Singapore, December 2–5.

Jong, T. D. (2010). Cognitive load theory, educational research, and instructional design: Some food for thought. *Journal Instructional Science*, *38*, 105–134. doi:10.1007/s11251-009-9110-0

Kalyuga, S., Ayres, P., Chandler, P., & Sweller, J. (2003). The expertise reversal effect. *Educational Psychologist*, *38*(1), 23–31.

Kluge, S., & Riley, L. (2008). Teaching in virtual worlds: Opportunities and challenges. *Science and Information Technology*, *5*, 127–135.

Mayadas, F. (1997). Asynchronous learning networks: A Sloan foundation perspective. *Journal of Asynchronous Learning Networks*, *1*(1), 1–16.

Mayer, R. E., & Moreno, R. (2003). Nine ways to reduce cognitive load in multimedia learning. *Educational Psychologist*, *38*(1), 43–52.

McKerlich, R., & Anderson, T. (2007). Community of inquiry and learning in immersive environments. *Journal of Asynchronous Learning Networks, 11*, 35–52.

Moreno, R., Mayer, R. E, Spires, H. A., & Lester, J. C. (2001). The case for social agency in computer-based teaching: Do students learn more deeply when they interact with animated pedagogical agents? *Cognition and Instruction, 19*, 177–213.

National Broadband Plan. (2009). Retrieved from http://www.broadband.gov/plan/

Nelson, D., & Blenkin, C. (2007). The power of online role-play simulations: Technology in nursing education. *International Journal of Nursing Education Scholarship*, *4*(1), 1–12.

Nelson, B. C., & Erlandson, B. E. (2008). Managing cognitive load in educational multi-user virtual environments: Reflection on design practices. *Education Tech Research Development*, *56*, 619–641.

Paas, F., Renkl, A., & Sweller, J. (2003). Cognitive load theory andinstructional design: Recent developments. *Educational Psychologist*, *38*(1), 1–4.

Renkl, A., & Atkinson, R. K. (2003). Structuring the transition from example study to problem solving in cognitive skill acquisition: A cognitive load perspective. *Educational Psychologist*, *38(1)*, 15–22.

Roschelle, J. (2010). Learning in interactive environments: Prior knowledge and new experience. Retrieved from http://www.exploratorium.edu/IFI/resources/museameducation/priorknowledge.html

Sherer, M., & Maddux, J. (1982). The Self-Efficacy Scale: Construction and validation. *Psychological Reports*, *51*, 663–671

Sweller, J., Merrienborer, J. J. G., & Paas, F. G. W. C. (1998). Cognitive architecture and instructional design. *Educational Psychology Review*, *10(3)*, 251–295.

U.S. Department of Education, Institute of Education Sciences–National Center for Education Statistics. (2011). Fast facts: Distance education. Retrieved from http://nces.ed.gov/fastfacts/display.asp?id=80

Wang, Y., & Braman, J. (2010). Extending the classroom through Second Life. *Journal of Information Systems Education*, *20*(2), 235–247.

Warburton, S. (2009). Second Life in higher education: Assessing the potential for the barriers to deploying virtual worlds in learning and teaching. *British Journal of Educational Technology*, *40*(3), 414–426.

What is a Virtual World? (n.d.). Retrieved from http://www.virtualworldsreview.com/info/whatis.shtml

Yee, N. (2006). The psychology of MMORGs: Emotional investment, motivations, relationship formations, and problematic usage. In R. Schroeder and A. Axelsson (Eds.), *Avatars at work and play: Collaboration and interaction in shared virtual environments* (pp. 187–207). London, UK: Springer-Verlag.

Meeting Professional Competencies through Specialized Distance Education: The McMaster University Addiction Studies Program

RICK CSIERNIK
School of Social Work, King's University College, University of Western Ontario, London, Ontario, Canada

CHRISTIE McGAGHRAN
Addiction Studies Program, McMaster University, Hamilton, Ontario, Canada

Historically, addiction has been an area in which Canadian social workers have received limited formal education. This reality led to the development of 18 core technical competencies through the auspices of the Canadian Centre on Substance Abuse in 2006. A survey of Canadian schools and faculties of social work found that social work students might obtain a grounding in many of these competencies, however, there was no certainty of this. An option now for those interested in becoming more proficient in this field of addiction is a specialized distance education program developed by McMaster University in Hamilton, Ontario. Along with meeting the majority of the core competencies, there are several other attributes that make this program unique. It offers 27 distinct addiction-specific course options at both an introductory and an advanced level; has continuous enrollment allowing students to begin a course at the beginning of any month; has no minimum course load requirement; and meets the academic requirements for optional certification through the Canadian Addiction Counselors Certification Federation. In a nation like Canada, with a small population spread across a large geographic area, the Addiction Studies Program may serve as a template for offering specialized distance education to enhance professional competencies and thus better prepare social workers to serve community needs.

INTRODUCTION

The moral model view of addiction remains pervasively attached to those misusing and abusing psychoactive drugs in our society. A disproportionate number of social work clients with addiction issues come from marginalized groups including First Nations, those involved with the criminal justice system, and individuals with mental health issues. It therefore has been argued that those with addiction issues are among the most oppressed groups with whom social workers engage (Csiernik & Rowe, 2010). Hence, it is not surprising that there has been a historic concern about the lack of sufficient education and training in the addiction field for professional social workers and other helping professionals (Fornili & Haack, 2005; Keller & Dermatis, 1999; Miller, Scarborough, Clark, Leonard, & Keziah, 2010). This realization may be one contributing factor to why there is more professional turnover in this practice area than in human services in general (White & Garner, 2011).

Those working in the Canadian addiction field come not only from social work but from a variety of professional backgrounds, including psychology, nursing, medicine, family counseling, child and community work, along with a small number who obtain specific degrees or diplomas in addiction studies. As well, there remains a portion of the Canadian addiction workforce who have as their primary employment credential their own personal experiences and recovery from the abuse of psychoactive substances (Ogborne & Graves, 2005). In the interdisciplinary field of addiction counseling, health promotion, and prevention, social work historically has not been the predominant profession. With the professionalization of the addiction field, more social workers have been entering this practice area over the past two decades. However, there is still no obligation or accreditation expectation for any social worker educated in Canada to have knowledge of psychoactive drugs or addiction. Presently, no faculty or school of social work mandates that either undergraduate or graduate level students take a course in the addictions (Graves, Csiernik, Foy, & Cesar, 2009).

COMPETENCY-BASED EDUCATION IN ADDICTION

Freeman and Lewis (1998) defined a competent learner as an individual who has reached a defined standard of performance. In 2006, the Workforce Development Division of the Canadian Centre on Substance Abuse (CCSA) collaborated with a range of stakeholders from across Canada to establish a set of core competencies in order to further enhance professionalism and evidence informed practice in the field (CCSA, 2007). However, competency-based education is not without controversy in social work (Csiernik, Vitali, & Gordon, 2000; Hancock, Echlin, Hallberg, Lewis, Liston, & West, 2003; Vitali, 2010). The traditional goal of professional programs in post-secondary settings has been to educate and enlighten, while competency-based education has been critiqued as being reductionist, technical, and bureaucratically driven, leading instead to deprofessionalization of a field of study (Csiernik et al., 2000; Hyland, 1995). Still, since social work education has a focus upon preparing students to engage in professional practice, competency-based education has been argued to be a good fit with social work, both as an academic discipline and a professional program (Clark & Arkava, 1979; Grant, 1979; O'Hagan, 1996; Phillips, 2011). It is an approach that advocates for and attempts to provide measurable knowledge, skills, and behaviors at the end of a course or an entire educational program (Richards & Rodgers, 2001). Competencies are specific, assessable skills, knowledge, and values needed to effectively perform a particular function that can be readily measured against an agreed benchmark of standards (Marrelli, 2001; Mirabile, 1997).

In the United Kingdom, National Occupational Standards for entry-level social workers have long been established (Training Organisation for the Personal Social Services, 2002). With respect to the addictions in the United States, in 1993 the Center for Substance Abuse Treatment created the Addiction Technology Transfer Center Program to better prepare the addiction treatment professional in America for the field, resulting in the development of 121 competencies for practice (Horavitch & Wergin, 1998). Using this as a foundation, the U.S. Substance Abuse and Mental Health Services Administration (1998) developed an outline of the knowledge, skills, and attitudes required for providing competent addiction counseling. The report (which has since been updated) identified eight practice dimensions that would be critical in order for future addiction counselors to be competent in the field of practice: clinical evaluation (screening and assessment); treatment planning; referral, service coordination (implementing the treatment plan, consulting, ongoing assessment); counseling (individual, family, and group); client, family, and community education; documentation; and professional and ethical responsibility. The document's intent was not to provide a proscriptive curriculum but rather to identify the knowledge, skills, and attitudes that could point to outcomes which the curricula might embrace (Center for Substance Abuse Treatment, 2006).

In Canada, the development of the core competencies for the substance abuse field began in 2006. It entailed the identification and comparative analysis of existing and emerging Canadian and international addiction workforce competencies. The process involved workshops and consultations with a National Advisory Group on Workforce Development. Using focus

TABLE 1 Technical Competencies Summary Table

Competency	BSW Required Courses $N = 32$	BSW Addiction Electives $N = 23$	MSW Required Courses $N = 28$	MSW Addiction Electives $N = 5$
1. Case Management	6	3	0	0
2. Community Development	25	4	9	1
3. Conflict Management	3	0	0	1
4. Counselling	25	9	13	3
5. Crisis Intervention	9	0	3	0
6. Diversity & Cultural Responsiveness	32	12	24	3
7. Ethics & Professionalism	30	2	8	1
8. Family & Social Support	21	8	6	4
9. Group Facilitation	24	2	7	0
10. Mental Health	6	3	2	2
11. Outreach	0	3	0	0
12. Pharmacology	0	16	0	2
13. Prevention & Health Promotion	4	15	2	3
14. Program Development, Implementation, & Evaluation	13	1	28	0
15. Screening & Assessment	11	11	3	2
16. Teamwork	5	2	1	0
17. Treatment Planning	0	12	0	3
18. Understanding Substance Abuse & Dependency	0	21	0	4
Average	6.7	5.6	3.8	5.8
Median	7	5	3	5
Range	2–11	2–13	1–7	3–9
Standard Deviation	2.2	2.4	1.7	2.6

Source: Graves et al., 2009.

groups, in-depth interviews, e-mail communication, and a blog, subject-matter experts (including both academics and practitioners) were engaged in order to gather additional feedback (Canadian Centre on Substance Abuse, 2007). The end product was 18 specific technical competencies (Table 1) deemed critical for mastery by any professional working in the substance abuse field in Canada. Upon publication of the standards, a study, course outlines, and objectives were examined to determine the extent to which the 18 core competencies for the substance abuse field were taught in the general and addiction-specific curricula in schools and faculties of social work throughout Canada (Graves et al., 2009).

It was discovered that a majority of social work undergraduates in Canada receive formal education in the following one-third of the core competencies: diversity and cultural responsiveness, ethics and professionalism, counseling, community development, group facilitation, and family and social support. Topic areas not mentioned in any required course outline were outreach, pharmacology, treatment planning or understanding substance use, abuse, and dependency. On average, 6.7 competencies

(*SD* = 2.2) are part of the mandated curriculum for a Canadian BSW student with a range of 2 to 11. Moreover, 23 of 32 (71.9%) of undergraduate social work programs offer an addiction elective to their students. However, the curriculum within these electives varies greatly, with the number of competencies being taught ranging from 2 to 13, with a mean of 5.6 and an *SD* of 2.4. The most commonly taught competencies in these electives are understanding substance abuse and dependency (91.3%), pharmacology (69.6%), and prevention and health promotion (65.2%). What is interesting to note is that of the 23 addiction-specific elective offerings, not 1 had conflict management or crisis intervention as part of their stated objectives, and only 1 had program development. Two taught team work, and three offered case management, mental health, or outreach. Thus, while most undergraduate social work students do gain introductory knowledge in many of the core competencies, there remain many areas in which they would still need ongoing education or professional development (see Table 1).

Another means for obtaining additional education is to pursue an MSW after earning a BSW, though there remain many social workers whose education in the profession is only at the master's level. In examining the course objectives of required MSW courses, it was discovered that they actually covered *fewer* of the 18 core addiction competencies than did the mandated BSW courses (3.8 versus 6.7; *SD* 1.7 versus 2.2). The focus at the master's level of every graduate social work program in Canada is on research. Thus, each MSW student would receive some formal training in program evaluation along with a continued emphasis on diversity and cultural competency. The only other core competency taught with any consistency at the graduate level in social work is counseling, and even that is only a requirement of 13 of the 28 MSW programs (46.4%). Fewer than one-fifth of Canadian graduate programs have a specific addiction elective as part of their curriculum, and of those five programs, two do not have a corresponding undergraduate program, and one does not list an undergraduate BSW elective as an option (Graves et al., 2009).

RESPONDING TO THE NEED

Canada is a huge nation geographically. It has nearly double the land mass of the United States with only one-tenth the population. Whereas there are 740 accredited schools of social work in the United States (CSWE, 2012), there are only 37 programs in Canada, of which only 8 currently offer any type of distance education offering (CASWE, 2012). Thus, not only are there substantive geographic issues in attending a program in social work; once you are admitted, there is no certainty that a student will obtain any specific education or clinical experience in the addiction field, a practice area the majority will encounter and in which some will specialize upon graduation.

McMaster University, located in Hamilton, Ontario, has offered an Addiction Education Program through the Centre for Continuing Education since the 1980s. It began modestly by hosting campus-based summer residential conferences for anyone associated with addiction service provision but has grown to a program now offering 27 undergraduate-level credit courses through both in-class and distance formats on an array of addiction specific topics (Table 2). Given that addiction is a specialized area of practice, despite so many social work clients having addiction issues, the only way to be able to provide such a diversity of educational options was to broaden the scope of the program, and thus an active outreach campaign accompanied the program's expansion until students from all 10 provinces and three territories were enrolled.

TABLE 2 Technical Competencies Covered by McMaster Addiction Studies Program

Competency	Course
1. Case Management	620-462 Case Management and Report Writing
2. Community Development	None
3. Conflict Management	611-428 Problem Management Skills for Helpers
4. Counseling	611-122 Counseling Techniques in Addiction Practice
	611-421 Working with Problem Gamblers
	611-430 Solution Focused Approaches in Addiction Counseling
	620-492 Working with Women and Addiction
	620-494 Youth and Addictions
	620-865 Working with Older Canadians
5. Crisis Intervention	620-899 Crisis Intervention
6. Diversity & Cultural Responsiveness	611-811 Diversity and Special Issues in Addiction Counseling
7. Ethics & Professionalism	611-831 Professional Ethics and Helping
8. Family & Social Support	620-879 Working with Families and Addiction
	611-832 Co-Dependency as an Addiction
	620-498 Self-Help/Mutual Aid: Roles and Realities
9. Group Facilitation	611-429 Concepts and Dimensions of Group Work
10. Mental Health	620-476 Concurrent Disorders in Addiction
11. Outreach	None
12. Pharmacology	620-474 Pharmacology and Drug Abuse
13. Prevention & Health Promotion	611-427 Introduction to Addiction
14. Program Development, Implementation, & Evaluation	611-406 Program Development
15. Screening & Assessment	620-488 Assessment of Addictive Behavior
16. Teamwork	611-429 Concepts and Dimensions of Group Work
17. Treatment Planning	620-495 Treatment of Addictive Behavior
18. Understanding Substance Abuse & Dependency	611-427 Introduction to Addiction
	611-412 Understanding and Preventing Relapse

This has been accomplished by acknowledging the flexibility required by adult learners and allowing students to begin any distance course in any month of the year. Applications are accepted throughout the year with continuous intake. All of the distance courses are available the first of every month. Students can complete one course and enroll in another immediately, or they can take a break and start up again when they are ready. This flexibility allows students to dictate their study schedule, which is important for adult learners who are often juggling work, study, and family obligations. The distance format is, of course, crucial for students who live in remote areas as the addiction studies program allows them to pursue a specialization without relocating. This has also greatly contributed to the program's utility nationally as relationships have been fostered with employers across the country, particularly those in remote geographical settings with limited options in training their staff or enhancing their professional competencies. As well, in class sessions are offered in condensed weekend blocks staggered throughout the term to accommodate both working schedules and those more distant from campus. Weekend block classes have also been moved off campus into different communities where there are sufficient numbers of students interested in a particular course. Tuition costs are based solely upon the actual courses a student registers for; thus there is no enrollment cost for any term, which makes their ongoing education more financially feasible, particularly for those still paying off student loans. Needless to include is the fact that the faculty must consist of seasoned addiction professionals combining both practice skills and extensive post-secondary training who, like their students, must be very flexible in terms of providing relevant, timely feedback.

In an era when simultaneous chat functions and live video-teleconferencing have become the norm, it may seem odd that the addiction education program is thriving in a less electronic format. In fact, it is the adherence to this delivery method that makes the program popular. Students have been surveyed several times to determine whether they would prefer to have the program as a more term-based online classroom format, but the majority have said they prefer it in the individual-led arrangement. Students indicated that they enjoyed the simplicity and unencumbered nature of the digital/electronic course material and that they value not having to deal with technological issues such as workplace fire-walls and computer limitations, dial-up Internet connections, and older software that cannot be updated due to budget limits or purchasing agreements. They also, due to shift work and Canada's size, prefer not to have specified chat requirements as Canada spans six distinct time zones. Course graders are always available through e-mail for clarification and assistance. The philosophy of the distance offering is that the most critical aspect of the education process is the transfer of new skills and knowledge. If technology becomes an encumbrance that prohibits learning transfer, it is not an asset for distance students.

Currently, students may enroll in either the Certificate in Addiction Studies (15 units) or the Addiction Careworker Diploma (24 units) or simply take a course for professional development or to assist with certification or recertification. Courses include many specialized topics not offered by any other institution and thus are able to meet almost the entire range of competency requirements as developed by the CCSA (see Table 2). Of the 18 technical competencies, only 2 are not met by the McMaster curriculum, Community Development and Outreach.

As well, not only is a student able to meet the competencies that are sometimes difficult to find as a full course elsewhere but, in doing so, the program meets the educational component for Canadian addiction certification. Creating a niche, and offering the courses via both in-class and distance formats, have allowed for greater flexibility than a traditional social work program can offer. However, the addiction studies program's affiliation with a school of social work has ensured that education standards are current, evidence-informed, and pertinent to client and community needs. Offering nearly 30 courses around the theme of addiction also provides flexibility and allows students to customize their learning needs. Those entering with a BSW, for example, will likely have a different course selection than those entering with a MSW, and both may have needs and interests different from those who are using the program as an entry point to gaining acceptance into a school of social work. In this way, the program has been structured to serve as both a pre- and post-program educational opportunity, due to the audience it needs to serve, both student and employer.

DISCUSSION

Given accreditation demands placed upon social work education programs, it is not possible to meet all the educational and professional needs that a social worker may encounter upon graduation, a fact that has been regularly lamented in the literature (Bosma et al., 2010; Csiernik, 2000; Fredriksen-Goldsen, Woodford, Luke, & Gutiérrez, 2011; Sheridan, 2009). Despite the lack of mandated addiction education, Canadian social work students can obtain a grounding in many of the CCSA core competencies that should provide them with basic skills to provide addiction counseling. Nonetheless, there typically remain many gaps in graduates' knowledge and skills; this is where a specialized program has great utility. However, the nature of specialization makes it difficult for any traditional classroom-based program to attract sufficient students to make the initiative economically feasible, especially in a nation like Canada, with large geographic areas relative to its population.

What also makes the addiction studies program of value is that the University views it as an initiative that can both support graduates and recruit new students. A university strives to have its name carried across the country, and with over 400 active students nationwide in the program at any given time (and approximately 75 graduates of the program each year), professionals in the field are carrying the McMaster name on their resumes and websites. Without the distance education option, in fact, many would never have considered attending the University. The addiction studies program also provides an opportunity for undergraduate students to remain at McMaster upon convocation and enhance the value of their degree with a specialized certificate or diploma. Finally, those students who choose to complete the certificate or diploma concurrently with their undergraduate degree are presented with increased elective options and the chance to gain skills and knowledge that are not commonly available at other universities. Moreover, employers across Canada have come to view this educational option as a means of meeting the professional development and training needs of their staff. The online education format provides employers with a flexible and affordable option to training staff at their own pace, preparing for both certification and required re-certification through CACCF while meeting the ongoing professional development hours requisite to maintaining membership in their professional college. Each group is able to attain a different value and service. Once an adult learner makes the decision and commitment to pursue an education, it is important to be available to them on their terms.

> *After completing my Bachelor degree I was looking for a program that offered specialization in my field of interest and the Addiction Careworker Diploma Program more than exceeded my expectations. The format of this course allows you to work at your own pace, which is fantastic. Since most courses are offered in distance, I was able to maintain full-time employment while also furthering my career.* (C. Plater, Ontario)

The key to the program's success lies in its unique market-captured niche and flexibility provided. Topics are specialized enough that it is set apart from the other addiction counseling programs. No other program, for example, offers 27 addiction-specific courses. The flexibility of continuous new student intake, staggered course dates, distance study, and the ability for students to determine their own course and unit load allow the program to meet the needs of a wide range of students. In this way, students can complete requirements for certification while they continue to work and take care of their family. Courses meet the needs for professional accreditation, recertification, and ongoing professional development and can be used as a post-degree education or transferred into a new degree. The program can also be used as a specialty for a wide variety of professional fields and not just those working directly in addictions or only in Canada. It, therefore, appeals to a broad range of prospective students and thus responds to a broad range of community need.

> *In Hong Kong we don't have any academic courses related to addiction. I found I was not competent before because I lacked relevant academic knowledge. However, the Addiction Careworker Diploma provided me with practical knowledge and skills. I enjoyed this program because it is flexible and has many course choices that fit my own needs. I could study this program without flying to Canada and could adjust it according to my own personal learning pace.* (Cheuk-yan Li, Executive Director, Zion Social Services, Hong Kong)

CONCLUSION

Social work graduates are fortunate in that they possess skills, knowledge, and competencies that are sought after in a variety of settings. Should they find themselves in a position where they wish to build upon these skills in a specialized direction, such as addiction, it is important that they have access to programs that meet their needs as learners and working professionals. A flexible distance learning model, based on practitioner and industry need, is the key to promoting a well-trained workforce able to respond to the expectations of clients and community.

REFERENCES

Bosma, H., Johnston, M., Cadell, S., Wainwright, W., Abernethy, N., Feron, A., . . . Nelson, F. (2010). Creating social work competencies for practice in hospice palliative care. *Palliative Medicine, 24*(1), 79–87.

Canadian Association of Social Work Educators. (2012). Institutional members: Universities. Retrieved from http://www.caswe-acfts.ca/en/Universities_37.html

Canadian Centre on Substance Abuse. (2007). *Core competencies for Canada's substance abuse field (version 1).* Ottawa: Canadian Centre on Substance Abuse.

Center for Substance Abuse Treatment. (2006). *Addiction counseling competencies: The knowledge, skills, and attitudes of professional practice. Technical Assistance Publication series 21. DHHS Publication No. (SMA) 06-4171.* Rockville, MD: Substance Abuse and Mental Health Services Administration.

Council on Social Work Education. (2012). *Directory of accredited programs.* Retrieved from http://www.cswe.org/Accreditation/Accredited-Programs.aspx

Clark, E., & Arkava, M. (1979). *The pursuit of competence in social work.* San Francisco, CA: Jossey-Bass.

Csiernik, R. (2000). The state of the nation: EAP education in Canada. *Employee Assistance Quarterly, 15*(3), 15–22.

Csiernik, R., & Rowe, W. (Eds.). (2010). *Responding to the oppression of addiction* (2nd ed.). Toronto: Canadian Scholars Press.

Csiernik, R., Vitali, S., & Gordon, G. (2000). Student and field instructor perceptions of a child welfare competency based education and training program. *Canadian Social Work, 2*(2), 53–64.

Fornili, K., & Haack, M. (2005). Promoting early intervention for substance use disorders through interdisciplinary education for health professionals. *Journal of Addiction Nursing, 16*(3), 153–160.

Fredriksen-Goldsen, K., Woodford, M., Luke, K., & Gutiérrez, L. (2011). Support of sexual orientation and gender identity content in social work education: Results from national surveys of U.S. and Anglophone Canadian Faculty. *Journal of Social Work Education, 47*(1), 19–35.

Freeman, R., and Lewis, R. (1998). *Planning and implementing assessment*. London, UIK: Kogan Page Limited.

Grant, G. (Ed.). (1979). *On competence: A critical analysis of competence-based reforms in higher education*. San Francisco, CA: Jossey-Bass.

Graves. G., Csiernik, R., Foy, J., & Cesar, J. (2009). An examination of Canadian social work program curriculum and the addiction core competencies. *Journal of Social Work Practice in the Addictions, 9*(4), 400–413.

Hancock, K., Echlin, C., Hallberg, R., Lewis, M., Liston, J., & West, T. (2003). A child welfare competency-based education and training (CBET) pilot project. *Canadian Social Work, 5*(1), 54–64.

Horvatich, P., & Wergin, J. (1998). Building a new profession: Defining and measuring the competence of addiction counselors. Paper presented at the Annual Meeting of the American Educational Research Association, San Diego, CA, April 13–17.

Hyland, T. (1995). Morality, work and employment: towards a values dimension in vocational education and training. *Journal of Moral Education, 24*(4), 445–457.

Keller, D., & Dermatis, H. (1999). Current status of professional training in the addictions. *Substance Abuse, 20*(3), 123–140.

Marrelli, A. F. (2001). *Introduction to competency modeling*. New York, NY: American Express.

McMaster University. (2013). Summary of total enrollment. Retrieved from http://www.mcmaster.ca/avpira/statistics/mcmaster_statistics_total_enrolment0812.html

Miller, G., Scarborough, J., Clark, C., Leonard, J., & Keziah, T. (2010). The need for national credentialing standards for addiction counselors. *Journal of Addictions & Offender Counseling, 30*(2), 50–57.

Mirabile, R. (1997). Everything you wanted to know about competency modeling. *Training and Development, 51*(8), 73–78.

Ogborne, A., & Graves, G. (2005). *Optimizing Canada's addiction treatment workforce: Results of a national survey of service providers*. Ottawa: Canadian Centre on Substance Abuse.

O'Hagan, K. (Ed.). (1996). *Competence in social work practice: A practical guide for professionals*. London, UK: Jessica Kingsley Publishers.

Phillips, A. (2011). Service-learning and social work competency-based education: A "goodness of fit?" *Advances in Social Work, 12*(1), 1–20.

Richards, J., & Rodgers, T. (2001). *Approaches to methods in language and teaching* (2nd ed.). Cambridge, UK: Cambridge University Press

Substance Abuse and Mental Health Services Administration. (1998). *Addiction counseling competencies: The knowledge, skills, and attitudes of professional practice*. Rockville, MD: Author.

Sheridan, M. (2009). Ethical issues in the use of spiritually based interventions in social work practice: What are we doing and why. *Journal of Religion & Spirituality in Social Work: Social Thought*, *28*(1–2), 99–126.

Training Organisation for the Personal Social Services. (2002) *The national occupational standards for social work*. Leeds, UK: Author.

Vitali, S. (2010). Can we measure and track the acquisition of competency on a professional social work degree? In H. Burgess & J. Carpenter (Eds.), *The outcomes of social work education: Developing evaluation methods* (pp. 62–72). University of Southampton: Higher Education Academy Subject Centre for Social Policy and Social Work.

White, W., & Garner, B. (2011). Staff turnover in addiction treatment: Toward science-based answers to critical questions. *Counselor*, *12*(3), 56–59.

Increasing MSW Students' Information Competencies through Online Tutorials, Application Exercises, and Course Assignments

JOHN A. KAYSER
Graduate School of Social Work, University of Denver, Denver, Colorado, USA

JENNIFER BOWERS
University Libraries, University of Denver, Denver, Colorado, USA

LIN JIANG and MARIAN BUSSEY
Graduate School of Social Work, University of Denver, Denver, Colorado, USA

Increasing MSW students' information competencies was achieved through a 2-year project in which online video tutorials, in-class exercises, and course assignments were created and integrated into two required foundation courses. Tutorials demonstrated basic and advanced search techniques, online databases, and online course-specific research guides. Tutorials were viewed during and outside of class. In-class exercises and course assignments enabled students to immediately apply what they had learned. Results indicate a significant increase in the adequacy of students' search for online information and ability to critically examine sources and evidence. Implications for social work education are discussed.

This paper describes the development and evaluation of a two-year project at the University of Denver Graduate School of Social Work designed to advance students' critical thinking and information skills, whereby they could effectively and efficiently search for, evaluate, and use online information in their social work practice. The information literacy skills were integrated into two foundation courses, *History of Social Welfare and Social Work* and *Research Methods and Design*. As Brustman and Bernnard observe (2007), effective social workers must develop advanced information competencies:

> Social work is a knowledge-intensive profession where information is essential in decision-making and practice. Information must be evidence-based, relevant, current, clear, accurate, conveniently accessed, and easily communicated. Innovations in information-technology (IT) have dramatically affected our profession. IT affects what we collect, how we collect it, how we express it, and how it is communicated. (p. 90)

With the widespread use of the Internet, traditional library instruction to introduce students to the general and discipline-specific resources found in college and university libraries (e.g., journals, books, media) has expanded. Students now are introduced to the vast array of electronic journals, online databases, and websites; are provided with strategies for searching effectively and efficiently; and offered criteria for evaluating the credibility of this vast new wealth of information. The Association of College and Research Libraries (2000) has conceptualized this expanded learning as a form of *information literacy provision*, which librarians recently have incorporated into face-to-face instruction with social work students (Brustman & Bernnard, 2007; Johnson, Whitfield, & Grohe, 2011; Sizemore & Marcum, 2008).

In a parallel manner, the increased emphasis on practice effectiveness in social work has heightened the need for students to develop sophisticated critical thinking and online search skills as components both of successful evidence-based practice and advanced information competence. Social work educators are calling for students to become proficient in these areas, whether they be identified as *information literacy skills* (Johnson et al., 2011; Walker, Briggs, Koroloff, & Friesen, 2007; Wheeler & Goodman, 2007); more generally as *research and critical thinking skills* (Drake, Hovmand, Jonson-Reid, & Zayas, 2007; Mirabito, 2012); or as *critical appraisal skills* (Smith, Cohen-Callow, Hall, & Hayward, 2007).

From their case study of student reference lists, Silfen and Zgoda (2008) found that graduate social work students require library instruction targeting how to identify and evaluate high-quality research publications. Lynch, Vernon, and Smith (2001) emphasized the need for these students to develop evaluation skills, specifically for freely available Web resources. Conducting successful reviews of the literature, analyzing sources critically, data searching proficiently, and preventing plagiarism are additional areas of concern (Culpepper, 2008; Hiller, Wernecke, & McKelvey, 2005; Plionis, Thompson, & Eisenhower, 2005).

Nontraditional social work students face specific challenges in today's complex research environment, since typically they have been out of academia for several years and may be unfamiliar with current disciplinary databases and may need more assistance finding and accessing relevant literature (Bellard, 2005; Ismail, 2009). These findings and needs are similar to the information competencies required of graduate students in affiliated social and health sciences disciplines (Catalano, 2010; Harrington, 2009; Holler, 2009; Jacobs, Rosenfeld, & Haber, 2003; Monroe-Gulick & Petr, 2012).

The technological advances of high-speed Internet connectivity and video streaming have prompted several libraries and schools of social work to develop online tutorials to provide video demonstration and/or text-based instruction. However, only a few publications in the relevant library literature describe these social work tutorials to date (Johnston, 2010; Lawler, 2003; Xu, 2009), and only Johnston has included an evaluation of these tutorials.

Lawler (2003) employed Web-based tutorials, including one focused on historical social policy research and critical thinking skills, integrated with library instruction. Xu (2009) describes a blended instructional approach using topical, Web-based tutorials focused on finding books and articles, specific research skills (evidence-based practice, demographic data, tests and measurements), along with in-class library sessions. Although neither author evaluated the efficacy of these tutorials, library surveys to incoming students (Xu) and surveys both before and after library instruction (Lawler) measured social work students' information competencies.

At James Cook University in Queensland, Australia, Johnston (2010) created an online information literacy tutorial to serve the needs of both on- and off-campus graduate social work students. The tutorial covered effective search strategies for finding information in databases and on the Internet, evaluating sources, and using APA style. The effectiveness of this instruction was assessed both via a survey and student focus groups in order to solicit feedback about satisfaction with the tutorial and the perceived need for information literacy instruction. In addition, a post-module test evaluated students' acquisition of information literacy. Johnston concluded that although the tutorial was somewhat successful in improving information literacy skills, additional instruction was needed, especially with respect to database search techniques.

Online library tutorials also have been developed for graduate students in affiliated social sciences and health sciences. Studies in these disciplines used a wider variety of assessment methods to gauge the effectiveness of the tutorials, including *faculty feedback sessions* (Appelt & Pendell, 2010); *pre- and posttests* (Anderson & Wilson, 2009; Grant & Brettle, 2006; Lechner, 2005; Shaffer, 2011); *surveys* (Harkins, Rodrigues, & Orlov, 2011; Kumar & Ochoa, 2012; Mages & Garson, 2010; Schroeder, 2010); or a *combination of methods* (Beile & Boote, 2004). Findings varied but suggested that online tutorials work best when they are integrated into the curriculum, provide an interactive component, means for students to apply the skills presented, and are supplemented with opportunities to consult with a librarian, such as through discussion boards, e-mail, or chat.

Our project adds to the literature on literacy instruction and evaluation through (1) explicit development of in-class exercises and assignments; (2) extensive faculty participation; and (3) the triangulation of diverse assessment measures, including a pre-post literacy skills test, an evaluation of students' papers in two courses, and an end-of-year survey of student attitudes toward the literacy content.

DEVELOPMENT OF THE ONLINE TUTORIALS

Beginning in academic year 2008–2009, a general orientation to library services was discontinued in favor of providing online video tutorials. However, it soon became apparent that the tutorials were not used uniformly across all foundation course sections. Some instructors regarded the tutorials merely as an adjunctive tool available for student review on their own time, whereas others made the tutorials a more central feature of their course. Given that most section instructors had not participated in the development of the tutorials, a lack of uniform buy-in was understandable.

In 2010, funding was obtained from the University of Denver's Office of Teaching and Learning for a 2-year project to develop a comprehensive approach to increasing students' information literacy in their foundation year. This project was implemented through the following steps.

First, we adopted the information literacy model developed by the Social Work/Social Welfare Committee (Education and Behavioral Sciences Section) of the American Association of College and Research Libraries (1997), which conceptualized information literacy as the developmental progression of six skills, to wit, the ability to (1) precisely define a client or program problem and the type of information needed to solve the problem, (2) conduct efficient searches in multiple databases to tap all relevant data sources, (3) evaluate the trustworthiness and credibility of the evaluation, (4) extract the information and apply it to client or program, (5) communicate with others about the information, and (6) use the information in an ethical and legal manner. Table 1 provides examples of how the information competencies in the two foundation courses were adapted and operationalized.

These information competencies are congruent with the practice behaviors specified by the Council on Social Work Education (CSWE) Educational Policy and Accreditation Standards (2008), specifically, (1) critical thinking to inform and communicate professional judgments, (2) research-informed practice, and practice-informed research, and (3) knowledge of human behavior and the social environment with individuals, families, groups, organizations, and communities.

Second, we developed 31 brief online video tutorials covering the following content areas: overview of library services and resources, basic search techniques, and using the bibliographic management program, RefWorks

TABLE 1 Information Literacy Competencies Operationalized

Information Literacy Component	Social Welfare History	Research Methods/Design
Define Information Needed	Define the type of information needed to complete a historical analysis, such as: "What primary and secondary sources of information will best help in understanding historical events?"	Define the type of information needed to complete a review of research literature, such as: "What kind of client factors best predict positive outcomes?"
Locate and Access	Use basic search techniques (i.e., key words, subject headings, truncation, Boolean operators) to identify primary source material in the library catalog. Use contemporary language for topics when searching the full text of historical newspapers and periodicals.	Use advanced search techniques (i.e., controlled vocabulary, thesaurus, searching in multiple databases) to identify peer-reviewed articles on practice outcomes. Search for information about the evidence of practice effectiveness.
Evaluate	Identify discrepancies and contradictions in the historical record. Critically evaluate, compare, contrast, and synthesize the oral and written historical record.	Evaluate the articles according to an EBP hierarchy of research evidence.
Manage	Use RefWorks and database individual account and folder options to organize information.	Use RefWorks and database individual account and folder options to organize information.
Create and Communicate	Create history research paper and presentations disseminating the results of history research.	Create an annotated bibliography of research studies located, and write evidence-based practice guidelines for the client population or problem under study.

(9 tutorials); core databases in social work (2 tutorials); finding primary and secondary historical sources, government statistics, historic newspapers, Congressional records, legislative hearings, and public opinion polls (10 tutorials); evaluating sources and evidence (2 tutorials); and using advanced search techniques to locate and evaluate evidence-based practice articles and reviews (8 tutorials). Table 2 summarizes the tutorial content.

Third, we convened separate focus groups for the six history instructors and six research instructors (including both full-time and adjunct faculty) who collectively were covering 17 course sections. The video tutorials were shown to the teaching faculty in each course in order to increase instructor buy-in and to ensure uniformity of use across course sections. Faculty discussed whether the tutorials would be more effective if viewed by students on their own or whether they should be shown in class. In the end, both options were permitted.

TABLE 2 Information Literacy Tutorial Content

Techniques	Databases
Key Word & Descriptors	Core Databases
Library of Congress Subject Headings	*Social Work Abstracts*
Thesaurus Search for Alternate Terms	*Social Services Abstracts*
Truncation	*PsycInfo*
Facets, Tags, & Limiters	*Sociological Abstracts*
Times "Cited By"	*ERIC*
Pros & Cons of Searching Multiple Databases Simultaneously	*UlrichsWeb*
	Other Databases and Resources
Evidence-based Searches: for Population, Literature Reviews, Type Of Methodology	*America: History and Life*
	America's Historical Newspapers
Locating Full-Text Articles	*Google Scholar*
Evaluating Journals' Authority	*Medline/PubMed*
Finding Measures	*Oral History Sources*
Creating a Bibliography through RefWorks	*ProQuest Congressional*
	ProQuest Historical Newspapers
	Readex US Congressional Serial Set
	Roper Public Opinion Archives
	US Census & Statistical Sources

Fourth, the tutorials were also shown to separate focus groups of 10 to 12 advanced concentration–year students who already had completed these two foundation courses. Student feedback emphasized the need to make the tutorials concise and focused on the skills requisite to complete course assignments. Finding time for viewing the tutorials outside of class was a particular concern. These focus group students who previously had been out of school for a number of years indicated that they would have benefited from the tutorials had they been available at the very start of their studies.

Fifth, the tutorials were revised, based on the faculty and student focus group feedback, and then subsequently indexed with title slides—listing the content of each tutorial along with time signatures, noting where particular content could be found in the video. The history course video tutorials were recorded using Camtasia Relay, a screen capture program, and then embedded into Blackboard, the online course management program. For the research course, tutorials were uploaded into YouTube but made secure, so that only viewers with the appropriate URLs would be able to access the video. The advantage of YouTube was that students could retain access to the tutorials after the research course was completed, and the Blackboard site was no longer accessible.

TUTORIAL INCLUSION IN THE CURRICULUM

Twenty-one of the tutorials were used in the fall semester history course covering library services and catalogs, core social work databases, bibliographic management, basic search techniques, and history-specific databases. Ten modules were used in the spring research course, focusing on evidence-based practice and criteria to evaluate sources and findings. Students were expected to have reviewed the online tutorials prior to class sessions. Instructors also had the option to show excerpts of tutorials in class, as part of the demonstration of skills.

Course syllabi were redesigned in order to tie the search skills and databases, demonstrated in the online tutorials, to written assignments. Both the history and research courses contained a literature review assignment in which students had to define, locate, evaluate, and ethically use sources found online. In addition, in-class exercises and worksheets were developed, which required students to actually apply what they had seen demonstrated in the tutorials.

Evaluation of Student Progress

In order to assess the effectiveness of the project in increasing students' information competencies, a multi-measure assessment plan was developed. Two research questions were posed:

- Do course-specific online library tutorials increase foundation students' ability to locate, evaluate, and use information obtained from electronic databases and other digital sources in their course assignments?
- How do students assess the usefulness of specific literacy skills modules, exercises and assignments?

Subjects for this study were the 185 students in the Foundation Year of the MSW program, fall quarter 2011 through spring quarter 2012. The study was approved by the University's IRB.

Assessing Skills

The first question was measured in two ways: Rubrics were developed to rate the literacy skills demonstrated in relevant assignments from the history and research courses, and students were invited to participate in the anonymous survey.

The literacy survey drew items from the library science and social work literature as well as new items created to cover content on social work history, social welfare policy, and social work intervention research. The 40-item survey included 7 items from Brustman and Bernnard's (2007) published literacy assessment; 16 questions from the Albin O. Kuhn Library Information Literacy Survey (2003) about familiarity with and use of search strategies; and 15 additional literacy content questions created specifically

TABLE 3 Sample Literacy Skills Survey Items

From Brustman & Bernnard (2007)	From Albin O. Kuhn Library (2003)	Developed by Project Faculty
Internet sites need to be evaluated for: (a) Authority (b) Bias (c) Currency (d) Accuracy (e) All of the above	How comfortable are you with the following information literacy skills: Formulating questions; Developing successful search strategies	The best source for finding an official count of the number of women living below the poverty level in the Denver metro area would be: (a) LexisNexis Congressional for house and senate documents (b) The US Census website (c) A recently published book about women in Colorado (d) A *Denver Post* article about a homeless shelter (e) Not sure

for this survey. We also asked about age range (in 5-year increments) and undergraduate major to see whether either of those factors would affect students' level of preparation in literacy skills. No other demographic questions were included, in order to preserve participant anonymity. Each question was reviewed, debated, and revised before a decision was made to include it in the final version of the survey. The final result assessed both conceptual and skill domains, using a variety of testing formats including multiple choice questions, fill-in-the-blank items, and queries incorporating screen shots from the University's library website, external agency websites, and historic newspaper articles. Table 3 provides examples of survey questions.

The survey was pilot-tested with nine advanced concentration–year students. Confusing questions were revised, and then incoming students were invited to participate in a pre–post literacy assessment at the start of the 2011–2012 academic year. They received an initial e-mail (with an informed consent document) describing what this component of the literacy skills project would involve, and when needed, two follow-up e-mails. Participation in the anonymous survey was voluntary, and students were offered modest gift card amounts as an incentive. Approximately one third of the incoming class (33.5%, $n = 62$) chose to participate and complete the online pre-test assessment.

Students who had taken the pretest survey were reminded about taking the online posttest survey at the end of spring quarter. (While 62 students began the posttest survey, as noted, only 52 actually chose to provide responses.) The University's online testing system linked each student's pre- and posttest survey scores prior to sending the results to project staff; thus, analysis of the results was done using paired samples *t*-tests.

TABLE 4 Literacy Skills Survey: Results of Pre- and Posttest ($N = 52$)

Literacy Skill Domains–Survey	Pretest Means (*SD*)	Posttest Means (*SD*)	*p* Value
Familiarity with Literacy Concepts	3.84 (.67)	4.10 (.82)	.005
Specific Search Strategies Used	2.23 (.67)	3.05 (.61)	.000
Competency in Literacy Skills	8.75 (2.68)	11.90 (2.58)	.000

Results based on the 52 students with completed data showed that *familiarity with information literacy concepts, specific search strategies used,* and *competency in information literacy skills* increased significantly across the year. Table 4 shows the means, standard deviations, and significance levels of the change.

Specific items from the survey with the largest gains over the year included *developing search strategies; accessing information; using truncation*; and *locating systematic reviews*. There were no significant relationships between age or undergraduate major and the outcome variables. There was also no relationship between number of library research classes the student had taken and the questions in our survey derived from the Albin O. Kuhn Library Survey (2003), which assessed familiarity with information literacy skills and use of search strategies; however, there was a modest positive correlation between library classes attended and number of *application questions* answered correctly (.273, $p = .023$), representing questions that required students to apply tutorial content to correctly answer the question.

It also should be noted that since the Kuhn Survey posted the results of its measures of literacy skills familiarity and use of search strategies for 262 University of Maryland (UM) undergraduates online, we were able to compare our students' results with this non-equivalent (undergraduate) group. Incoming MSW students were much less familiar with search strategies than UM undergraduates but very similar in their familiarity with information literacy and more comfortable with two specific skills: *formulating questions based on information needs*, and *organizing information for practical application*.

In addition to the quantitative survey, procedures were developed to rate a random selection of student papers from the history and research courses. While the two assignments had different content and thus different rubrics, there were three items common to both assignments and rubrics: *adequacy of the search, critical appraisal of the sources found*, and *percent of scholarly sources* (academic books or peer-reviewed articles) used. Copies of papers were received from five history sections ($N = 72$) and eight research sections ($N = 147$). Three faculty and two graduate assistants read six history papers in common, using and revising the rubrics until the language was clear and the inter-rater reliability was .80. After that, one professor and two graduate assistants rated an additional 74 papers

TABLE 5 Comparison of History and Research Papers' Search Adequacy and Appraisal of Evidence ($N = 52$)

Literacy Skill Domains–Papers	History Papers Mean (*SD*)	Research Papers Mean (*SD*)	*p* Value
Adequacy of Search	3.85 (.71)	3.75 (.57)	NS
Appraisal of Quality of Evidence	1.85 (1.15)	3.33 (.69)	.000
Percent of Scholarly Sources Used	89%	96%	.001

(27 history, 47 research, randomly selected) for a final sample size of 80. Since the history and research papers had been de-identified, results were analyzed using independent samples *t*-tests. As noted in Table 5. while the adequacy of students' search did not change significantly, the research papers showed a significantly higher rating in the area of *appraisal of the quality of the evidence* and used a higher percentage of *scholarly sources*.

Assessing Attitudes

The second question, measuring student attitudes about literacy skills learning, was assessed via open-end questions. At the conclusion of spring quarter 2012, foundation students completed an online exit survey, inquiring about their educational experiences and satisfaction during their first year of graduate studies. Two specific questions were asked with respect to the information literacy and online search modules: "What did you learn that was new to you?" and "Has it been useful?"

For ease of analysis, responses were divided into two categories: *Positive or Neutral Responses* and *Negative Responses*. Positive responses were those indicating that the modules were helpful or something new was learned. Neutral responses were those in which students endorsed the need for training in library research skills/information literacy but expressed a preference for another method of instruction—usually a face-to-face meeting with a librarian or an in-person class presentation. Negative responses were those in which the modules were seen as not being helpful or useful.

Student comments about the modules used for the fall history course were 65% positive or neutral (of 110 responding) and 76% positive or neutral for the modules used in the spring research methods course (of 102 answers). Examples of positive or neutral comments about the history course literacy modules included the following:

- *I learned a lot about searching databases using subject headings, truncating terms, etc. It was one of the most useful aspects of the course.*
- *I am embarrassed to say that it took me until graduate school to learn about truncating key words! Much of what I learned in the modules was either new or an imperative refresher.*

- *Although the videos were useful, it was a lot of extra time outside of class, on top of all our other homework. I do not think I learned anything new; it just helped me to navigate the system better.*

Examples of negative comments included the following:

- *I would have learned more if someone came into our class and physically taught us search strategies.*
- *I learned most of what I know from appointments with the research librarians.*
- *I am just as successful using Google Scholar.*

Positive responses about the research course information literacy modules included comments about their immediacy, as seen in this sample:

- *My research instructor showed modules in class and then guided us through the same material that we could follow along on our laptops. This interactive approach allowed me to learn the material better.*
- *Learning the modules during this class was particularly useful because we practiced them in several different ways both within class activities and the assignments for the class.*

Negative responses often referred to the fact that the student already knew the material, such as these comments:

- *I already know how to do literacy searches and had conducted full-blown research projects in the past.*
- *By the time this class was offered, most students already had figured out how to have search strategies.*

DISCUSSION

The results of the pre–post administration of the information literacy survey (see Table 4) show a statistically significant increase in information literacy competencies, even though the overall gain was modest. In addition, analysis of individual item-responses indicates a broad, across-the-board increase in information competencies as students, on average, answered 13 of the 21 factual questions correctly. Importantly, these gains were most noted in key information competency areas, such as searching by subject headings and key words, deploying limiters to narrow a search, using "Cited By" to expand and extend a search, and employing a thesaurus to generate alternative search terms.

These results provide preliminary evidence that we are on the right track in developing an integrated instructional design that combines online tutorials with in-class applications to increase information literacy. Three main factors appear most relevant to this successful outcome: First, separate faculty and student focus groups had the opportunity to review the tutorials and give feedback, which increased their relevancy and usefulness; second, in-class exercises and course assignments allowed for repeated application of the search strategies (and database content) demonstrated in the tutorials; and third, the online video tutorials could be viewed as many times as needed by students, allowing for a consolidation of specific information literacy skills. Although we implemented this integrated instructional design by adding a major online component to traditional face-to-face instruction, it is important to note that this design could be readily adapted to distance/online-only or hybrid/blended courses.

At the same time, it is clear that we have a considerable way to go before we are likely to see marked increases in overall information competencies. Students likely will need systematic exposure and sustained practice in several foundation courses in order to see greater overall gains. Skills for searching and locating information may be more quickly mastered in fact than skills needed to critically evaluate evidence and sources of information. Hence, sequencing of skill-building activities must be addressed in order to maximize retention and promote generalization of competencies across courses.

There also were several limitations to the evaluation of this project. Since taking the literacy survey was voluntary, our sample of 62, reduced to 52 usable posttests due to unanticipated missing data, represented less than a third of the foundation year class. This response rate was lower than expected but may be explained by the fact that students were busy with orientation and by the trend (seen in higher education) of dwindling student response rates to e-mailed surveys, from 70% 20 years ago to closer to 20% today (Lipka, 2011). It is also difficult to know why 10 of the participants provided no responses on the posttest of the literacy survey, though we could read that as a sign of survey wariness, information literacy fatigue, or end-of–the-year stress.

The age ranges of students who participated were comparable to, though slightly higher than, those of the 185 incoming students: 40% of participants were 20 to 24 years old (compared to 42.4% for the class); 38.5% were 25–29 (compared to 38%); 12.3% were 30–34 (compared to 10.9%); 6.2% were 35–39 (compared to 4.9%); and 3.1% were 40–49 (compared to 3.8%).

In addition, although we pilot-tested and revised the survey, there is still the possibility, especially with newly created items, that they were unclear or confusing. We also had a much larger sample of student papers to read and rate using the rubrics, but even though the written assignments were completed by all students, not all section instructors participated by making de-identified copies available for analysis. Moreover, because the papers had been de-identified, we could not track student progress in literacy skills by linking their fall history paper with their spring research paper; instead, we had to analyze the papers as two groups. If all sections and students had used a coded ID, we would have been able to track their growth more accurately.

It should be noted as well that one of the main drawbacks to using online video tutorials for library instruction is the challenge in keeping them current. Database vendors frequently alter the look of their search interfaces, and library and other websites also frequently change their layout and organization. Even though the search techniques and profiled databases tend to remain fairly constant, students get confused if what they see demonstrated in the tutorial is not precisely mirrored on their computer screen. Ideally, new videos would be created every time an interface is changed, but this is not always feasible, and replacing outdated sections with new material can require a significant time and financial commitment. Although it becomes imperative to update video tutorials when major changes occur to a database's search functionality or scope, updating tutorials for minor alterations must be considered and balanced with time and fiscal constraints. An additional drawback involves the extensive amount of training required to teach instructors in multi-section courses. Section instructors' commitments range greatly from lukewarm to strong. This speaks to the need for developing ongoing faculty training in information literacy for both adjuncts and full-time faculty.

An unanticipated benefit of the tutorial instruction was that the social work students were better prepared for their consultation appointments with the research librarians. Since the tutorials gave students a strong foundation in research skills and introduced them to key resources for their discipline, they were able to focus on more challenging questions when they met with the librarians. The tutorials gave them ownership of a baseline competency that they not only could apply to their history and research course assignments but found useful for their other courses and projects.

CONCLUSION

The findings of this study are congruent with the emerging principles derived from the science of learning. As noted by Ambrose, Bridges, DiPietro, Lovett, and Norman (2010), learning involves a process of active discovery rather than merely memorization of content. When significant learning experiences are aligned with the educational goals of formal courses, the search for, critical evaluation of, and ethical use of online information can be transformed into a coherent framework of critical thinking (Fink, 2003). Through the process of guided discovery, students can develop an integrated system of thinking, feeling, and meaning-making that is essential for effective social work practice.

REFERENCES

Albin O. Kuhn Library and Gallery. (2003). Information literacy survey. Retrieved from http://aok.lib.umbc.edu/informationliteracy/umbcsurvey.pdf

Ambrose, S., Bridges, M., DiPietro, M., Lovett, M., & Norman, M. (2010). *How learning works: Seven research-based principles for smart teaching*. San Francisco, CA: Jossey-Bass.

Anderson, R. P., & Wilson, S. P. (2009). Quantifying the effectiveness of interactive tutorials in medical library instruction. *Medical Reference Services Quarterly, 28*(1), 10–21. doi:10.1080/02763860802615815

Appelt, K., & Pendell, K. (2010). Assess and invest: Faculty feedback on library tutorials. *College and Research Libraries*, *71*(3), 245–253.

Association of College and Research Libraries. (2000). Information literacy competency standards for higher education. Retrieved from http://www.ala.org/acrl/standards/informationliteracycompetency

Beile, P. M., & Boote, D. N. (2004). Does the medium matter? A comparison of a web-based tutorial with face-to-face library instruction on education students' self-efficacy levels and learning outcomes. *Research Strategies, 20*(1), 57–68. doi:10.1016/j.resstr.2005.07.002

Bellard, E. M. (2005). Information literacy needs of nontraditional graduate students in social work. *Research Strategies, 20*(4), 494–505. doi:10.1016/j.resstr.2006.12.019

Brustman, M., & Bernnard, D. (2007). Information literacy for social workers. *Communication in Information Literacy*, *1*(2), 89–101.

Catalano, A. J. (2010). Using ACRL standards to assess the information literacy of graduate students in an education program. *Evidence Based Library and Information Practice*, *5*(4), 21–38.

Council on Social Work Education. (2008). *Educational policy and accreditation standards*. Alexandria, VA: Author.

Culpepper, J. (2008). An interdisciplinary approach to preventing plagiarism: A librarian–social work educator collaboration. *Journal of Social Work Values and Ethics, 5*(1). Retrieved from http://www.socialworker.com/jswve/content/view/76/55/

Drake, B., Hovmand, P., Jonson-Reid, M., & Zayas, L. (2007). Adopting and teaching evidence-based practice in master's-level social work programs. *Journal of Social Work Education, 43*(3), 431–446. doi:10.5175/JSWE.2007.200600625

Fink, L. D. (2003) *Creating significant learning experiences: An integrated approach to designing college courses*. San Francisco, CA: Jossey-Bass.

Grant, M. J., & Brettle, A. J. (2006). Developing and evaluating an interactive information skills tutorial. *Health Information and Libraries Journal*, *23*(2), 79–86.

Harkins, M. J., Rodrigues, D. B., & Orlov, S. (2011). "Where to start?" Considerations for faculty and librarians in delivering information literacy instruction for graduate students. *Practical Academic Librarianship: The International Journal of the SLA Academic Division, 1*, 28–50.

Harrington, M. R. (2009). Information literacy and research-intensive graduate students: Enhancing the role of research librarians. *Behavioral & Social Sciences Librarian, 28*(4), 179–201. doi:10.1080/01639260903272778

Hiller, A., Wernecke, M., & McKelvey, H. (2005). Removing barriers to the use of community information systems. *Journal of Community Practice, 13*(1), 121–139.

Holler, C. (2009). Client-based projects and the ACRL information literacy standards for higher education. *Behavioral and Social Science Librarian, 28*, 7–22.

Ismail, L. (2009). What they are telling us: Library use and the needs of traditional and non-traditional students in a graduate social work program. *The Journal of Academic Librarianship, 35*(6), 555–564.

Jacobs, S. K., Rosenfeld, P., & Haber, J. (2003). Information literacy as the foundation for evidence-based practice in graduate nursing education. A curriculum integrated approach. *Journal of Professional Nursing, 19*(5), 320–328.

Johnson, O. J., Whitfield, J. S., & Grohe, B. (2011). Improving social work students' information literacy skills: A faculty and librarian collaboration. *Journal on Excellence in College Teaching, 22*(3), 5–21.

Johnston, N. (2010). Is an online learning module an effective way to develop information literacy skills? *Australian Academic & Research Libraries, 41*(3), 207–218.

Kumar, S., & Ochoa, M. (2012). Program-integrated information literacy instruction for online graduate students. *Journal of Library & Information Services in Distance Learning, 6*(2), 67–78.

Lawler, S. H. (2003). Information literacy competencies in social work. *Academic Exchange, 7*(3), 125–131.

Lechner, D. L. (2005). Graduate student research instruction: Testing an interactive web-based library tutorial for a health sciences database. *Research Strategies, 20*(4), 469–481. doi:10.1016/j.resstr.2006.12.017

Lipka, S. (2011). Want data? Ask students. Again and again. *Chronicle of Higher Education, 57*(43), A1–A6.

Lynch, D., Vernon, R., & Smith, M. (2001). Critical thinking and the web. *Journal of Social Work Education, 37*(2), 381–386.

Mages, W. K., & Garson, D. S. (2010). Get the cite right: Design and evaluation of a high-quality online citation tutorial. *Library and Information Science Research, 32*(2), 138–146. doi:10.1016/j.lisr.2009.10.004

Mirabito, D. M. (2012). Educating a new generation of social workers: Challenges and skills needed for contemporary agency-based practice. *Clinical Social Work Journal, 40*(2), 245–254. doi:10.1007/s10615-011-0378-6

Monroe-Gulick, A., & Petr, J. (2012). Incoming graduate students in the social sciences: How much do they really know about library research? *Portal: Libraries and the Academy, 12*(3), 315–335.

Plionis, E. M., Thompson, M. A., & Eisenhower, C. (2005). The scholarship crash on the Internet highway: Implications for faculty-librarian collaboration. *Journal of Baccalaureate Social Work, 11*(1), 101–114.

Schroeder, H. (2010). Creating library tutorials for nursing students. *Medical Reference Services Quarterly, 29*(2), 109–120. doi:10.1080/02763861003723135

Shaffer, B. A. (2011). Graduate student library research skills: Is online instruction effective? *Journal of Library & Information Services in Distance Learning, 5*(1–2), 35–55.

Silfen, K., & Zgoda, K. (2008). Evidence-based practice and information literacy in social work: An assessment of students' reference lists. *Behavioral & Social Sciences Librarian, 27*(2), 104–115. doi:10.1080/01639260802202082

Sizemore, L., & Marcum, B. (2008). Social policy and constructivism: Using constructivist learning theory in teaching social work students research skills. *Southeastern Librarian, 56*(3), 17–20.

Smith, C., Cohen-Callow, A., Hall, D., & Hayward, R. (2007). Impact of a foundation-level MSW research course on students' critical appraisal skills. *Journal of Social Work Education, 43*(3), 481–495. doi:10.5175/JSWE.2007.200600644

Social Work/Social Welfare Committee, Education and Behavioral Sciences Section, Association of College and Research Libraries. (1997). Information competencies for social work students. Retrieved from http://www.ala.org/acrl/aboutacrl/directoryofleadership/sections/ebss/ebsswebsite/social/swkpyramid/pyramid

Walker, J., Briggs, H., Koroloff, N., & Friesen, B. (2007). Implementing and sustaining evidence-based practice in social work. *Journal of Social Work Education, 43*(3), 361–375.

Wheeler, D. P., & Goodman, H. (2007). Health and mental health social workers need information literacy skills. *Health & Social Work, 32*(3), 235–237.

Xu, F. G. (2009). Social work information center 2.0: A case study. *Public Services Quarterly, 5*(1), 1–14. doi:10.1080/15228950802461707

The Pathway Program: How a Collaborative, Distributed Learning Program Showed Us the Future of Social Work Education

TERESA MORRIS
School of Social Work, California State University, San Bernardino, San Bernardino, California, USA

CHRISTINE MATHIAS
California Social Work Education Center, UC Berkeley School of Social Welfare, Berkeley, California, USA

RONNIE SWARTZ
Department of Social Work, Humboldt State University, Arcata, California, USA

CELESTE A. JONES and MEKA KLUNGTVET-MORANO
School of Social Work, California State University, Chico, Chico, California, USA

This paper describes a three-campus collaborative, distributed learning program that delivers social work education to remote rural and desert communities in California via distance learning modalities. This "Pathway Program" provides accredited social work education for a career ladder beginning with advising and developing an academic plan and leading to BSW and MSW degrees. The paper offers assessment data on the Pathway Program and also suggests the potential for major changes in social work education. Questions about the nature of the university, the role of the faculty member, and the future of social work students in the twenty-first century are discussed.

This paper focuses on a statewide collaborative social work distance education program in California with an exploration of how such programs may be incubating major changes in social work education. The new initiative is called the Pathway Program. It offers social work education at three stages of a professional pathway: (1) pre-BSW advising, (2) accredited BSW education, and (3) accredited MSW education. The Program offers asynchronous online curriculum content combined with some synchronous online class sessions and occasional on-campus and off-campus student meetings. It also includes extensive student advising, faculty development and community outreach. The Pathway Program currently is offered by the three California State Universities of Chico, Humboldt, and San Bernardino and is supported, coordinated, and funded by the California Social Work Education Center (CalSWEC) through a federal Title IVE child welfare grant.

The original goal for this program seemed simple. It was to offer social work education to those living in remote rural and desert communities who were unable to attend on-campus degree programs because of geography or family commitments as part of an overall workforce development strategy for such underserved regions. While this remains the goal, as the program has matured, its leaders have developed a broader mission—to become advocates for change in social work education. We realized that programs such as these lead to a reconsideration of what a university, faculty member, and student actually are and how learning takes place. Here we offer an assessment of the progress of our program and our understanding of changes that are coming to social work education. The paper is structured in three parts. Part One presents the initial needs assessments for the Pathway Program and our reflections on the changing nature of universities. Part Two discusses the implementation of the Pathway Program and our reflections on the need for a redefinition of faculty and student identities and roles. Part Three reviews outcomes of the Pathway Program and our concurrent reflections on its implications for the future.

PART ONE: STARTING THE PROGRAM

The Pathway Program: Initial Needs Assessment

Social work programs have had limited success in reaching remote regions of California that are not proximate to 4-year university campuses. This finding is supported by CalSWEC's annual analysis of graduate retention data. Over the past 15 years, the percentage of counties in which MSW graduates have been employed has increased from 67% to 86%. Despite these gains, the most remote rural and desert areas of the state generally still lack MSW graduates. These data prompted interest from county social service directors for a study of workforce development issues and needs in the remote regions of California. The mobilizing concepts were (1) that rural counties face a markedly greater challenge in recruiting and retaining a quality workforce than their large urban counterparts and (2) that distance education strategies might offer an opportunity to address the educational needs of human service agency staff in these remote areas.

This project involved a two-part needs assessment. Part One determined whether counties perceived a need for workforce development. Part Two assessed the ability of social agencies, tribal groups, and community colleges to partner with 4-year universities to build the professional social work workforce. During the first phase, focus groups were held, and surveys were conducted asking about staff educational levels, vacancy rates, turnover, and overall staff needs. These were implemented with county leaders who are members of the "20 Small" consortium of counties in California, which is a committee within the California County Welfare Directors organization that represents the concerns of the 20 smallest counties in the state. In Phase Two, the three state university campuses that are in closest proximity to many of California's rural and desert counties embarked upon a needs assessment process that included interviews and surveys with community colleges, county and tribal leadership, and potential students for the program.

The data collected confirmed that the social work education level in the remote regions was either at or below state regulatory standards for child welfare staffing; vacancy rates ranged from 16% to 33%; staff turnover ranged from 6% up to 62%; many agencies had not been fully staffed for several years; and it frequently took a year to fill open positions. The majority of the counties agreed that there was a need for more education of their current staff, citing that social work knowledge and skills were necessary components to improving agency practice and, by extension, service to children and families. The barriers to educating staff related to travel time required to gain access to the education, lack of financial support, and the limited ability of the employing agencies to cover job duties while staff took time to fulfill course requirements. To address these barriers, the county leaders recommended a multi-pronged approach that would include increasing the availability of online classes while maintaining an in-person component, supporting student engagement in the educational program, and removing financial barriers to student attendance at classes.

Such findings demonstrated to us that we could not continue "business as usual" if we wanted to serve these communities. Clearly, we needed to take social work education to the students rather than assume that these students could come to us. As we considered the design of such social work education, we realized that the solution would not be campus-based (in terms of a physical campus) but would be campus-based conceptually, with courses delivered directly to the students' home or office. We concluded that the university is not just a location; it is a medium that can deliver education in a range of other settings. As traditional university faculty with what we thought were clearly defined positions, this realization made us feel a little insecure but led us to reflect fruitfully on the question: What is a university?

The Redefinition of the University

We asked ourselves the core question, where does learning take place? If we believe that learning takes place when learners gather around a teacher, then we will develop contexts that center the teacher and create physical space for the learners to observe, Whether it is in a central square in Athens, a wall-papered lounge in New Haven, or a cinder-block classroom in Northern California, this has been the traditional method of higher education in Western and European culture for a very long time. The age of modernity, however, has provided technologies for the distribution of knowledge across multiple contexts of people's lives. While learning often may very well continue to occur in the classroom, learning also takes place in the family, among peers, at work, and in the community. Post-modern education looks mighty different than lectures delivered in imposing structures at a traditional university campus.

How many students use e-mail? How many students have a cell phone? How many students go online at least once a day? New technologies present us with an opportunity to re-think education as a process and re-think the architecture of learning environments. This is not to suggest a narrative of progress or educational evolution (Gergen, 2000) or a de-valuing of traditional higher education structures. Rather, distributed learning is a response to the grounded experiences and activities of interconnected learners. Relationships are not formed because of real-time, face-to-face, corporeal contact between people. Relationships are formed out of common and shared meaning. We can create such meaning synchronously or asynchronously, face to face or online. If learning is conceived as an outcome of social interaction, relationships, and construction, then a physical campus is not required. Instead, multiple vehicles for interaction—or opportunities to make shared meaning—are required (such as student to instructor, instructor to student, student to student, student to community, students with family members, students with colleagues, etc.).

We postulated that a program of learning that builds on synchronous and asynchronous social relations and multi-modal interaction would not be limited to a university campus and would likely utilize very few mechanisms of traditional power, like awe-inspiring edifices and ceremonial pomp (White, 2002). Distributed learning could emerge from the use of university learning management systems, video-conferencing tools, cell phones, hand-held video cameras, case management systems, and other electronic and/or networked tools. Such distributed learning would be interactive, locally based, networked, student-centered and, yes, online. However, online education is only a component of distributed learning. It is a thin description. It is shorthand for communicating a central feature of the educational model, much like a diagnosis is a heuristic for describing much more complicated and rich stories. The Fielding Graduate University (2012), an innovator of nonprofit distributed education, suggests that activities for distributed learning integrate day-to-day life (work and non-work) and involve an emphasis on collaborative learning via peer and community interaction. Prospectively, this would be a clear departure from competitive and atomistic campus environments that are grounded in the proud modernist tradition of individualism.

In a distributed learning context, the "campus" is developed within the conceptual framework of universal design (Dukes, Koorland, & Scott, 2009). This educational model also is inclusive of people with disabilities because of the use of accessible technologies. Distributed learning does not make *accommodations* for people with disabilities; it is *accessible* from the onset. While not everyone will avail themselves of it, the opportunity for further education is now at least a possibility for all. Distributed learning brings education to people so they can strengthen their own communities without needing to leave their neighborhoods, jobs, and families.

With these ideas in mind, we came to the conclusion that we can no longer assume that our campuses are the sole centers of higher education. A university can usefully be conceptualized as both a *physical place* and a *virtual world* of learning. This emerging reality applies to social work education. Without distributed learning, social work programs may risk losing their standing as centers for professional education.

PART TWO: IMPLEMENTING THE PROGRAM

The Pathway Program: Building the Infrastructure

The three campuses tasked with responding to the unmet needs identified in the assessment came together and developed a career Pathway Program, rooted in Morris's recent discussion of a social work ladder of learning (Morris, 2005). Considerable community outreach, student recruitment, faculty advising, and course conversion to the online environment were carried out. Each of the three social work programs began developing the "distributed learning wing" of their programs. While building this capacity, process journals were kept that recorded data on student, faculty, and community member experiences in opening up the new Pathway. These formative data were reported in Pathway Program in Review (CalSWEC, 2011) and documented the characteristics of the new faculty members and new students.

Identifying a core group of faculty members interested in developing new courses and converting existing courses for delivery at a distance was perceived as essential to success. At first there were just a few champions of the program and significant resistance from those who questioned the validity of teaching social work knowledge, skills, and values at a distance. We felt it was important to make sure that faculty members committed to the traditional, on-campus model would not feel disenfranchised. Nonetheless, we wanted to create an inviting and creative environment for faculty members who might wish to try out the new model. Concerns about quality and standards were debated in faculty meetings, while incentives (such as course releases and funding for conferences) were offered to faculty interested in experimenting with the new course delivery modes. As noted in the Pathway Program in Review (CalSWEC, 2011) report:

> One site successfully won the buy-in of several members of their faculty, leading to a committee focused on creating an online Bachelor's program, and the development of online courses for Pathway students. The other sites also successfully developed online courses, with one site to offer both Bachelor's and MSW degree programs completely online. One coordinator successfully submitted a conference proposal, with a Pathway student, who presented on the Pathway Program at the California Conference for American Indian Education. Prospective students at all the sites progressed forward, with several successfully completing general requirement courses at their community college. Program growth led to one site hiring a full-time program coordinator solely dedicated to Pathway. (p. 4)

At the end of the first year, there were 26 students enrolled in the program. Most were completing lower-division requirements for entry into the BSW, but there were some who were starting to take BSW courses. These 26 students were very different from traditional undergraduates. They were older and had family commitments and full-time positions as child welfare workers. They lived in small communities and usually worked in modest agency settings that had a limited capacity to give employees free time for further education. Also, they generally had been away from school for a long time. As noted in the Pathway (CalSWEC, 2011) report:

> . . . all students in the program are existing public or tribal service workers, working full-time, and pursuing their education on top of lives already full of work and family responsibilities. The challenges they face often differ from those of most post-secondary education students. In addition to balancing full workloads and familial commitments, many of the Pathway students live and work far distances from school campuses, some up to "a 4½ hour drive away" and "need different kinds of help in staying organized for what they need [in terms of school]". A lot of participants in the program have "also been away from a school setting for a while and really struggle with [math] and writing.
>
> Indeed, when asked what they see as their biggest challenges to completing their degree, almost all students who were interviewed reported time management as the biggest challenge. Students shared that juggling family and work responsibilities while also attending school is a significant

> challenge for them. Other challenges students listed include health problems, mastering math, and having internet access at home. One student noted that attending school as a public child welfare employee is particularly challenging, citing an instance when she almost missed a midterm exam due to being in the midst of a detention case at work. (p. 3)

Experiencing changes in faculty roles while working with this new kind of student brought us to a consideration of how we need to deconstruct and reconstruct our current definitions of faculty and students in the context of a distributed learning program. Our traditional notion of a student who comes to us almost from high school, attends full-time, lives on or near campus, has few family responsibilities, enjoys parental support, and may work in low-skilled temporary jobs is no longer valid. A Pathway student would probably require a reconceptualization of the faculty role, from a leader at the front of learning adventures to a facilitator following at the rear of learning discoveries. The students in the Pathway Program were learning in distant, sometimes isolated, settings where they were taking charge of their learning and asking faculty members to follow their lead and give them the knowledge, skills, and values they needed to address the often-novel and unexpected issues that frequently emerged for them as they made progress through their courses.

What is the Faculty Member's Role?

We realized that teaching students of the twenty-first century would demand that faculty members shift to a new paradigm that would embrace technological advances, a focus on learning outcomes, systematic assessment, and a new approach to teaching. Yet, not all faculty like change, and there is an inevitable pushback if it is imposed. Even though 67% of academic leaders would appear to perceive the quality of online education to be comparable to traditional face-to-face teaching (Allen, Seaman, & Sloan, 2011), many faculty members remain fearful and skeptical about the efficacy of online education. Like others, social work faculty members often may be unconvinced about the new roles of technology in the delivery of the social work curriculum and may well reject (or delay) programs that embrace online/blended education (Ayala, 2009). Concerns about computer-based teaching, especially of practice skills, frequently provides a platform for these skeptics. Their doubts may persist even though there is evidence, for example, that when online-based tutorials are compared to face-to-face instruction in practice courses teaching crisis intervention skills, evidence-based assessment demonstrated that the online-based program actually out performed face-to-face instruction (Seabury, 2005).

Allen et al. (2012) noted that faculty members who are exposed to (and begin to utilize) online technologies are more likely to see the usefulness of these new modalities than those without such experience. It has generally been found that once faculty members have an experience with online options they will likely appreciate the possibilities. One psychological barrier to exploring how new technologies might be integrated into program curricula stems from faculty socialization, acculturation, and training. For many, it would seem intuitive that face-to-face instruction cannot be equaled, much less exceeded, by online options. Although most faculty members have basic computer skills, they may have difficulty thinking of course development and delivery as happening in a setting other than the physically bound educational world. Within this environment, faculty members build relationships and "know" students through seeing them each week, from additional conversations before and after class. After all, physical space traditionally dictates what faculty members do, how they do it, and how they evaluate student learning. Online and blended programs challenge, and perhaps threaten, traditional ideas of educational space, engagement, relationships, and assessment. While having some (or even considerable) technology skills, many faculty members remain committed to traditional pedagogies until coaxed to incorporate new technologies into their teaching.

Teaching in an online environment is not for everyone. However, creating new educational options for students who work or live in remote, isolated areas brings basic social work values of economic and social justice into the educational decision-making matrix (Mathias & Benton, 2011). Social work faculty members support educational access to a broader swath of the population and thus generally support the idea of alternative program delivery. It is certainly the case that distance education has been a part of social work for several decades. However, past distance education programs usually tried to emulate traditional place-based instructional modes. Responsive innovations in twenty-first-century social work education, therefore, demand more investment and confidence in technology.

Faculty members will need to deconstruct their face-to-face teaching in order to re-think how assignments, engagement, assessment, and the transfer of knowledge can be delivered in an online environment. They also may need "in-time" paced training, one-to-one experience with trainers, and opportunities to collaborate on course development. They need permission to see each new or redesigned course as a pilot project with a growth and design trajectory. Ultimately, faculty may have to dare to put themselves in the uncomfortable position of being students themselves.

Historically, nontraditional students have been principally defined by age and part-time enrollment and seen as being most likely to drop out of school. This limited definition has left many unaccounted for in data collections and studies. In 1996, with great awareness of the changing student demographics, the National Center for Education Statistics (NCES) developed a more comprehensive definition for the nontraditional student that moved away from a purely age or enrollment status definition and shifted to "choices and behaviors that may increase the students' risk of attrition" (Horn & Carroll, 1996, p. 3). These included: delayed entry, part-time enrollment, being a single parent, full-time employment, lack of financial independence, and not having a high school diploma. The more of these characteristics a student poses, the more likely he or she would be defined as nontraditional (Horn & Carroll, 1996). Of course, by this definition, the nontraditional student is becoming far more the norm than the exception. In fact, nearly three-fourths of all students meet criteria for being nontraditional (Choy, 2002).

While the NCES did develop a more realistic definition of the nontraditional student, missing are several other features, specifically challenges and barriers. These may include being a first-generation student or from a special population (e.g., foster care, homeless, veteran), low-income status, and lack of physical access to a college. Arguably, there are more. However, it is here, in the often-minimized attributes of what it means to be nontraditional, that students frequently need more supports and options. No longer can universities automatically assume that long-prescribed campus norms represent equity and best practices for the majority.

Hence, a significant increase in demand has emerged for alternative options for the pursuit of higher education. One way this can be seen is through participation in distributed (or distance) learning opportunities that use new technologies. In 2008, for example, nearly 20% of all undergraduate students were enrolled in at least one distributed learning course, up from 8% in 2000. A higher portion of these students was "nontraditional" in some respect. For example, those who were over the age of 30, worked full-time, were married, or had dependents participated in distributed learning more than their peers (Radford & Weko, 2011).

Harrell (2008) identified three main categories of services needed by such students: student readiness (assessments tools and preparedness resources), student orientation (technological, course, and university expectations), and student supports (help with technology, access to online communities, and mentoring programs). Without question, distance students also will benefit from online libraries, financial assistance, and counselors. However, as undergraduate students become increasingly ready for courses within their chosen majors, access to one-to-one advising could prove to be the pivotal source of support. A consistent presence by a committed faculty person may serve an integral role in solidifying a distance learner's satisfaction and continued enrollment.

PART THREE: PROGRAM ACHIEVEMENTS

Current Outcomes

The Pathway Program is now in its third year. There are 26 students in the Title IVE funded part of the program, and on each campus, the Title IVE program was a catalyst to expand BSW and MSW education. Each campus now has a fully developed "Pathway" to which any social work student meeting the admission requirements can apply.

Comments from program coordinators offered in the process evaluation confirm the unexpectedly speedy success of the program:

> . . . I would never have projected that half of our group would be coming to [our university] after only a year and half. I'm so excited about that. And just the fact that we have all of our undergraduate classes online. Sometimes I have to pinch myself and ask how this all happened in such a short period of time. (p. 4)

In addition, students seem to be satisfied with how the program meets their needs. The Pathway Program in Review (CalSWEC, 2011) report illustrates this:

> Some of the interviewed students noted changes in their practice and everyday lives that they attributed to their participation in the Pathway program. One student reported being more likely to advocate for change "in the way [they] do business" by making "services more easily accessible and culturally appropriate," while another student values the connections she has made with others working in social services and how Pathway "has definitely opened doors" for her. Another indicated that, since returning to school, she engages in more critical thinking and is more confident at work, while also being proud that she can be a role model for her daughters and others in her community. This same student also noted having a greater appreciation for the social work profession's Code of Ethics since discussing them in greater detail during her classes. Finally, one student reported a greater awareness and interest in issues relevant to Native American populations, while another is appreciative of the new connections she has with others working in tribal communities. (p. 5)

Of course there have been challenges, the major one being the complexity of the task. As coordinators noted:

> . . . the whole process, the different grants, the approval processes needed for accreditation, have been very time consuming" and ". . . making trips, doing things face-to-face, it was a lot to get things up and running." And ". . . I thought conceptually that it's such a simple idea, of finding people where they are and helping them through a ladder of learning. And that is just hard. We are struggling to get that to happen. Just getting it started . . . we're building infrastructure . . . (p. 5)

Overall, there were a number of "lessons learned' that are the focus of future development. One of these is the need for intensive communication with participating community colleges; a faculty summary of student comments noted that,

> The degree of coordination with participating community colleges had a great impact on students' experiences in the program. Students sometimes encountered advisors who were unaware of or didn't understand the program, and so were unable to appropriately advise them. Students also found challenges in finding classes at community colleges with available spots as well as finding classes that work with their schedules, and noted that maintaining motivation and endurance to complete their degree through the Pathway Program will require considerable effort. This is also due to the slightly longer time to completion for a Bachelor's or Master's degree through Pathway. (p. 8)

Also, there is a need to address problems with coordinating Title IVE student funding with campuses' bookstores and tuition fee payments:

> This was a struggle for the site coordinators, "because [the students] are ready, but they can't pay the funds. So now we're hitting roadblocks with community colleges, the bookstore, and other entities when the students are ready." Ultimately, the site coordinators developed an agreement with the bookstore where "as the coordinator I need to call them and set things up. And I have to do that for each individual student. But . . . the students don't understand the process and they just show up at the bookstore and say they want their books . . . The students get frustrated. We are trying to stay a few steps ahead of them to make it work.

And a need to address the complexities of transferring from community colleges to 4-year institutions and time delays that may extend the length of students' programs:

> Another challenge is [state university] admissions. I've written a two-page letter about why these students should be admitted and I've had someone from admissions helping me . . . If they aren't admitted, the challenge is going to be around the advocacy we'll need to do. And then working with the students to keep them committed, taking classes . . . I mean, when is the best time for a student to come in? Should they wait a year if they are only short one course?

Future development of the Pathway Program will include the need to develop curriculum protocols for field placements; further faculty development; coordination with partnering institutions; student mentorship; community building; meeting the specific student academic needs; and identifying and refining program procedures and logistics.

Social Work Programs in the Future

To create social work distributed learning programs, we ought to begin with thoughtful preparation that includes designing the delivery model, addressing curriculum needs, and course redesign. We need to brainstorm, process the emerging ideas, and be patient. Shifting from face-to-face courses to online/blended courses will generate excitement as well as frustration. Effective change is a long-term developmental process that can only be accomplished through systematic evaluation of learning outcomes, guidance from social work colleagues, and knowledgeable support from university technology departments. Several online schools note that course development and redesign often shift the focus from faculty teaching *per se* to student centered pedagogies (Moloney & Oakley, 2010). Nonetheless, faculty input and feedback in program development and curriculum redesign remain the *sine qua non* of successful pedagogical change.

Learning about evolving technologies and different tools can ignite innovation in course redesign. Anderson (2007) defines Web 2.0 as involving new technologies that may enable individuals to socially connect through a variety of methods, including blogs, podcasts, virtual worlds, avatars, and wikis. Tunks (2012) states, "Web-based tools enable instructors to demonstrate their presence and allow students to communicate easily without sharing the same physical space. The exploration and application of Web 2.0 tools removes the barriers typically associated with online classes" (p. 6). These technologies can fuel innovation as faculty conceptualize and extend their perspectives of what constitutes an academic setting.

We continue to develop our Pathway Program and have converted our BSW and MSW courses to the distributed learning environment. Orientation and training programs have been developed for students and faculty who consider and format the changing nature of learning. We have increased community outreach via information sessions and our attendance at employing agencies' meetings. Developing support services for our nontraditional students so that barriers to access to higher education are removed is a continuing commitment. We have a long way to go, both practically and conceptually, but we are learning all we can about twenty-first-century social work education and the strengths inherent in collaborative distributive learning.

REFERENCES

Allen, I., Seaman, J., & Sloan, C. (2011). Going the distance: Online education in the United States, 2011. Retrieved from Sloan Consortium. ERIC, EBSCOhost.

Anderson, P. (2007). What is Web 2.0? Ideas, technologies and implications for education. Technical report, JISC. Retrieved from www.jisc.ac.uk/media/documents/techwatch/tsw0701b.pdf

Ayala, J. S. (2009). Blended learning as a new approach to social work education. *Journal of Social Work Education, 45*(2), 277–288.

CalSWEC. (2011). The pathway program in review. Retrieved from http://calswec.berkeley.edu/pathway-program-distance-education

Choy, S. (2002). *Nontraditional undergraduates: Findings from the condition of education 2002* (NCES 2002-012). Washington, DC: U.S. Department of Education, National Center for Education Statistics. Retrieved from http://nces.ed.gov/pubsearch/pubsinfo.asp?pubid=2002012

Dukes, L. III, Koorland, M., & Scott, S. (2009). Making Blended Instruction better: Integrating the principles of universal design for instruction into course design and delivery. *Action in Teacher Education, 31*(1). 38–48.

Fielding Graduate University. (2012). What is the distributed learning model. Retrieved from http://fielding.edu/whyFielding/distributed.aspx

Gergen, K. (2000). *The saturated self*. New York, NY: Basic Books.

Harrell, I. L. II. (2008). Increasing the success of online students. *Inquiry, 13*(1), 36–44.

Horn, L. J., & Carroll, C. D. (1996). *Nontraditional undergraduates: Trends in enrollment from 1986 to 1992 and persistence and attainment among 1989–1990 beginning postsecondary students* (NCES 97-578). Washington, DC: U.S. Department of Education, National Center for Education.

Mathias, C., & Benton A. D. (2011). Social justice through the education of a rural and tribal child welfare workforce. *Journal of Public Child Welfare, 5*(2–3), 282–296.

Moloney, J. F., & Oakley, B. (2010). Scaling online education: Increasing access to higher education. *Journal of Asynchronous Learning Networks, 14*(1), 55–70.

Morris, T. (2005). Social work professional education and workforce development: A ladder of learning. *Professional Development: The International Journal of Continuing Education, 8*(2–3), 108–115.

Radford, A. W., & Weko, T. (2011). *Learning at a distance: Undergraduate enrollment in distance education courses and degree programs*. Washington, DC: U.S. Department of Education, National Center for Education Statistics. Retrieved from http://nces.ed.gov/pubsearch/pubsinfo.asp?pubid=2012154

Seabury, B. E. (2005). An evaluation of online, interactive tutorials designed to teach practice concepts. *Technology in Social Work Education and Curriculum, 25*(1–2), 103–115.

Tunks, K. W. (2012). An introduction and guide to enhancing online instruction with Web 2.0 Tools. *Journal of Educators Online*, 9(2). Retrieved from ERIC, EBSCOhost.

White, M. (2002). Responding to personal failure. *The International Journal of Narrative Therapy and Community Work, 3*, 4–14.

Conclusion

CONCLUSION

Toward the Future

R. PAUL MAIDEN
School of Social Work, University of Southern California, Los Angeles, California, USA

The response to the Call for Papers for a special issue on Distance Learning and Online Education in Social Work far exceeded the editors' expectations, and these 18 papers represent the crème de la crème. Conceptually, most fell into one of four categories: (1) organizational and administrative issues, (2) teaching practice in an online environment, (3) teaching and conducting research, and (4) creating intimacy and interaction. Anyone who has more than a year or two of experience, of course, can attest to the challenges social work educators face in each of these areas. Online social work education is still in the early stages of exploration, discovery and creativity, as demonstrated by the varied approaches schools of social work and their faculty members are taking in the use of technology and social media in the classroom and in online platforms.

CLASSROOMS WITHOUT WALLS

My first exposure to this brave new world occurred 14 years ago when I joined the faculty of the School of Social Work at the University of Central Florida (UCF). The smart classroom where I taught my first social policy class was equipped with an amazing array of technology, including the capacity to televise my lecture for a group of students at one of the school's satellite locations. The School had no online classes at that time, and the thinking of the faculty was still in the mode of "YOU CAN'T TEACH SOCIAL WORK PRACTICE IN AN ONLINE ENVIRONMENT." (In the Web world, writing in all caps is the equivalent of yelling, which would capture the intensity of faculty reaction!) Social work educators likely have all heard some variation of such strident discussions in faculty and curriculum committee meetings. I believed much the same. However, the UCF incentivized faculty to develop online courses with a free laptop, a $2,500 stipend, and extensive individual consultation with an instructional designer. I was curious about how these courses actually worked and took the leap. I joined a work group of six faculty, none of whom were social work colleagues, thus providing me with different perspectives, and together we entered the "brave new world" of online education.

The following semester, my 15-week Substance Abuse Interventions course was converted into a fully Web-based format and added to the university schedule. (Faculty who developed Web courses were required to teach them at least once.) I had enjoyed "storyboarding" the contents of each of my class sessions, collaborating and engaging with colleagues outside my own discipline, and receiving a highly accelerated education on available technology. Inwardly, I was a bit skeptical about how well it would really work. Would social work students be interested in taking an online course? I expected to feel relieved if just 8 to 10 students registered. To be truthful, I was not ready to relinquish the "stage" on which I had successfully performed for many years with wit and wisdom, to mostly adoring students. Within an hour of the opening of registration, students began requesting overrides into this new online class, which had already reached capacity and closed with an enrollment of 25 students. My second surprise came when students started posting brief bios on the class website, and I learned that some were not my own MSW students but students from MSW programs at Florida State, Florida International, or the University of South Florida. I was not aware of the existence of the Florida University Consortium, which granted students throughout the state full credit for courses taken beyond the university where they were admitted. And then I had an epiphany! It was a moment that changed my concept of the"classroom." It really was not a matter of thinking outside the box; rather, the four sides of my box collapsed, giving me a strikingly new 360-degree view of the pedagogical landscape. By the time I left UCF to take a position at the University of Southern California we were teaching more than 40 BSW and MSW fully Web-based or 50/50 hybrid courses—alternating weeks in the classroom and online, thereby doubling the use of available classroom space.

By comparison, the University of Southern California's Virtual Academic Center (VAC) offers no hybrid courses that would require a campus presence. As noted in the opening paper, all courses in the VAC are via distance learning and include both synchronous and asynchronous dimensions. Matriculating students attend a full schedule of live, interactive classes each week on a platform where all students and the instructor have visual and voice contact with one another, using a highly developed synchronous and asynchronous learning management system that is strikingly similar in appearance to "Hollywood Squares." Remarkably, the primary difference is that the students are located across the United States, Canada, Western Europe, and Asia. In addition to virtual classroom instruction, they can receive individual tutoring and writing instruction, schedule a personal consultation with a dedicated VAC social work librarian, participate in study group sessions with other VAC students, and join the campus meetings and other events organized by the Social Work Student Organization.

The "Faculty Lounge" in the VAC uses the same technology platform for new faculty orientation, private faculty development consultations, VAC faculty meetings, webinars, and chats among faculty colleagues for both full- and part-time teaching exclusively in the VAC and scattered throughout the United States. The UCF and USC examples are only two versions of Web-based platforms that have been developed. One approach gave current students an alternative to attending a traditional 3-hour lecture/discussion course every week while helping to relieve classroom shortage at a rapidly growing university. The other resulted in more than doubling graduate enrollment and the national expansion of a school's well recognized MSW program. Both generated new revenue. Given the recent surge of MSW programs now offering online content, there are a considerable number of other iterations, and the papers presented here hopefully have given the reader a sense of the possibilities and permutations.

IS ONLINE LEARNING A PARADIGM SHIFT?

As the papers in this issue demonstrate, schools of social work have developed a variety of approaches to online learning. Does this constitute a paradigm shift in social work education? It may appear so to the tradition-bound classroom instructor who primarily relies on a lecture/discussion format. Certainly, online learning provides a different lens through which to view the social work classroom, sometimes reflected in the comments of faculty who say that they are "old school" and prefer teaching without learning or using the new technology. Nevertheless, the reality is that even traditional campus-based programs today are technology-enhanced, and rely increasingly on Blackboard, Ares, and other internet resources as instructional and smart classroom management tools.

Some schools now offer "technology boot camps" as part of acculturation and on-boarding of new full- and part-time faculty because the broad array of technological tools used in Web-based instruction can be overwhelming to the new user. It does take practice to master the virtual classroom, especially those environments that combine asynchronous and synchronous elements. These complex venues require the instructor to create live class sessions on Adobe Connect, activate webcams, set up dial-ins for voice activation, move students in and out of small groups on the learning management system, receive, read, and grade assignments, provide feedback in the online environment, and hold virtual office hours for student consultation. Nonetheless, however different the presentation may have become, the core content of the curriculum remains the same. As social work educators, I think we might all agree that what we do in our classrooms is so much more: the teacher/student interaction; the mentor/mentee relationship; and conveying the essence of who we are and what we do in the practice of a profession to which we have dedicated our hearts and souls.

Yet, though I have taught in the campus classroom for many years and online classes on numerous occasions, I surprisingly have discovered an enhanced sense of intimacy and personal interaction with my students in the online environment. It is one experience to stand before a class of 20 students engaged in spirited lecture and discussion. In the online classroom, both synchronous and asynchronous, the interaction is more singular. Whether by face-to-face interaction via a webcam or the back-and-forth threads of an e-mail chat, the faculty/student interaction that occurs over the course of a semester often achieves an unexpected level of intimacy. The "collapsing of the box" seems to help us to discover new and different ways of creating and maintaining meaningful instructor-to-student and student-to-instructor relationships that transcend the brick-and-mortar setting. When, on the day of graduation, a student I had in one or two online courses but had never met in person walked up to me, beaming in cap and gown, the recognition was instantaneous, and the physicality and emotionality of the moment was powerful! Herein lies the future inquiry of online social work education: the quality of campus to cloud course conversion, the richness of instruction, the authenticity of instructor-student interaction, the assurance of faculty and student satisfaction, and, most important, measurement of student learning outcomes, professional competence, and professional socialization. Attention to these dimensions is, and always will be, the hallmark of social work education, on the ground and in the cloud.

Index

Note: Page numbers in **bold** type refer to **figures**
Page numbers in *italic* type refer to *tables*
Page numbers followed by 'n' refer to notes

For Product Safety Concerns and Information please contact our EU representative GPSR@taylorandfrancis.com Taylor & Francis Verlag GmbH, Kaufingerstraße 24, 80331 München, Germany

Batch number: 10726294

Printed by Printforce, the Netherlands